Clinical Procedures in THIRD EDITION
PRIMARY EYE CARE

For Elsevier:

Commissioning Editor: Robert Edwards
Development Editor: Rebecca Gleave
Project Manager: Morven Dean
Designer: Charles Gray
Illustrator: David Graham

Clinical Procedures in
PRIMARY EYE CARE

THIRD EDITION

Edited by

David B. Elliott PhD MCOptom FAAO
Professor of Clinical Vision Science, University of Bradford, UK

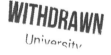

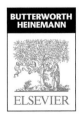

ELSEVIER

Edinburgh   London   New York   Oxford   Philadelphia   St Louis   Sydney   Toronto   2007

BUTTERWORTH
HEINEMANN
ELSEVIER

First edition 1997
Second Edition 2003
Third edition 2007

ISBN 13: 9780750688963
ISBN 10: 0750688963

British Library Cataloguing in Publication Data
A catalogue record for this book is available from the British Library

Library of Congress Cataloging in Publication Data
A catalog record for this book is available from the Library of Congress

Knowledge and best practice in this field are constantly changing. As new research and experience broaden our knowledge, changes in practice, treatment and drug therapy may become necessary or appropriate. Readers are advised to check the most current information provided (i) on procedures featured or (ii) by the manufacturer of each product to be administered, to verify the recommended dose or formula, the method and duration of administration, and contraindications. It is the responsibility of the practitioner, relying on their own experience and knowledge of the patient, to make diagnoses, to determine dosages and the best treatment for each individual patient, and to take all appropriate safety precautions.

To the fullest extent of the law, neither the publisher nor the editors assumes any liability for any injury and/or damage.

The Publisher

Printed in China

CONTENTS

CONTRIBUTORS

Brendan Barrett PhD DipOptom FAOI
Senior Lecturer, Department of Optometry, University of Bradford, UK

David B. Elliott PhD MCOptom FAAO
Professor of Clinical Vision Science, Department of Optometry, University of Bradford, UK

John G. Flanagan PhD MCOptom FAAO
Professor, School of Optometry, University of Waterloo, Ontario, Canada
Professor, Department of Ophthalmology and Vision Sciences, University of Toronto, Ontario, Canada

Patricia Hrynchak OD FAAO
Clinical Lecturer, School of Optometry, University of Waterloo, Ontario, Canada

C. Lisa Prokopich OD MSc
Clinical Lecturer, School of Optometry, University of Waterloo, Ontario, Canada

Contributors to the electronic ancillary

Edward Mallen PhD MCOptom
Senior Lecturer, Department of Optometry, University of Bradford, UK

Konrad Pesudovs BScOptom PhD PGDipAdvClinOptom MCOptom FVCO FAAO FCLSA,
Associate Professor of Ophthalmology, Flinders University and Flinders Medical Centre, South Australia, Australia

PREFACE

This textbook was written primarily as a teaching aid for undergraduate optometry students and for practitioners wishing to review their clinical practice. Although it is not intended to be inclusive of all techniques that can be performed in primary eye care examinations, most popular procedures are covered. For each test, brief background information is provided, then a discussion of the function or state assessed, the advantages and disadvantages of the particular test, the measurement procedure, how to record the results, how to interpret them and a list of errors most commonly made by students, with an attempt to put the most common first. The recommended tests and procedures are explicitly based on evidence from the research literature whenever possible, rather than just clinical experience. Chapter 1 includes a review of how clinical tests and procedures are assessed in the research literature and how such reports should be critiqued. It also discusses the theory behind the use of screening tests and their use in primary eye care exams. Test procedures are grouped within the following six chapters. Chapter 2 compares the various formats of an eye examination and introduces the communication skills needed in primary eye care. A discussion of the case history and how it should be performed completes the chapter. Tests are subsequently grouped together in terms of which system they assess: visual function (Chapter 3), refractive correction (Chapter 4), binocular vision (Chapter 5) and ocular health (Chapter 6). This layout was chosen because the organisation of the book is directed towards the assimilation of a problem-oriented approach (Section 2.1.3) that is built upon a systems examination (Section 2.1.2). Grouping the tests in this way, rather than in the order they are typically used in an eye examination, may also help students to better appreciate the relationship between the various tests that assess a particular system. The book is completed in Chapter 7 with an introduction to some physical examination procedures that may be used in primary care eye

examinations. A list of key references and a Bibliography/Further reading section is provided at the end of each chapter. References have been kept to a minimum, with the most recently published references often chosen as these will usually cite earlier published reports.

The third edition differs from the second edition in several ways:

- Video-clips of various clinical procedures and fundus and slit-lamp photographs are provided on the website .

- Significantly more diagrams and photographs have been included within the textbook, including several colour panels.

- There is one new chapter that introduces physical assessment procedures that could be used in primary eye care, including sphygmomanometry and carotid artery assessment. In addition, there are new sections that introduce communication skills and variations in appearance of the normal, healthy young and elderly eye.

- The book has a new format with numbered sections and subsections and similar headings for subsections to allow easier manoeuvring around the book.

COMMENTS AND SUGGESTIONS FOR FUTURE EDITIONS

The advantages and disadvantages of each procedure are provided and where possible, the measurement procedure is based on evidence from the research literature. However, there is no doubt that tests and test methodologies have been included which may reflect our biases due to our particular training, research and clinical experience. There may also be errors and omissions. We therefore welcome any comments and suggestions that would improve any further editions of this textbook. Please write to the editor, Professor David Elliott at the Department of Optometry, University of Bradford, Bradford, BD7 1DP, UK (e-mail: d.elliott1@bradford.ac.uk).

INFORMATION RELEVANT TO STUDENTS

The recommendations in this manual are just that and not hard and fast rules. There are many ways of conducting an eye examination and different ways to properly perform various tests or procedures. Any methods or tests that are not included in this manual are not in any way 'wrong'. Indeed, the tests and test methodologies included no doubt reflect our biases due to our particular training, research and clinical experience. In particular, in university primary care clinics it is the supervising clinician's decision as to which techniques or tests should be used in an eye examination. They are taking legal responsibility for the examination. If they indicate that a particular test needs using, use it! Once the patient has left and you are discussing the case with your supervisor, to further your learning, you should ask them about the advantages and disadvantages of their suggested technique.

ACKNOWLEDGEMENTS

We wish to thank Kathy Dumbleton, Ken Hadley, Natalie Hutchings, Edward Gilmore (University of Waterloo), Matt Cufflin, Elizabeth Richardson, Sem Sem Chin and Annette Parkinson (University of Bradford) for help with the video clips; the University of Bradford, Flinders Medical School and University of Waterloo eye clinics, Ketha Sivasegaran and Graham Mouat for help with the photographs; Anne Weber (University of Waterloo) for several of the figures; Walter Mittelstaedt for recording the Korotkoff sounds; Mary Elliott, Niall Strang (Glasgow Caledonian University) and Cathy Starling for valuable comments on earlier versions of the third edition; Anya Bykar for collating many useful suggestions regarding additions to the text and new formatting and Mark Hurst and Barry Winn for their contributions to earlier editions of the book and the students and retired volunteer patients of the University of Bradford for sitting as subjects for many of the photographs and video clips. Finally we wish to especially thank our families and partners for their support and their understanding of the time commitment required to produce this textbook.

EVIDENCE-BASED PRIMARY EYE CARE

DAVID B ELLIOTT

1

Evidence-based primary eye care means integrating individual clinical expertise with the best currently available evidence from the research literature. What should always be avoided is the use of exam procedures purely because of tradition or habit.

1.1 REVIEWING THE RESEARCH LITERATURE

The research literature should be regularly reviewed. There may be reports of newly developed techniques or instruments that are superior to the ones you typically use or even studies indicating that old and forgotten tests are actually better than commonly used ones (e.g. Rainey et al. 1998).

1.1.1 What makes a good research report?

Unfortunately, not all research reports necessarily provide accurate information. A study could be flawed for a variety of reasons (Harper & Reeves 1999, Lai et al. 2006), including a lack of exploration or misinterpretation of previous literature, poor study design, a subject group that is too small or biased, poorly or inappropriately performed tests, an unreliable or inappropriate gold standard test, inappropriate or limited statistical analyses and exaggerated conclusions. In theory, all of this should be picked up in the review process. All papers submitted to academic journals are sent to two or three reviewers with expertise in the area. They send comments to the editor, who decides whether to accept the paper, accept it with minor revision, accept after major revision and a re-review or reject the paper. However, this process cannot always be perfect and it is useful to be able to critique a research paper, rather than just accept its conclusions. Various criteria can be used to assess the methodological quality of research articles (e.g. Harper & Reeves 1999, Lai et al. 2006) and a high quality paper should include the following:

- The paper should be easy to read and understand. Particularly in the area of the assessment of clinical techniques, there should be little that a clinician cannot understand. The rationale behind any complicated statistical analyses should be explained in a simple way. A paper that is difficult to understand often indicates a poorly written paper rather than any lack of understanding on the part of the reader.

- The introduction of a paper should include the purpose of the study and discuss pertinent previous work.

- The methods section should be clear and precise. Another researcher should be able to replicate the study from the information provided in the methods section. It is usually necessary to randomise the order in which tests are performed to ensure that there are no significant learning or fatigue effects that could affect the data.

- In studies where tests are compared against a gold standard, the clinicians should be blind to the results from the other test.

- The subject sample should be clearly outlined: Why was that particular group of subjects chosen and how were they recruited? A description of the demographics of the group should be provided. A sufficiently large sample and a broad spectrum of subjects should be used to ensure no recruitment bias.

■ The authors may highlight the limitations of the study. The majority of research studies have some limitations and it is very helpful to the reader if the authors indicate them. It also suggests that the authors are not exaggerating the findings of their study.

The research literature that describes a clinical test's usefulness often uses assessments of validity, discriminative ability and/or repeatability and these are discussed in detail below.

1.1.2 Assessment of validity

A test is valid if it measures what it says it measures. This is often indicated by how closely the test's results match those from a 'gold standard' measurement. For example, the validity of new tonometers has usually been determined by how similar the results are to Goldmann Applanation Tonometry (GAT) readings. This highlights the possible problem with validity measurements in that they are only as good as the gold standard. If the gold standard is flawed, an excellent instrument could be reported to have poor validity. For example, the GAT is known to give high intraocular pressure readings on thick corneas and low readings with thin corneas (Doughty & Zaman 2000). This has tended to be ignored until recently when significant reductions in IOP have been found after refractive surgery (see section 6.13). If a tonometer that was resistant to corneal thickness effects had been compared to GAT, it would have been shown to be variable. The conclusion would have been that the new tonometer was somewhat variable compared to GAT. Inappropriate gold standards can also be chosen. For example, Calvin et al. (1996) used the von Graefe phoria measurement as the gold standard test to assess the usefulness of the cover test and suggested that the cover test was occasionally inaccurate. The gold standard in this area should be the cover test and not the von Graefe. The cover test is the only test that discriminates between strabismus and heterophoria, it is objective and not reliant on subject responses and a subsequent study has shown it to be far more repeatable than the von Graefe, which appears to be unreliable (Rainey et al. 1998). The 1996 study should have used the cover test as the gold standard and they would then have reported the limitations of the von Graefe. The gold

standard test must also be appropriately measured. For example, Salchow et al. (1999) compared autorefraction results after LASIK refractive surgery against the gold standard of subjective refraction. Subjective refraction was an appropriate choice of gold standard, but was inappropriately measured. The authors concluded that autorefraction compared very poorly against subjective refraction post-LASIK. However, inspection of the results clearly indicates that the majority of the subjective refractions (particularly of the hyperopes) provided a result of plano. This suggests that a normal or near normal visual acuity resulted in a 'brief' subjective refraction and a result of plano.

The approach of determining the validity of new tests by comparing them to a gold standard can lead to the invincibility of the gold standard. For example, the limitations of GAT have been known for many years (Doughty & Zaman 2000; see section 6.13), but these limitations have tended to be ignored. The use of subjective refraction as a gold standard assessment of refractive error has meant that there has been little or no comparison of the various methods used in subjective refraction. Subjective refraction is the gold standard, so how can we compare the various methods? Previous studies have tended to compare the various tests against each other. For example, West & Somers (1984) compared the various binocular balancing tests and found that they all gave similar results and concluded that they were therefore all equally useful. Johnson et al. (1996) reported a similar finding when comparing subjective tests for astigmatism. These are not surprising findings, and provide little information regarding which test is the most useful. A very good but under-utilised approach is to use some measure of patient satisfaction as the gold standard. If patients are happy with the results of subjective refraction using a particular test, then the test must be providing appropriate results. Hanlon et al. (1987) used this approach in a comparison of techniques used to determine the reading addition. They examined 37 patients that were dissatisfied with the near vision in their new spectacles. From the case history information in the review (recheck) examination, it was determined whether the improper add was too low or too high. For each patient, their reading addition was then determined using the four methods of age, ½ amplitude of accommodation, NRA/PRA (negative relative accommodation/positive relative accommodation) balance and binocular cross-cylinder. The percentage of adds for each test that gave the same result as the improper add or worse (higher than an improper add determined too high or lower than an improper add determined as too low) was calculated. The results are discussed in section 4.21. The study would have been even better if they had confirmed that the patients were subsequently satisfied with their changed spectacles (i.e. that it really was the gold standard). This technique of using patient satisfaction as the gold standard test could be usefully employed to compare the various techniques used in distance refraction, particularly those that assess astigmatism and binocular balancing.

A test's validity is often described by the correlation coefficient between the results from the test and the gold standard. However, care must be taken when considering such analyses as correlation coefficients are very much affected by the range of values used in the analysis (Bland & Altman 1986, Haegerstrom-Portnoy et al. 2000). If a small range of values is used in calculations (for example, visual acuity values between 6/4 and 6/9), the correlation coefficient is likely to be much smaller than if a larger range (e.g. 6/4 to 6/120) is used. This is highlighted in Figure 1.1, which shows a plot of correlation coefficients between visual acuity and other clinical measures of visual function versus the range of visual acuity of subjects used in the studies. Plotting frequency distributions of the differences between test and standard provides more useful information as well as being independent of the range of values. For example, although a correlation coefficient of 0.97 between the equivalent sphere predicted by an autorefractor and subjective refraction does indicate that the two provide very similar results, knowing that 83% of autorefractor results are within ±0.50D of subjective refraction and 96% are within ±1.00D is much more meaningful (Elliott & Wilkes 1989). A similar analysis, commonly known as a Bland–Altman plot (Bland & Altman 1986) shows the 95% confidence limits of the difference between the test and the gold standard (Fig. 1.2). Of course, this analysis can be used only if the gold standard and test are measured in the same units.

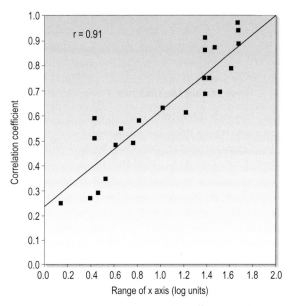

Fig. 1.1 Correlation coefficients from the literature between high contrast visual acuity and other spatial vision measures are plotted as a function of the range of high-contrast acuities in those studies. The solid line is the regression line and the correlation coefficient for the plotted data points is 0.91. (Redrawn from Haegerstrom-Portnoy et al. 2000, with permission of The American Academy of Optometry).

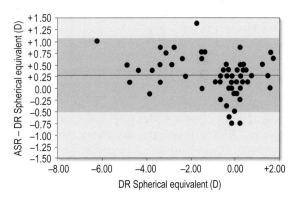

Fig. 1.2 A Bland–Altman plot of test – gold standard differences showing the validity of automated subjective refraction (ASR) using a comparison against optometrist subjective refraction. (Reprinted from Sheedy et al. 2004, with permission of The American Academy of Optometry).

1.1.3 Discriminative ability

Discriminative ability indicates how well a test discriminates between normal and abnormal eyes. In

published results of clinical studies, it is often reported that a significant difference was found between a group of patients with an ocular abnormality and a control group. It should be noted that this only indicates that there is a difference between the averages of the two groups. It does not indicate how well the test predicts whether an individual patient has the abnormality or not. Sensitivity and specificity values and plots of one against the other for a range of cut-off values in receiver operating characteristic (ROC curves, Fig. 1.3) or kappa functions (Gilchrist 1992) are usually presented to represent discriminative ability. Sensitivity is the proportion of abnormal eyes correctly identified, and specificity is the proportion of normal eyes correctly identified. They are discussed in detail in section 1.2.2. It should again be noticed that to determine whether a test can correctly identify 'abnormal' or 'normal' eyes, a 'gold standard' test (or battery of tests) must have been used to classify eyes as abnormal or normal. The assessment of discriminative ability is therefore also dependent on the validity and reliability of the gold standard test. For example, new instruments or techniques that attempt to identify primary open-angle glaucoma are typically assessed against classifications of patients into glaucomatous and control groups by clinical evaluation of optic nerve head assessment, visual fields and tonometry (e.g. Hutchings et al. 2001). This classification will therefore differ depending on the type of visual field assessment and tonometer used and the skill/experience of the clinician.

1.1.4 Repeatability

Repeatability assesses the variability of results between testing occasions. Reliability, also called precision (the ability of a measurement to be consistently produced) or repeatability, has most often been described in terms of correlation coefficients. The limitations of correlation coefficients have already been discussed in section 1.1.2 and it can often be better to assess repeatability in terms of the coefficient of repeatability (COR). This represents the 95% confidence limits of the difference between the test and retest scores (Bland & Altman 1986, Fig. 1.4). For example, correlation coefficients between test and retest visual acuity scores have been found to be 0.95 (unaided) and 0.90 (aided), respectively (Elliott & Sheridan 1988). This suggests that the repeatability of the two tests is similar and may be slightly better for unaided

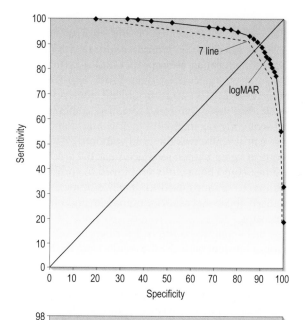
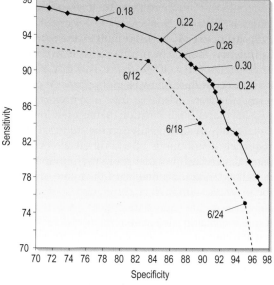

Fig. 1.3 Receiver-operating characteristic (ROC) curve showing the discriminative ability of visual acuity systems. (Redrawn from Tong et al. 2004, with permission of The American Academy of Optometry)

acuity. However, COR results were ±0.07 logMAR (test and retest scores generally differ by less than a line) for aided acuity and ±0.21 logMAR (test scores can differ by up to two lines on retest) for unaided acuity, showing a much better repeatability for aided acuity (Elliott & Sheridan 1988). The high

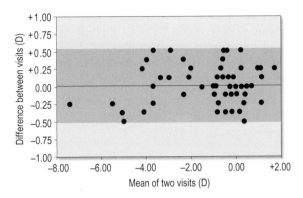

Fig. 1.4 A Bland–Altman plot of test-retest differences showing the repeatability of subjective refraction. (Reprinted from Sheedy et al. 2004, with permission of The American Academy of Optometry)

correlation coefficient found for unaided acuity is in part due to the much larger range of values used in its calculation (6/60, 20/200 to 6/4, 20/13), compared with the calculation involving aided acuity (6/6, 20/20 to 6/4, 20/13) (Elliott & Sheridan 1988). Correlation coefficients can be used when comparing tests that do not use the same units, but their limitations need to be realised. In particular, a large range of values should be used, so that correlation coefficients are not artificially low. Concordance values (the percentage of patients getting exactly the same score on test and retest) have also been used to indicate that a test is repeatable. However, a high proportion of patients often obtaining exactly the same score on follow-up visits indicates that the step sizes on the test are too big rather than that the test is repeatable (Bailey et al. 1991). For example, a visual acuity chart containing only 20/20 (6/6) and 20/200 (6/60) lines would provide very high concordance but would be of very little value.

Coefficients of repeatability results are also of value because they indicate the size of a clinically significant change. Repeatability studies providing COR data indicate the size of the change in score due to chance. A significant change in score would then be anything larger than the COR (at least for tests with a continuous scale). More studies are required that indicate the size of a clinically significant change for optometric tests. Repeatability appears to be the most important quality of a test, as it influences the others. For example, if a test has poor repeatability and test results correlate poorly with retest results, it is unlikely that results from

the test correlate highly with a gold standard measure. Therefore, its validity is poor. If a test correlates poorly with itself, how can it correlate well with something else? Similarly, a test with poor repeatability is likely to have a large range of scores in patients with normal, healthy eyes. For an abnormal eye to be outside this large normal range would be more difficult, so good discriminative ability is less likely. Optical companies should be encouraged to provide repeatability data with any newly available test, so that it can be compared with the currently available tests.

1.2 ROUTINE SCREENING

Another area of the primary eye care examination that has been discussed in detail in the research literature is the issue of using tests for screening purposes. This issue has become more pertinent to optometry with the increasing use of clinical assistants to routinely perform various automated or simple tests as part of a screening process prior to the primary eye care examination.

1.2.1 The use of clinical assistants in routine screening

The rationale behind the use of clinical assistants in pre-examination screening is twofold:

- These procedures generally become more routinely performed.

- As clinical assistants perform certain tests that the optometrist would previously have performed, some of the optometrist's time is freed up. They could use this time to perform additional procedures or examine more patients per day. The pros and cons of clinical assistants performing ocular health screening tests routinely are further discussed in the following sections.

What procedures and tests can a clinical assistant perform? After a period of training, they should be able to competently perform any automated procedure, such as automated visual fields and focimetry, autorefraction and non-contact tonometry. In addition, other simple tests could be performed such as colour vision and stereopsis screening and interpupillary distance (PD) measurement. It is not possible for a clinical assistant to complete the full case history, since history taking continues throughout the examination. However, assistants could record a baseline history that could be reviewed and augmented by the clinician. However, this approach provides less likelihood of a good rapport being established between patient and clinician, which is vital for an optimal examination result (Ettinger 1994). Clinical assistants could also measure visual acuity with the patient's spectacles. However, important information can be obtained during visual acuity measurement in addition to the acuity score and, as an important part of the subjective refraction is to compare the final visual acuity (which the optometrist measures) with the habitual acuity, it appears best to have both measurements made by the clinician.

1.2.2 False positives and the positive predictive value

The decision to use any screening test/procedure routinely is more complicated than boldly stating 'I want to catch all patients with . . . glaucoma, a retinal detachment, a brain tumour, etc. . . . so I am going to perform this test on everybody'. To understand the advantages and disadvantages of screening, it is important to understand sensitivity and specificity. How good do you think your screening tests are? If a test indicates that a patient has an eye disease, what are the chances that they actually have the condition? When considering this question, you must not only consider how good the test is at identifying the disease, but you must also consider how good the test is at correctly identifying someone as normal. Unfortunately, all tests provide false positives: patients with normal, healthy eyes which the test results suggest are abnormal. There

are four possible outcomes from the results of a screening test (Table 1.1) and this information is used to quantify how well the test discriminates between 'normal' and 'abnormal' eyes, by providing sensitivity and specificity values.

- Sensitivity is the ability of the test to identify the disease in those who have it.
- Sensitivity = TP/(TP + FN)
- Specificity is the ability of the test to correctly identify those who do not have the disease.
- Specificity = TN/(TN + FP)

- The false positive rate is simply 1 minus the specificity.
- Another important term to understand is the Positive Predictive Value (+PV). This is the proportion of people with a positive test result who have disease.
- +PV = TP/(TP + FP)

The reported sensitivity and specificity of a test will differ depending on the pool of patients examined, the gold standard used to determine the presence or absence of disease and the cut-off criteria used.

The ability of a screening test to correctly identify patients with disease is highly dependent upon how prevalent the condition is (Bayes Theorem). For example, let us consider primary open-angle glaucoma (POAG), which has a prevalence in the over-40 population of approximately 1%, and assume that we have a screening test for glaucoma with 95% sensitivity and 95% specificity. Out of 1000 patients, 10 (1%) could have POAG and it is likely that 9 or all 10 would be detected, as the test sensitivity is 95%. With a false positive rate of 5% (1–0.95), the screening test would also suggest that about 50 of the remaining 990 patients with normal healthy eyes actually had POAG. In total, 60 patients would give positive results, of which only 10 would have the disease (+PV = 17%). If the

Table 1.1   Possible outcomes of a screening test.

	Diseased eye	Normal eye
Test says diseased	True positive, TP (hit)	False positive, FP (false alarm)
Test says normal	False negative, FN (miss)	True negative, TN

sensitivity and specificity of the screening test was an amazing 99%, there would be 10 true positives and 10 false positives, and there is still a 50% chance that a patient with a positive result is normal.

Now let us consider the likely outcomes using the same test on patients with a family history of POAG where the prevalence of the disease is higher at about 10%. For the screening test with 95% sensitivity and specificity, out of 1000 patients, 100 would have POAG and it is likely that 95 would be detected. With a false positive rate of 5%, the screening test would also suggest that 45 of the remaining 900 patients with normal healthy eyes actually had POAG. In total, 140 patients gave positive results, of which 95 had the disease (+PV = 68%). For the 99% sensitivity and specificity screening test, there would be 99 true positives and 9 false positives and a +PV of 92%.

1.2.3 Are false positives so important?

Elmore et al. (1998) reported the false positive rate of breast cancer screening tests to be 6.5% and 3.7% respectively. These translate to very good specificity values of 93.5% and 96.3%, which are similar to the specificity of screening tests used in primary eye care (Bullimore 1998a). Despite this good specificity, over a ten-year period, nearly one-third of the women screened had at least one false positive mammogram or clinical breast examination. It has been shown that these false positive results have negative psychological effects on these women (Brett & Austoker 2001) and likely their families. Imagine being told that you or one of your family has received a positive screening test and has to undergo further tests for breast cancer.

Similarly, there is considerable and unnecessary worry and stress caused by a false positive result leading to referral to a secondary eye care system, in that some patients worry that they might be going blind. Patients should not be referred to secondary eye care on the basis of a slightly high intraocular pressure using a non-contact tonometer or a single positive visual field screening or because one clinician judged an optic disc to be suspicious (Bullimore 1998a). In addition to the psychological effects on patients and their families, the cost of all the subsequent clinical tests prompted by a positive screening result should also be considered.

1.2.4 Screening all patients

It is important to understand the limitations of screening. Realise that one positive screening result does not mean somebody has the disease being screened for and in many cases the chances that they have the disease remains small (Bullimore 1998a). Screening tests used to detect diseases with a low prevalence should have a reasonable specificity (typically >95%) and yet retain good sensitivity (typically >90%). However, even then, if a positive result is obtained, the test should be repeated. For example, as part of the ocular hypertension treatment study, Keltner et al. (2000) found 703 Humphrey visual field test results that showed abnormal (positive glaucoma hemifield test and/or Corrected Pattern Standard Deviation, $p < 0.05$), and reliable visual fields. On retesting, abnormalities *were not* confirmed for 604 (86%)! The vast majority of visual field abnormalities were not verified on retest and confirmation of visual field abnormalities is essential for distinguishing reproducible visual field loss from long-term variability.

Because of false positive results, if you test a healthy eye often enough, it will sooner or later give a positive result. The poorer the specificity of a test, the more likely this is to happen. Elmore et al. (1998) estimated that the cumulative risk of having at least one false positive result after 10 mammogram screenings was nearly 50% ($= 1 - 0.935^{10}$).

Similarly, when screening for POAG visual field defects every year for 10 years with a test with a specificity of 95%, the cumulative risk of having at least one false positive result is 40% ($= 1 - 0.95^{10}$). Even if the test specificity is 99%, at least one annual assessment over a 10-year period would be a false positive.

1.2.5 Overcoming the problem of false positives: repeat tests

The best way to keep false positive referrals to a minimum is to repeat positive results. For example, the 95% sensitive and specific glaucoma screening test discussed in section 1.2.2 would produce positive results in 60 patients if 1000 were screened, yet only 10 would have the disease (+PV = 17%). If all these 60 patients were retested, 9 or all 10 of the glaucoma patients would be identified. However, 95% of the false positives (47 or 48) would now give a normal result. On retesting, positive results are found for 13 patients, of whom 10 have the disease ($+PV = 77\%$).

This approach is further improved by only screening those patients that are 'at risk'. In these patients, the prevalence of the disease is much higher than in the general population. Let us consider the likely outcomes using the same tests on patients with a family history of POAG where the prevalence of the disease is about 10%. For example, the 95% sensitive and specific glaucoma screening test discussed in section 1.2.2 would produce positive results in 140 patients if 1000 were screened and 95 would have the disease ($+PV = 68\%$). On retesting the 140 patients, 90 of the glaucoma patients are detected. Of the 45 false positives, 43 of them now give a normal field. After the repeat test, 92 give positive results, of which 90 have glaucoma ($+PV = 98\%$). Of course, 5 glaucoma patients will now not be referred, so that a patient with a positive field test, even when followed by a normal field, should be closely monitored. The positive predictive value is also improved if you just perform screening on all patients over 75 years of age (prevalence of POAG $\approx 5\%$; $+PV = 50\%$, after repeat testing, $+PV = 96\%$) or patients over 40 years of age who are African American, diabetics or have high myopia or those with suspicious optic discs, high intraocular pressure, etc.

1.2.6 Routine fundus dilation?

There has been considerable debate about whether a primary care eye examination should routinely include a dilated fundus examination or DFE (Siegel et al. 1990, Parisi et al. 1996, Batchelder et al. 1997, Bullimore 1998b). Two main arguments, supported by clinical data, are proposed in favour of the DFE. The first is that a DFE increases the number of posterior pole anomalies detected (Siegel et al. 1990, Parisi et al. 1996). In these studies, a non-dilated fundus examination with direct ophthalmoscopy was compared to a DFE using headband binocular indirect ophthalmoscopy (BIO) and direct ophthalmoscopy. Siegel et al. (1990) also used a monocular indirect ophthalmoscope examination as part of the non-dilated exam. The poor field of view of the direct ophthalmoscope was

particularly blamed for missing anomalies in the posterior pole as it is too small to examine the area quickly and easily. For further clarification of the need for a DFE to detect posterior pole anomalies, it would be useful if these studies could be repeated to compare an undilated fundus examination with fundus biomicroscopy to a DFE. It is possible that the better field of view and stereoscopic image provided by fundus biomicroscopy would limit the advantage of a DFE for the posterior pole in a patient with a reasonable pupil size. The second argument in favour of a DFE is that significant anomalies would otherwise be missed in the peripheral retina. However, many of the anomalies found in the peripheral retina are benign and do not need treatment (Siegel et al. 1990, Parisi et al. 1996, Batchelder et al. 1997). The question is how often does a routine DFE detect a peripheral lesion that requires treatment beyond those detected by DFEs prompted by symptoms, signs and/or risk factors. Although Siegel et al. (1990) and Parisi et al. (1996) found important peripheral lesions in patients who were asymptomatic, it is unclear whether they considered clinical risk factors that would have prompted clinicians to perform a DFE. The majority of patients with peripheral retinal disease reported by Batchelder et al. (1997) had important risk factors including previous anterior segment surgery, previous retinal detachment, strong family history of retinal detachment and high myopia. In summary, Siegel et al. (1990) suggest that a routine DFE should be part of a primary care examination. Parisi et al. (1996) support this viewpoint, particularly for paediatric examinations. Batchelder et al. (1997) suggested that pupillary dilation is only required when signs, symptoms or risk factors suggest a peripheral lesion. Finally, another aspect to consider is the legal one. It is possible that in the US, the case of *Keir vs. United States* will make a DFE the standard of care for paediatric examinations, particularly for the initial visit (Classé 1989).

1.3 BIBLIOGRAPHY AND FURTHER READING

Greenhalgh, T. (2006) *How to read a paper: the basics of evidence-based medicine*, 3rd edn. Oxford: Blackwell.

1.4 REFERENCES

Bailey, I.L., Bullimore, M.A., Raasch, T.W. et al. (1991) Clinical grading and the effects of scaling. *Investigative Ophthalmology and Visual Science* **32**, 422–432.

Batchelder, T.J., Fireman, B., Friedman, G.D. et al. (1997) The value of routine dilated pupil screening examination. *Archives of Ophthalmology* **115**, 1179–1184.

Bland, J.M. and Altman, D.G. (1986) Statistical methods for assessing agreement between two methods of clinical measurement. *Lancet* **1**, 307–310.

Brett, J. and Austoker, J. (2001) Women who are recalled for further investigation for breast screening: psychological consequences 3 years after recall and factors affecting re-attendance. *Journal of Public Health* **23**, 292–300.

Bullimore, M.A. (1998a) The true and false negatives of screening. *Optometry and Vision Science* **75**, 461.

Bullimore, M.A. (1998b) Is routine dilation a waste of time? *Optometry and Vision Science* **75**, 161–162.

Calvin, H., Rupnow, P. and Grosvenor, T. (1996) How good is the estimated cover test at predicting the von Graefe phoria measurement? *Optometry and Vision Science* **73**, 701–706.

Classé, J.G. (1989) The eye-opening case of Keir v. United States. *Journal of the American Optometric Association* **60**, 471–476.

Doughty, M.J. and Zaman, M.L. (2000) Human corneal thickness and its impact on intraocular pressure measures: a review and meta-analysis approach. *Survey of Ophthalmology* **44**, 367–408.

Elliott, D.B. and Sheridan, M. (1988) The use of accurate visual acuity measurements in clinical ant-cataract formulation trials. *Ophthalmic and Physiological Optics* **8**, 397–401.

Elliott, D.B. and Wilkes, R. (1989) A clinical evaluation of the Topcon RM-6000 autorefractor. *Clinical and Experimental Optometry* **72**, 150–153.

Elmore, J.G., Barton, M.B., Moceri, V.M. et al. (1998) Ten-year risk of false positive screening mammograms and clinical breast examinations. *The New England Journal of Medicine* **338**, 1089–1096.

Ettinger, E.R. (1994) *Professional communications in eye care*. Oxford: Butterworth-Heinemann.

Gilchrist, J. (1992) QROC curves and kappa functions: new methods for evaluating the quality of clinical decisions. *Ophthalmic and Physiological Optics* **12**, 350–360.

Haegerstrom-Portnoy, G., Schneck, M.E., Lott, L.A. et al. (2000) The relation between visual acuity and other spatial vision measures. *Optometry and Vision Science* **77**, 653–662.

Hanlon, S.D., Nakabayashi, J. and Shigezawa, G. (1987) A critical view of presbyopic add determination. *Journal of the American Optometric Association* **58**, 468–472.

Harper, R. and Reeves, B. (1999) Compliance with methodological standards when evaluating ophthalmic diagnostic tests. *Investigative Ophthalmology and Visual Science* **40**, 1650–1657.

Hutchings, N., Hosking, S.L., Wild, J.M. et al. (2001) Long-term fluctuation in short-wavelength automated perimetry in glaucoma suspects and glaucoma patients. *Investigative Ophthalmology and Visual Science* **42**, 2332–2337.

Johnson, B.L., Edwards, J.S., Goss, D.A. et al. (1996) A comparison of three subjective tests for astigmatism and their interexaminer reliabilities. *Journal of the American Optometric Association* **67**, 590–598.

Keltner, J.L., Johnson, C.A., Quigg, J.M. et al. (2000) Confirmation of visual field abnormalities in the Ocular Hypertension Treatment Study. *Archives of Ophthalmology* **118**, 1187–1194.

Lai, T.Y., Leung, G.M., Wong, V.W. et al. (2006) How evidence-based are publications in clinical ophthalmic journals? *Investigative Ophthalmology and Visual Science* **47**, 1831–1838.

Parisi, M.L., Scheiman, M. and Coulter, R.S. (1996) Comparison of the effectiveness of a non-dilated versus dilated fundus examination in the pediatric population. *Journal of the American Optometric Association* **67**, 266–272.

Rainey, B.B., Schroeder, T.L., Goss, D.A. et al. (1998) Inter-examiner repeatability of heterophoria tests. *Optometry and Vision Science* **75**, 719–726.

Salchow, D.J., Zirm, M.E., Stieldorf, C. et al. (1999) Comparison of objective and subjective refraction before and after laser in situ keratomileusis. *Journal of Cataract and Refractive Surgery* **25**, 827–835.

Sheedy, J., Schanz, P. and Bullimore, M. (2004) Evaluation of an automated subjective refractor. *Optometry and Vision Science* **81**, 334–340.

Siegel, B.S., Thompson, A.K., Yolton, D.P. et al. (1990) A comparison of diagnostic outcomes with and without pupillary dilatation. *Journal of the American Optometric Association* **61**, 25–34.

Tong, L., Saw, S.M., Chan, E.S. et al. (2004) Screening for myopia and refractive errors using LogMAR visual acuity by optometrists and a simplified visual acuity chart by nurses. *Optometry and Vision Science* **81**, 684–691.

West, D. and Somers, W.W. (1984) Binocular balance validity: a comparison of five different subjective techniques. *Ophthalmic and Physiological Optics* **4**, 155–159.

INTRODUCTION TO THE PRIMARY EYE CARE EXAMINATION

DAVID B. ELLIOTT

2

What constitutes a primary eye care examination? The primary eye care examination must first and foremost adhere to the legal requirements of where you are working. However, legal requirements tend to be given in very broad terms. Some professional organisations that you belong to may also provide clinical guidelines of what your eye examination should include. These may be prescriptive or for guidance only. There are various types of format and these can essentially be separated into a data collection style of examination or one that concentrates on the patient's symptoms. In addition, the primary eye care exam could follow a clinician-centred approach or a patient-centred one.

2.1 THE FORMAT OF THE PRIMARY CARE EYE EXAMINATION

There are three main styles for a primary eye care examination, which could be used singularly or in combination: the database format, which uses a predetermined series of tests, the systems approach, which ensures an assessment of several systems and/or the problem-oriented approach, which focuses mainly on the patient's problems (Amos 1987, Elliott 1998). In addition, some parts of the eye examination could be performed by clinical assistants.

2.1.1 The database examination

A database examination style means using essentially the same set of clinical procedures in every examination. A large 'complete' database of information is collected to ensure that most patients' problems can be addressed using the information provided. This is the style of examination that will be used by students, because they need to practise the various clinical techniques to gain technical competence. Technical competence should be the aim for students after the first year's clinical teaching. A much greater task is gaining clinical competence. What do all the tests mean and how do they interact? How do you use test results to solve the patients' problems? Only once a student/practitioner has gained a high level of clinical competence should the database style of examination be abandoned and another approach used.

Although the database examination style is ideal for students, it is not for experienced practitioners. Often, if a large database is used, some data collected provide no useful information regarding the clinical diagnosis or treatment options. If patients require additional testing, because of the inflexibility of the approach, practitioners either perform the tests at the end of the examination, which can lead to them being late for subsequent examinations, or another appointment is made at a later date. At its worst, this style of examination could be said to provide some test data which are not used and of little value and provides a bias against performing additional procedures which may be of real benefit.

2.1.2 Systems examination

A systems examination style includes an assessment of visual function, the refractive and binocular systems and an ocular health assessment. The optometric examination is defined not by tests used, but by the systems that are assessed (Table 2.1). This approach is much more flexible as it does not demand that a certain collection of tests is used. In such an examination style, a minimum database has been gathered when each system has been tested. In summary, think in terms of assessing systems and not of using individual tests.

2.1.3 Problem-oriented examination

The problem-oriented examination aligns the examination around the problems reported by the patient. However, the examination does not only use tests that help solve the patient's problems as it is built upon a systems examination approach (Amos 1987, Elliott 1998). To perform a problem-oriented examination, the case history is critical as it guides the whole examination. From the information gained in the case history, the clinician should attempt to deduce a list of tentative diagnoses. For example, symptoms of blurred distance vision with normal near vision in a teenager could suggest the following tentative diagnoses (in order of likelihood): myopia, malingering and pseudomyopia. It is likely that visual acuity, retinoscopy and subjective refraction are all that is required to enable a differential diagnosis, although a cycloplegic refraction may be required if pseudomyopia is suspected. Other tests ensure an assessment of all the systems and depending on legal requirements and as a minimum these could include a cover test (binocular system), assessment of pupil reflexes, slit-lamp biomicroscopy and fundus biomicroscopy (ocular health assessment).

Although the problem-oriented examination requires a minimal database for legal reasons and to ensure that each system is assessed, this is not its major characteristic. Rather, it is distinguished by its variability. For example, if a 12-year-old patient complains of frontal headaches and eyestrain when reading, the most likely tentative diagnoses are uncorrected hyperopia or decompensated near heterophoria. Depending on results from other tests, tests used may include measuring fusional reserves, AC/A ratio, fixation disparity and cycloplegic refraction. If a 30-year-old patient is complaining of sudden painless vision loss in one eye (>24 hours), the most likely tentative diagnoses would include a unilateral change in refractive error (i.e. suddenly noticed rather than sudden onset), optic neuritis and idiopathic central serous choroidopathy. None of the additional tests used in the previous example would be used. Instead, fundus biomicroscopy, photostress recovery time, central visual field and contrast sensitivity testing may be used. In the latter case, an assessment of the refractive system may be limited to focimetry (lensometry), visual acuity and pinhole visual acuity. If the pinhole visual acuity suggests that visual acuity improvements are unlikely with an altered refractive correction, then a full objective and subjective refraction may not be necessary.

When using this style of examination, you must also be aware that any new or changed prescription should not produce symptoms. For example, the possible effect of an increased myopic correction on an esophoria should be determined prior to dispensing the spectacles: the increased myopia would likely increase the esophoria and you need to know whether it could become decompensated.

Table 2.1 Classification of tests/procedures into one of four clinical oculovisual systems.

Visual*	Binocular*	Refractive	Ocular health
Case history	Case history	Case history	Case history
Visual acuity	Cover test	Visual acuity	Visual acuity
Colour vision	Motility	Retinoscopy	Biomicroscopy
Visual fields	Convergence tests	Autorefraction	Ophthalmoscopy
Contrast sensitivity	Accommodation tests	Subjective	Tonometry
Disability glare	Suppression tests	Near add determination	Gonioscopy
	Pupil responses	Keratometry	Pupil responses
	Stereopsis		

* Other classifications discuss the sensory and motor systems rather than the visual and binocular systems and place suppression and stereopsis within the sensory system.

Disadvantages of the problem-oriented examination include its dependence on the patient's symptoms. Obviously if a case history is not possible for any reason, a problem-oriented approach cannot be used and a database style of examination is necessary. In addition, there are also a variety of reasons why some patients may not disclose all their symptoms (Ettinger 1994). These include:

- They might believe that their headaches are not associated with their vision or their eyes.

- They may assume that the clinician will identify a problem and would ask specifically about it if it was important.

- They could think that their slightly blurred vision is a normal consequence of ageing.

- They might not mention some symptoms such as flashes and floaters because they may think that they are not important and they may even believe that mentioning such symptoms would make them look foolish.

This further highlights the need to use the problem-oriented examination within a system assessment approach. It also indicates the importance of developing a good rapport with the patient to obtain a comprehensive case history (Ettinger 1994). A further disadvantage of the problem-oriented approach is its complexity. To perform a problem-oriented examination, excellent communication skills are required to obtain a complete case history, a competent grasp of the information provided in the case history and how it relates to various ocular abnormalities is needed, plus a knowledge of which tests are required to perform the huge variety of differential diagnoses. It is not suitable for the student clinician and can only be developed after significant experience has been gained in primary eye care.

2.1.4 Combination approach

Another approach is to gain a complete database of information during an initial examination of a patient, and then use a problem-oriented approach during subsequent examinations. This necessitates different appointment slots for first time and subsequent examinations, with the first time appointment slot being longer than for subsequent visits.

2.1.5 Test order

Table 2.2 provides a suggested order of testing for performing an efficient optometric examination. The exact testing to be performed will depend on the presenting complaint of the patient. Other test procedures should be inserted at appropriate

Table 2.2 Approximate order of testing for performing various procedures in a routine optometric examination of an adult patient.

1. Case history
2. Focimetry
3. Vision (Unaided visual acuity)
4. Unaided cover test
5. Habitual visual acuity
6. Aided cover test
7. Near point of covergence
8. Worth 4-dot
9. Motility testing
10. Interpupillary distance measurement
11. Retinoscopy (and/or autorefraction)
12. Subjective refraction
13. Distance modified Thorington (or alternative)
14. Distance fusional reserves (or associated phoria measurement)
15. Amplitude of accommodation
16. Reading add determination (if required)
17. Near modified Thorington (or alternative)
18. Near fusional reserves (or associated phoria measurement)
19. Stereoacuity
20. Pupil reflexes
21. Slit-lamp biomicroscopy
22. Undilated fundus biomicroscopy (if patient has large pupils)
23. Tonometry
24. Visual field screening (or analysis)
25. (If dilating the pupils): anterior angle assessment
26. Binocular indirect ophthalmoscopy (and fundus biomicroscopy)
27. Post-dilation tonometry
28. Discussion with the patient

times when the test result is not jeopardised by a preceding test and will not jeopardise tests that follow it in the eye examination. For example, refraction and pupil reflexes must be assessed prior to mydriasis and near muscle balance tests must be performed prior to cycloplegia.

2.1.6 Recording

In the descriptions of clinical procedures in the following chapters, a subsection on recording is included in each case. It is essential that all test results (including the 'results' from case history) are recorded. If they are not recorded, subsequent legal analysis of the records will conclude that they were not performed. Clearly, it is important to write legibly on your record cards. Not only should they be legible to colleagues who may examine the patient subsequently, they should be legible in case of possible subsequent legal analysis. Illegible record cards are a significant source of error in primary eye care (Steele et al. 2006). Similarly, it is hugely important to ensure that record cards are stored in an efficient and organised manner. One study has suggested that missing record cards are one of the most common problems in optometric practice (Steele et al. 2006).

The format of record cards can vary hugely. Many include various designated areas for certain test results that are commonly performed. This is an attempt to save time, as you do not have to write down the test or procedure used, but merely the result. Figure 2.1 shows an example of a recording form from a university clinic. The problem-oriented examination uses the acronym SOAP for its record format (Weed 1968). The record card itself is a plain white sheet. This reflects the fact that this style of examination is distinguished by its variability, so there is little point in making boxes for individual tests. SOAP stands for Subjective, Objective, Assessment, and Plan. The subjective information is that obtained from the case history and the objective information is the various test results obtained during the examination. The assessment and plan refer to the problem-plan list that is described in detail in a later section. These sections must 'close the loop' and link the assessment and plan back to the complaints of the patient.

2.2 PATIENT-CENTRED OPTOMETRY AND COMMUNICATION SKILLS

2.2.1 Patient-centred optometry

Optometry, with its mixture of healthcare and consumer products, appears to have always practised some degree of patient-centred healthcare, even if it was not known by that name. Patient satisfaction, which is at the centre of patient-centred healthcare, is vital for a thriving optometric practice. For example, patient satisfaction is associated with greater patient retention, increased patient referrals, greater profitability and lower rates of malpractice suits (Dawn & Lee 2004), which suggests that the most successful optometry practices must use a patient-centred approach. The medical research literature consistently indicates that patients particularly want good communication from their healthcare practitioners and explanations of diagnoses, prognoses, treatment and prevention using clear, non-technical terms (Dawn & Lee 2004). In addition, patients expect eye care clinicians to be honest, empathic and be able to listen well and address their concerns (Dawn et al. 2004). Patient-centred healthcare also means that patients take an active partnership role in their healthcare rather than a passive recipient role (Fylan & Grunfeld 2002).

2.2.2 Communicating with patients

It is evident from the medical literature that patient satisfaction is strongly linked with good communication. Good communicators are able to make a patient feel relaxed and that they have been listened to, that the problems they have with their vision and/or eyes have been fully understood and that all the appropriate tests have been performed. Good communicators are also able to provide understandable diagnoses, prognoses and management plan(s) that will be adhered to (Dawn & Lee 2004).

All student optometrists are taught basic communication skills. You are taught which questions to ask during the case history, what instructions to give for each test, an explanation of why you are doing the test and what to record. In clinics, you will be taught

THE EYE CLINIC: EXAMINATION RECORD CARD   Date:

Family name:	Other names:
Address:	DOB:
	NI no:
	GP & surgery: Age 47
	Occupation/Dept:
Tel no: Postcode:	Graduation year:

Date last NHS test: NHS eligibility   *not*   Evidence seen? ☐

CC: NV blur, "Needs longer arms", last 6/12. PC is ok DV ✓ Never worn
glasses or CLs. No h/a's, diplopia or other symptoms.
OH - None. LEE - 4 years ago, Leeds D&A.
FOH - None, no glaucoma or cataracts
GH - good, no meds or allergies. LME - l yr ago, Dr Thomas
FMH - none, no high BP or diabetes
Px drives, PC - 4 hrs/day, hobbies, reading and squash (no eye protection)

	sph	cyl	axis	prism	ADD	Details:
R						No previous Rx
L						

Peliminary testing

Distance Vision/~~VA~~

R 6/5   L 6/5

Near Vision/~~VA~~

R N8   L N8   @40cm

Muscle balance:

CT NMD, D
      4° XOP, N

Convergence:
to nose

PD: 63 / 60   @ 40

Motility:

SAFE ✳

Refraction

Objective: *Technique:*
R) + 0.25 / –0.25 x 100   VA: 6/5   L) + 0.25 / –0.25 x 80   VA: 6/5

Subjective: *Technique:* Binocular
R) + 0.50 / –0.25 x 105   VA: 6/5   L) + 0.25 / –0.25 x 70   VA: 6/5
Vertex Distance: 10 mm   Binocular Add: None

Tentative Reading Add.   R) + 1.00   L) + 1.00   From: ☑Age   ☐ WD ☐ Accom ☐ Other

READING ADD @ 40 cm   R) + 1.00   VA: N5   L) + 1.00   VA: N5   Range: 30 to 65

Intermediate ADD @   cm   R)   VA: L)   VA: Range: to

Binocular vision

Muscle balance:

⊕   ⊖
            4° XOP,
Technique: Moddox rod   M, Wing

Amplitude of Accommodation:
3D binocular
Technique: push-up/down

Other motor/sensory status:

Fig. 2.1   A University clinic record form detailing a fictional patient.

Ocular health

Tonometry: Time: 10:30	Anterior angle:
R) 15 L) 16	R) IV T L) IV T
Instrument: Goldmann	*Technique:* Van Herick
Pupils:	Sensitivity to diagnostic drugs? ☐ YES ☒ NO
D&C 3+, R+L	Mydriatic used: Tropicamide 0.5%
−ve RAPD	Post-dilation IOP $_{16}T_{16}$

Supplementary

R   ⟨S-lamp⟩ / Direct ?   L

Anterior eye
(lids, conjunctive, sclera, iris)
NAD R + L, small pingueculae nasal R+L

Media
(cornea, lens, vitreous)
Clear R + L

Disc

CD 0.40 H + V
Healthy NRR,
obeys ISNT rule.

CD 0.40 H 0.35 V
Healthy NRR,
obeys ISNT rule.

Vessels
AV 60%   AV 60%
No AV crossing changes R + L

Periphery
NAD R + L

Macula — NAD R + L
Direct / ⟨Volk⟩ / BIO ?

(e.g. Visual fields, cycloplegic refraction, colour vision, contrast sensitivity)

SITA - Fast: WNL R + L

SUMMARY

PROBLEM *(i.e. diagnosis)*	PLAN *(i.e. action to be taken)*
1. Presbyopia	1. PALS

Final Rx

	sph	cyl	axis	prism	ADD	Rx advice:
R	+ 0.50	− 0.25	105			Needed for NV tasks only.
L	+ 0.25	− 0.25	70		+ 1.00	No need to use with PC.

Student name and signature:

Student name and signature:	Supervisor's signature:	Suggested re-examination time:
		24 months

Fig. 2.1   (Continued).

how to provide diagnoses, prognoses and management plans. All optometrists should therefore gain adequate communication skills. How do you become a better communicator? You can obviously read about what they are. A brief summary is provided here and further reading is suggested (e.g. Ettinger 1994). Video recording your case history and/or eye examination can be a valuable tool and will particularly highlight your non-verbal communication skills. A helpful quality about communication skills is that you can learn them anywhere and from anybody. Obviously, observing an optometrist or other health professional who is popular with patients could be particularly beneficial. You can also practise your own communication skills in any environment that involves working with the public. As a supervisor in student clinics it is very obvious from the level of communication skills, which students have had jobs that involved working with the general public and which ones have not. A summer job that involves working with the general public is therefore advisable if you have never had such a job before.

2.2.3 Patient anxiety

Patients expect eye care clinicians to be empathic (Dawn et al. 2004). This means that a patient expects you to be able to recognise and understand their emotions and be able to 'put yourself in their shoes'. To do this, you need to think about how a patient might feel when they attend for an eye examination. Note that a significant number of patients are anxious about attending an optometric practice (e.g. Fylan & Grunfeld 2005) and possible reasons include:

1. Being told they need spectacles. This can be a worry for both pre-presbyopic (Pesudovs et al. 2004) and presbyopic patients (Fylan & Grunfeld 2005) who are often concerned about the effect on their appearance.

2. Fear of vision loss. Particularly true of elderly patients where eye disease is a greater risk (e.g. Fylan & Grunfeld 2005). This could be due to the fact that a friend or family member has lost their vision due to eye disease and this could even have

been detected at a routine visit to their optometrists. Some patients are even aware that optometrists can detect conditions such as brain tumours and worry about this.

3. Cost issues. Some patients are very worried about the potential cost of spectacles and contact lenses (Pesudovs et al. 2004, Fylan & Grunfeld 2005) and even that they will be 'sold' spectacles that aren't necessary. This can manifest as a comment such as 'my glasses are fine and I don't need another pair' at the start of the case history.

4. Fear of making a mistake. Some patients are worried about making mistakes during the subjective refraction part of the examination. This may be because they believe that a mistake on their part could lead to the provision of an incorrect refractive correction in their spectacles and/or are worried about feeling foolish if they make a mistake (note that some patients can feel educationally inferior to the optometrist).

5. Fear of increased ametropia. Young ametropes can worry that the increasing myopia or hyperopia will mean thicker and less attractive spectacles. Vision-related quality of life has been shown to be reduced in pre-presbyopic spectacle wearers with high prescriptions (Pesudovs et al. 2006).

6. Being told that they cannot wear contact lenses any more. Young contact lens wearers typically report a better vision-related quality of life than spectacle wearers (Pesudovs et al. 2006) and some may worry about being told that they cannot wear contact lenses any more.

7. Adaptation problems. Many patients report concerns about being able to adapt to their new spectacles (Fylan & Grunfeld 2005).

8. Fear of looking foolish. Some patients are very tentative about admitting some of their concerns about their vision in case they are made to look foolish by raising the issue. Concerns about vitreous floaters are a typical example of this.

2.2.4 Relaxing the patient and building a rapport

It should be evident that an anxious patient is unlikely to provide a full case history and reveal all their visual problems, unlikely to attend appropriately to your instructions, could provide unreliable responses in the subjective refraction and could easily misinterpret or forget what you said about their diagnoses and management plans. A good communicator will be able to relax an anxious patient. There are many ways to relax a patient and build a rapport and these include:

1. Provide a comfortable and welcoming setting in the practice waiting room. Comfortable chairs, a selection of magazines, some low level music, etc. can all help to relax the patient. Framed copies of your qualifications, either in the waiting room or the examination room, can provide reassurance to some patients.

2. Welcome the patient. First impressions count and most patients prefer a conservative, smart, 'professional' appearance. Ideally you should enter the waiting room, greet your patient by name and escort them to the examination room.

3. Beware of making the examination room frightening to the patient. For example, a poster containing a cross-sectional diagram of the eye can be very useful for explanation purposes, but one that portrays a variety of eye diseases is not likely to relax the patient!

4. Change the chair height to ensure you are at the same eye level as the patient.

5. Some practitioners like to chat about non-clinical issues (weather, holidays, sports teams, parking, etc.) prior to the examination to help relax the patient. In this respect, it can be useful to make a note of any relevant information (a child's favourite sport, sports player, team, author; the patient's pets and their names, their children's successes, etc.) to allow you to start a relaxing conversation at subsequent visits.

6. Your posture and style should be relaxed but attentive. Maintain regular eye contact and use the patient's name at appropriate times during the eye examination.

7. An open question is typically used to start the case history (section 2.3.2, step 4) as this allows the patient to tell you about any problems with their vision or spectacles. A balance is required between allowing the patient plenty of time to discuss their problems and not rushing them but at the same time retaining control of the discussion. You need to ensure that the patient feels that you have fully listened and understood their problems and you may even need to allow the patient to talk about information that you know is not necessary from a diagnostic viewpoint. However, you also need to develop the skill of being able to interrupt an overly talkative patient without appearing rude.

8. Some patients are very shy and an open question provides little information and may make the patient feel uncomfortable. Closed questions can be useful at the beginning of the case history with such patients. An open question can be used later in the case history if the patient relaxes and conversation becomes easier.

9. Listening is a hugely important communication skill. It is vital that you have fully listened to the patient and understood their problems (e.g. Dawn et al. 2004). There are a variety of ways that indicate to the patient that you are listening and these include maintaining eye contact and demonstrating attention by nodding and/or using affirmative comments such as 'I see', 'I understand', 'OK, go on', etc. Listening is also indicated by using follow-up questions to comments, such as asking about the location, onset, frequency, etc. of headaches when the patient indicates that they suffer with them. Finally, summarising the patient's problems at the end of the case history (section 2.3.2, step 10) is a very useful way of indicating to the patient that you have listened to what they have to say and fully understand what problems they are having whilst it also provides the patient with an opportunity to inform you if you have missed anything.

2.2.5 Providing information regarding tests used, diagnoses, prognoses and management plans

Provide an explanation of each test that you use in an eye examination. Suggested information, in lay terms, is provided for each test described in later chapters. Patients expect you to provide information about the cause of their visual problems, the prognoses and any management plans, all in a clear non-technical language (Dawn & Lee 2004). Non-compliance with instructions regarding eye care (Edmunds et al. 1997) and contact lenses (40–90%, Claydon & Efron 1994) is common, but is improved by a better patient-practitioner relationship (Claydon & Efron, 1994).

1. Diagnoses: At the end of the examination, you must discuss your findings, particularly those that relate to the patient's chief complaint and other secondary complaints. Give a full explanation of the diagnoses in lay terms (unless your patient works in the medical field and has some knowledge). It can be very useful to have a cross-sectional diagram of the eye to help you in this explanation. Make sure you go back to the case history and try to explain each of the patient's symptoms. It is generally best to discuss your findings in order of the relative importance of the problems to the patient rather than your own opinion of the relative importance of the diagnoses.

2. Reassurance: Provide reassurance if the cause of any symptoms cannot be found (Blume 1987). Indicate to the patient what conditions you have not detected. An example is provided in section 4.25.2 for a patient with headaches and no obvious oculo-visual cause.

3. Treatment options: Provide the patient with all the possible treatment options and involve the patient in the decision of the most appropriate management. Most clinicians report tailoring spectacle lens information to match the patient's requirements, based on the patient's occupation and hobbies (Fylan & Grunfeld 2005). One study reported that some practitioners do not always recommend the highest specification, and usually most expensive, lenses and overestimate the importance to some patients of the price of spectacles (Fylan & Grunfeld 2005).

4. Instructions: Instructions regarding ocular disease management, contact lens care and maintenance, etc. should be clear and unambiguous, with appropriate emphasis placed on the importance of procedures from a safety viewpoint. Written instructions are essential. Checking compliance and repeating the instructions at follow-up visits can improve matters (Claydon & Efron 1994, Edmunds et al. 1997).

5. Prognoses: Explain what is the likely prognosis of the patient's condition(s) and highlight any possible adaptation problems. Be honest: if the condition is likely to get worse, you must inform the patient of this.

6. Next appointment: Finally, indicate to the patient when you would like to see them again and if this is less than a standard time interval, explain why.

2.2.6 Information leaflets

Information leaflets should be available if requested. They are viewed by patients as valuable additional information to that provided verbally and information that can be referred to at a future time and for discussion with family members (Fylan & Grunfeld 2002). They are seen to be particularly valuable given that patients are aware of the time limitations of clinical appointments.

1. What leaflets? Patients would prefer more information on eye examination procedures, an explanation of prescriptions and practical information about how to look after their eyesight (Fylan & Grunfeld 2002).

2. Leaflet style: Research has indicated that patients find the information in currently available information leaflets and websites to contain too much jargon, with a poor layout of diagrams and text and inadequate or

irrelevant explanations (Fylan & Grunfeld 2002). Patients reported that leaflets often included unexplained terms, such as 'accommodation' and 'macula', that were confusing, and that they relied on an excessively high level of previous knowledge.

3. Problem-solving approach: Patients prefer a problem-solving approach being taken with information pamphlets rather than an educational approach (Fylan & Grunfeld 2002). Information should be provided which is applicable and relevant to the patient's own eye care.

4. Links with adverse outcomes: Contact lens instruction leaflets that provide a rationale for various procedures and links with adverse outcomes may help compliance (Claydon & Efron 1994).

5. Lay terms: Leaflets should be interesting, concise and with simple explanation written in lay terms.

6. Sections: Different topics should be organised into clearly labelled sections so that patients can identify particular sections that they are interested in.

7. Diagrams: Diagrams should be provided in colour. Patients have reported that diagrams in currently available leaflets can be too small with difficult-to-read labels (Fylan & Grunfeld 2002). Patients appear to prefer a brief explanation of the function of different structures if included, rather than just labelling them (Fylan & Grunfeld 2002).

2.2.7 Giving bad news

Unfortunately, you will occasionally need to inform a patient that you cannot improve their vision because they have an ocular disease of some description. This may be a disease like cataract that is treatable and the patient needs to be referred to a secondary eye care setting or it may be a disease like dry age-related maculopathy and essentially untreatable. In both cases, the following information should be provided:

1. Indicate the eye examination has finished and you wish to discuss your findings. You may put down your pen and even turn off the projector chart. Make eye contact with the patient and make sure that the patient is comfortable and attentive.

2. Introduce your diagnosis by reminding the patient of their symptoms and then link them with the diagnosis.

3. Explain what the eye disease is in simple lay terms. Give the patient time to digest the information and encourage them to ask questions.

4. Present the various treatment options and/or referral options available, with advantages and disadvantages.

5. Provide the patient with an appropriate information leaflet, if available, and indicate that they can return or phone with any questions.

With patients with an untreatable condition, such as dry age-related maculopathy, you should use the previously described approach. In addition:

1. You need to be aware of the possible emotional responses to such news. Various models have been proposed and a common model suggests stages of denial, anger, bargaining, depression and acceptance. These stages are not universal and some patients skip stages while others get 'stuck' at a particular stage. In the denial stage, patients will often seek a second opinion. You should not see this as a slight on your ability as a clinician and you may even suggest it to a patient who is openly in denial when you first tell them the news.

2. You should explain that they will not go 'blind' and should keep their peripheral vision. However, at the same time you must be honest and do not attempt to avoid difficult questions or even 'sugar the pill' (Hopper & Fischbach 1989). Indicate that their central, detailed vision that allows them to drive, read and see faces, is likely to get worse.

3. Explain the prevalence of the condition. This indicates that they are not alone. It can be

useful at this point to discuss support groups and local agencies.

4. Discuss the availability of low vision aids and what help they could provide. In this respect, remember the stages of response to vision loss. Patients are unlikely to have the motivation to successfully use low vision aids when depressed. Do not give up on these patients. As and when they overcome the depression and accept their vision loss, low vision aids may usefully be provided.

5. It can be very useful to explain all this information to the patient's family if they are present and if the patient is happy for you to do so.

6. Information leaflets are particularly useful in these situations as the patient's shock at the initial news may mean that much of the remainder of your discussion is forgotten.

2.3 THE CASE HISTORY

The case history is the cornerstone of an eye examination. You must listen to the patient to determine what their problems are and ask appropriate questions to obtain the crucial details about their complaints. The case history puts you in the position of detective. There may be problems to discover and you must use all your skills of observation, listening, and questioning to identify them as completely as possible. Undoubtedly the case history can differentiate an experienced clinician from a novice. It is common for clinical supervisors to have to ask several additional questions of a patient after a student has completed the examination. As a student, you should not worry about this, as you will improve with experience. However, never underestimate the value of history taking and how much there is to learn to be competent at it.

2.3.1 Information provided

Here are a few important points that the case history provides:

- A general observation of the patient. For example, you should notice any peculiarities of a patient's gait, head position, facial asymmetry, skin colour, physiological appearance in relation to chronological age, ability to speak and articulate, intellectual level, emotional state, overall state of health.

- Age, gender and race information allows you to think about the most likely problems in the light of the prevalence of ocular disorders and their association with these factors.

- The patient's chief complaint allows you to mentally list the most likely tentative diagnoses and ask appropriate supplementary questions to begin differential diagnosis during the case history. Some differential diagnoses, such as a red eye, may rely heavily on case history.

- Information about the patient's happiness with their current spectacles and/or contact lenses helps you determine whether to prescribe new lenses when the refractive change is low. Similarly, the degree of symptoms, combined with your assessment of personality and the amount of detailed visual work performed helps you to determine whether to prescribe a low-power refractive correction.

- The ocular history indicates whether the patient has had previous ocular treatment or surgery. A history of an ocular abnormality allows you to look for the manifestations of the disorder and any secondary effects (for example, glaucoma following central retinal vein occlusion).

- The medical history may indicate that you should particularly look for certain ocular disorders which manifest in certain systemic disease (most commonly diabetes) and whether it is safe to use certain diagnostic drugs such as phenylephrine.

- The medication information may alert you to possible adverse effects of systemic medications (e.g. dry eye in an elderly hypertensive taking beta-blockers).

- Family history information determines if there are any hereditary ocular and/or medical conditions in the patient's family.

Common examples include a family history of diabetes, hypertension, myopia, strabismus, amblyopia and glaucoma.

■ Information regarding the patient's occupation and hobbies is very useful when you are prescribing spectacles, particularly for near work. For example, you want to know whether the reading addition needs to provide clear vision for computer work, reading, sewing or all three, whether the patient uses protective eyewear when playing sports and whether the patient drives with spectacles or not.

■ Using the problem-orientated examination means that the case history decides to some degree which tests/procedures you are going to perform.

2.3.2 Procedure

1. Make sure that the room lights are on before the patient enters the examination room.

2. Observe the patient's appearance: Observe their stature, walking ability and overall physical appearance. Pay particular attention to any head tilt or obvious abnormalities of the face, eyelids and eyes that will require further investigation, such as facial asymmetry, lid lesions, ptosis, epiphora, entropion, ectropion, a red eye or strabismus.

3. You should sit about 1 m from the patient at eye level. Try to avoid long silences while writing notes and attempt to develop the ability to write down answers as the patient is talking, while retaining intermittent eye contact. Try to avoid long periods without making eye contact with the patient.

4. Chief Complaint (CC) or Reason For Visit (RFV): Determine the chief complaint by asking a very general open-ended question such as 'Do you have any problems with your vision or your eyes?' or 'Is there any particular reason for your visit, Ms Smith?' With some patients, you may get a good description of the problem with little prompting. However, you are

unlikely to obtain all the information you require and so will have to ask some questions to 'fill in the holes' in what the patient has already told you. The order of the type of questions you would generally ask is given below, to provide a reasonable acronym LOFTSEA for students, rather than a logical sequence. Examples of questions to ask are provided for symptoms of blurred distance vision, headaches and diplopia.

a) Location/laterality. Examples:
   ■ 'Is the blurred vision in both eyes or just one?', 'Is the blurred vision greater in one eye or the other?'
   ■ 'In which part of the head is the headache located?' *For a frontal headache, ask* 'Is it above one eye more than the other?'
   ■ 'Is the double vision in all directions of gaze or just one?'

b) Onset. Examples:
   ■ 'How long have you had blurred distance vision?'
   ■ 'When did the headaches start?'
   ■ 'When did you first get double vision?'

c) Frequency/occurrence. Examples:
   ■ *If the blurred vision is variable ask* 'How often do you get the blurred vision?'
   ■ 'How often do the headaches occur?', 'How long do the headaches last?'
   ■ 'How often do you get double vision?'

d) Type/severity. Examples:
   ■ 'Is the blur constant or intermittent?', 'Did the blurred vision start suddenly or gradually?' *If sudden vision loss, ask* 'Was the vision loss partial or total?'
   ■ 'Is it a throbbing, sharp or dull headache?'
   ■ 'Is the double vision one-on-top-of-the-other or side-by-side?'

e) Self-treatment and its effectivity:
   ■ 'Does anything make the blurred vision go away?' (*possibly a family member's spectacles for example*)
   ■ 'Does anything make the headaches go away?'
   ■ 'Does anything make the double vision go away?'

f) Effect on the patient:
  - 'Is your poor vision affecting how well you can do your job/schoolwork?'
  - 'How badly do the headaches affect you?' 'Have you been to see your GP about the headaches?'
  - 'Do you ever get the double vision when driving?' 'Have you seen a physician about the double vision?'

g) Associated factors: 'Are there any other symptoms associated with the problem?'

5. Symptom check:
  a) In a patient who has a chief complaint, you then need to ask about other visual problems (unless they were disclosed when discussing the chief complaint). For example, if a patient has a chief complaint of headaches, once you have a complete description of the headaches, you need to ask about their distance vision, near vision, eyestrain, pain or discomfort and diplopia. If a positive response to any of these questions is obtained, you then need to obtain a complete description of that complaint.
  b) In a patient stating they have no complaints to the general question asked above and who has just attended for their regular annual/biannual examination, ask the following questions:
    - 'How is your distance vision?' This can be adapted to suit the patient. For example, a student could be asked 'Any problems reading from the whiteboard?' and 'Is everything clear on the TV?'
    - 'Any problems with reading?' This can also be adapted to suit the patient. For example, a secretary could be asked: 'Can you see the computer screen clearly?'
    - 'Do you get any eyestrain?'
    - 'Do you get any headaches?'
    - 'Do you ever get any pain or burning/discomfort in your eyes?'
    - 'Do you ever see double?'

- Direct questioning regarding haloes, flashes and floaters can lead to longwinded and unnecessary descriptions of normal entoptic/light scatter phenomena (flashes of light when you press on the eye or the halo seen around candles) and are generally best not asked routinely, but should be asked of patients with high myopia or with other risk factors for retinal detachment.

6. Ocular History (OH) and Family Ocular History (FOH):
  a) If you are unsure, ask if the patient wears spectacles. If they do, then you need a complete description of the spectacles used. This may include:
    - 'How many pairs of spectacles do you have?'
    - 'What type are they and what do you use them for?'
    - 'Do you wear your spectacles all the time?' (if you suspect that they should) or 'When do you wear your spectacles?'
    - 'How old are your spectacles?'
    - 'Where did you get these spectacles from?'
    - 'How old were you when you first wore spectacles?'
    - 'Do you have prescription sunglasses?'
    - Particularly in a patient who has no visual complaints: 'Are you still happy with the fashion and fit of your spectacle frame?'
  b) If you are unsure, ask if the patient wears contact lenses. If they do, then you need a complete description of the contact lenses used:
    - 'What type of lens are they?' (soft, gas permeable, toric, bifocal, etc.)
    - 'How old are your contact lenses?'
    - 'Who prescribed the lenses?'
    - 'How long do you usually wear the lenses each day?' and 'How many days per week?' Also: 'What is the longest that you will wear your lenses?'

- 'When did you put your contact lenses in today?'
- 'What cleaning solutions do you use?'
- 'When was your last contact lens aftercare?'
- 'When is your next aftercare check scheduled?'
- 'Have you had to stop contact lens wear for any reason, even for a short time?'
- 'When did you first start wearing contact lenses?'

c) If the patient wears both spectacles and contact lenses, you will have to ask about visual symptoms (i.e. distance blur, near blur, headaches, eyestrain, etc.) in both situations.

d) Ask whether the patient has had any previous eye injuries, infections, surgery or treatment. Follow up any positive responses by asking the patient how old they were at the time, who managed the condition and over what period and what treatment they received. For example, if a patient indicates they have amblyopia, discover the age they were diagnosed (the later the diagnosis, the higher the likely degree of amblyopia) and whether and at what time they had an 'eye-patch', 'eye exercises', spectacles or surgery.

e) If you do not already know, ask the patient when their last eye examination (LEE) was and by whom it was done.

f) Family Ocular History (FOH): An open-ended question such as 'Has anybody in your family had any eye problem or disease?' should be asked. This can be clarified by providing examples of common hereditary conditions such as cataract or glaucoma for older patients, or spectacles, squint or lazy eyes with children.

7. General Health Information: A general question of 'how is your general health?' can be misleading because some patients think that systemic diseases are not relevant when they are borderline or are controlled by medication. It is better to follow up the initial question and give some examples of what is being specifically sought after, such as 'any high blood pressure or diabetes?' If you get a positive response to this question, you must ask the patient how long they have had the condition as ocular effects of systemic diseases are more likely the longer the patient has had the condition. For example, the duration of diabetes is a major risk factor for diabetic retinopathy (Moss et al. 1998). If the patient has diabetes or hypertension, ask how well the condition is controlled. The risk of diabetic retinopathy is greatly reduced with good glycaemic control in diabetic patients (Shamoon et al. 1993) and by good blood pressure control in a patient with diabetes and hypertension (Stearne et al. 1998). An alternative or additional question for a female who may be pregnant is to ask the patient if they see their GP or a practice nurse regularly. It is important to ask patients whether they are taking any medication even if they indicate that their general health is fine. Patients may believe their general health is fine because it is controlled by medication. Patients may also be taking medications, but be unsure why, because the medical diagnosis was not properly explained or was poorly understood. It is important to determine any medications that the patient is taking as some can have adverse ocular effects. For example, it is well known that beta-blockers prescribed for systemic hypertension can cause dry eyes and oral corticosteroids can cause posterior subcapsular cataracts. Typically, the higher the dosage of the drug and the longer the patient has been taking them, the more likely are adverse ocular effects. Therefore it is important to ask about the dosage and number of tablets taken per day and how long they have taken the drug. Note that patients may not consider 'over-the-counter' tablets, such as travel sickness pills, antihistamines, sleeping pills and painkillers as medications, so it can be useful to ask about them specifically, particularly with patients with unexplained symptoms. Similarly, female patients may not consider birth control pills to be medication, yet the

drugs in these pills can have adverse ocular effects. Ask the following questions:

   a) 'How is your general health?' and add a follow-up question such as 'any high blood pressure or diabetes?'

   b) If you receive a positive response, ask the patient how long they have had the condition. For some conditions, such as diabetes and hypertension, ask whether the condition is well controlled.

   c) 'Do you take any medication?'

   d) If you receive a positive response, ask the patient how long the medication has been taken, the present dosage and the number of tablets taken per day.

   e) 'Any allergies?'

   f) Ask the patient when they last visited their GP (last medical examination, LME) and obtain the name of the GP.

   g) Family Medical History (FMH): Ask an open-ended question, clarified by examples, such as 'Has anybody in your family had any medical problem?' This can be clarified by providing examples of common hereditary conditions such as 'any diabetes or high blood pressure in the family?'

8. Vocation, sports, hobbies, computer use and driving: Determine the patient's visual demands, including the safety hazards/ protection for the patient's vocation as well as their sports and hobbies. For presbyopic patients, you need to discover the distance used for reading and other near tasks and the use of any additional reading lights (e.g. anglepoise or goose-neck lights, etc.; section 4.23). Question whether they use a computer on a regular basis and determine approximate weekly usage. Determine whether the patient drives and whether they wear contact lenses or spectacles when driving.

9. History of falls: It can be useful to ask patients who are at risk of falling (over 75 years of age, using more than three medications, antidepressant use, systemic conditions that reduce mobility, cardiac problems, etc.) or who may be more dependent on their vision

for balance control (elderly patients with somatosensory system dysfunction such as diabetes and/or peripheral neuropathy or those with vestibular system dysfunction, such as Ménière's disease), whether they have a history of falling. A history of falls increases their risk of falling again. Patients at high risk of falling need to be identified as they should have more regular eye examinations, earlier cataract surgery and an altered spectacle prescribing strategy (section 4.24.5; Buckley & Elliott 2006).

10. Summarise the case history: Summarise the pertinent information from the case history and allow the patient to clarify any misunderstanding on your part or to add any additional information that has been missed. For example, 'So Mrs Jones, the main reasons for your visit are that reading has become a little difficult, even with your glasses, and that you particularly want me to perform all the glaucoma diagnostic tests because your mother has glaucoma. Is that correct?'

11. Remember that a case history continues throughout the examination. Certain signs or test results during the examination may suggest the need for further questioning.

Box 2.1   Summary of case history procedure

1. Determine the chief complaint. Use LOFTSEA or similar to collect all the appropriate information

2. Symptom check: Check the following if not part of the chief complaint: distance vision, near vision, headaches, eyestrain, pain or discomfort and diplopia

3. Ask about the patient's ocular history, family ocular history and LEE

4. Obtain general health information: All systemic diseases, medications, allergies, family medical history and LME

5. Vocation, sports, hobbies, computer use and driving

6. Summarise the case history

7. Remember that a case history continues throughout the examination

2.3.3 Recording

Both positive and negative patient responses must be recorded. Remember that from a legal viewpoint, if the response was not recorded the question was not asked. Use standard abbreviations (Table 2.3) and avoid personal ones. Using the patient's own words, recorded in quotation marks, can be useful. Here are some examples:

1. 12-year-old Px. Caucasian. Student.
   CC: 'Can't see blackboard' $\bar{c}$ Rx last 6/12 in both eyes, gradual onset. TV = OK $\bar{s}$ Rx, sits close. NV good $\bar{s}$ Rx. No H/A. No other Sxs.
   OH: Wears Rx for school only (w/board, not outside). 1st wore age 10, this Rx 2 years old. F&F = OK, no other OH. LEE: 2 yr, Dr Hurst, Oldham. FOH: mum and dad both myopic. GH = OK, no meds. No allergies. LME: 6/12, Dr Jarse, Saddleworth. FMH: mat grandfather has IDDM.
   Hobbies: football (no Rx worn), computer games. Uses PC ≈ 1 hour/day.

2. 48-year-old Caucasian female (secretary).
   RFV: NV blurred OU, grad ↓ last 4/12. PC work OK, although gets dull frontal h/as after ≈ 1 hr, last 2/12, gen. pm, goes if rest eyes & better on weekend, not seen GP. DV = fine. No other Sxs.
   OH: No specs. Has 'squint' and 'lazy eye' OD; Rx age 18/12 for strab; can't remember eyepatch; had surgery age 15 yrs and did eye exercises before and after surgery. Stopped wearing Rx after surgery. LEE: ≈ 5 yrs, Dr Bullimore, Ohio. FOH: Mother cataracts aged 65.
   GH: Good, no meds. Allergic to penicillin. LME: 4/12, Dr Who, Main Street, Ohio. FMH: Mother and sister high BP, no other.
   Hobbies: reading, cycling. Drives. Uses PC ≈ 5 hrs/day.

3. Case Hx: 68-year-old Asian female (retired).
   CC: Routine 2yr exam. DV & NV = fine $\bar{c}$ Rx. No h/as. Eyes sl. red last 9/12, 'Eyes burn', no pain, no discharge, no itching. Not had prev. Worse with reading & stops reading after 30 mins. No other Sxs.

Table 2.3   Abbreviations that could be used during the recording of a case history.

Abbreviation	Stands for	Abbreviation	Stands for
Px (or Pt)	Patient	OK or ✓	Okay
Rx	Prescription/spectacles	Sxs	Symptoms
CC(or PC or RFV)	Chief complaint or	CLs	Contact lenses
	Presenting complaint	OH	Ocular history
	or Reason for visit	FOH	Family ocular history
DV	Distance vision	FMH	Family medical history
NV	Near vision	GH	General health
R	Right	BP	Blood pressure
L	Left	IDDM/NIDDM	Insulin-dependent/
RE (or OD)	Right eye		non-insulin-dependent
LE (or OS)	Left eye		diabetes mellitus
B (or binoc)	Binocular	meds	Medication
BE (or OU)	Both eyes	Ung.	Ointment
$\bar{c}$ (or c)	With	o.d.	Once daily
$\bar{s}$ (or s)	Without	b.i.d. (or b.d.)	Twice a day
1/7, 3/7	1 day, 3 days	t.i.d.	Three times a day
1/52, 3/52	1 week, 3 weeks	q.i.d.	Four times a day
1/12, 3/12	1 month, 3 months	p.r.n.	When needed
H	Horizontal	q.h.	Every hour
V	Vertical	LEE	Last eye examination
H/as	Headaches	LME	Last medical examination
↑	Increase	F & F	Fit and fashion (of spectacles)
↓	Decrease		

OH: Bifs, worn all time. Happy *c* them. 1st wore age 50, this Rx 2 years old. F&F = OK, no other OH. Never worn CLs. LEE: 2 yr. D&As, Hull. No FOH.

GH = NIDDM for 15 yrs, Metformin 500 mg b.i.d, well controlled; High BP for 15 yrs, Propranolol 100 mg b.i.d, well controlled, check-up every 6/12; High cholesterol, last 2 yrs, 'Statins' 40 mg o.d now under control; Takes aspirin o.d, last 3 yrs to 'thin blood' & 'help avoid heart attack', check-up every 6/12; LME: 2/12, Dr Pesudovs, Second Place, Hull. No allergies, FMH: None. Hobbies: Walking, watching TV. No PC use. Doesn't drive.

2.3.4 Interpretation

Once all verbal information is accurately collected the examiner should have a list of tentative diagnoses in mind for each of the identified problems. The remainder of the eye examination is based on testing to differentiate which of the tentative diagnoses is correct as well as gathering information so that each system (visual function, refractive and binocular systems and an ocular health assessment; Table 1.1) has been assessed.

2.3.5 Most common errors

- Not fully investigating the patient's chief complaint.

- Not recording all information obtained from the patient.

- Failing to identify a drug name and dosage or identify possible side effects.

- Recording personal abbreviations that will not be universally understood.

- Not following through the case history in an organised manner.

- Forgetting that the case history taking can continue throughout the examination.

- Taking the confidential case history in public (e.g. waiting room).

- Assuming the same information is still current from the previous case history.

- Repeating questions.

- Leaving a record card on view to the public, such as on the reception desk.

2.4 BIBLIOGRAPHY AND FURTHER READING

Amos, J.F. (1991) Patient history. In: *Clinical procedures in optometry* (eds J.B. Eskridge, J.F. Amos and J.D. Bartlett). Philadelphia: J.B. Lippincott.

Elliott, D.B. (1997) The problem-oriented examination's case history. In: *The ocular examination: measurements and findings* (ed. K. Zadnik). Philadelphia: W.B. Saunders.

Ettinger, E.R. (1994) *Professional communications in eye care.* Boston: Butterworth-Heinemann.

2.5 REFERENCES

Amos, J.F. (1987) The problem-solving approach to patient care. In: *Diagnosis and management in vision care* (ed. J.F. Amos). Boston: Butterworths, pp. 1–8.

Blume, A.J. (1987) Reassurance therapy. In: *Diagnosis and management in vision care* (ed. J.F. Amos). Boston: Butterworths, pp. 715–718.

Buckley, J.G. and Elliott, D.B. (2006) Ophthalmic interventions to help prevent falls. *Geriatrics and Ageing* **9**, 276–280.

Claydon, B.E. and Efron, N. (1994) Non-compliance in contact lens wear. *Ophthalmic and Physiological Optics* **14**, 356–364.

Dawn, A.G. and Lee, P.P. (2004) Patient expectations for medical and surgical care: a review of the literature and applications to ophthalmology. *Survey of Ophthalmology* **49**: 513–524.

Dawn, A.G., Santiago-Turla, C., Lee, P.P. (2004) Patient expectations regarding eye care: focus group results. *Archives of Ophthalmology* **121**, 762–768.

Edmunds, B., Francis, P.J. and Elkington, A.R. (1997) Communication and compliance in eye casualty. *Eye* **11**, 345–348.

Elliott, D.B. (1998) The problem-oriented optometric examination. *Ophthalmic and Physiological Optics* (suppl. **18**), S21–S29.

Ettinger, E.R. (1994) *Professional communications in eye care*. Boston: Butterworth-Heinemann.

Fylan, F. and Grunfeld, E.A. (2002) Information within optometric practice: comprehension, preferences and implications. *Ophthalmic and Physiological Optics* **22**, 333–340.

Fylan, F. and Grunfeld, E.A. (2005) Visual illusions? Beliefs and behaviours of presbyope clients in optometric practice. *Patient Education and Counseling* **56**, 291–295.

Hopper, S.V. and Fischbach, R.L. (1989) Patient-physician communication when blindness threatens. *Patient Education and Counseling* **14**, 69–79.

Moss, S.E., Klein, R. and Klein, B.E.K. (1998) The 14-year incidence of visual loss in a diabetic population. *Ophthalmology* **105**, 998–1003.

Pesudovs, K., Garamendi, E. and Elliott, D.B. (2004) The Quality of Life Impact of Refractive Correction (QIRC) Questionnaire: development and validation. *Optometry and Vision Science* **81**, 769–777.

Pesudovs, K., Garamendi, E. and Elliott, D.B. (2006) A quality of life comparison of people wearing spectacles or contact lenses or having undergone refractive surgery. *Journal of Refractive Surgery* **22**, 19–27.

Shamoon, H., Duffy, H., Fleischer, N. et al. (1993) The effect of intensive treatment of diabetes on the development and progression of long-term complications in insulin-dependent diabetes-mellitus. *The New England Journal of Medicine* **329**: 977–986.

Stearne, M.R., Palmer, S.L., Hammersley, M.S. et al. (1998) Tight blood pressure control and risk of macrovascular and microvascular complications in type 2 diabetes: UKPDS 38. *British Medical Journal* **317**, 703–713.

Steele, C.F., Rubin, G. and Fraser, S. (2006) Error classification in community optometric practice – a pilot study. *Ophthalmic and Physiological Optics* **26**, 106–110.

Weed, L.L. (1968) Medical records that guide and teach. *The New England Journal of Medicine* **278**, 652–657.

3

ASSESSMENT OF VISUAL FUNCTION
DAVID B. ELLIOTT AND JOHN FLANAGAN

3.1.1 Symptoms

Symptoms of blurred vision or an inability to see well enough for certain tasks (reading the whiteboard, schoolbooks or a newspaper, watching TV, driving, etc.) all suggest reduced vision due to ametropia or ocular disease. These symptoms should be explained by reductions in visual acuity and/or contrast sensitivity. If a patient has symptoms of poor vision, but the visual acuity is normal, contrast sensitivity must be measured. Symptoms including unexplained headaches, unexplained visual acuity or contrast sensitivity loss, positive or scintillating scotoma, bumping into things on one side and symptoms consistent with neurological disease, such as cluster headache, acquired migraine, dizziness or tingling of limbs, all suggest the need for visual field testing. Obviously, if a patient complains of colour vision changes, their colour vision should be assessed.

3.1.2 Ocular, family and medical history

The ocular history may indicate an ocular condition that requires monitoring using visual acuity, contrast sensitivity, colour vision and/or visual fields, such as cataract or glaucoma. The family history may indicate a hereditary condition, such as open-angle glaucoma, that should be carefully checked using visual field assessment. The medical history could indicate a systemic condition that requires particular assessment, such as diabetes, or systemic medication that could affect some aspect of vision, such as chloroquine.

3.1 CASE HISTORY

The case history can provide significant information about visual function and whether particular tests of visual function should be used for a particular patient.

3.2 DISTANCE VISUAL ACUITY USING LOGMAR CHARTS

LogMAR visual acuity (VA) charts (Fig. 3.1) use the design principles suggested by Bailey & Lovie (e.g.

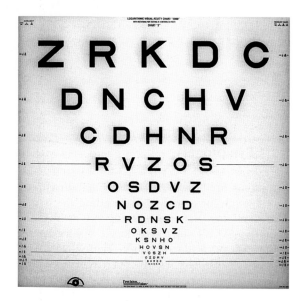

Fig. 3.1   A printed panel logMAR chart.

0.1 logMAR progression of letter size, five letters per line; Bailey & Lovie 1976). These charts contain more lines than a typical Snellen chart, particularly at poor VA levels and are not truncated to 6/5 (20/15) or similar.

3.2.1 Distance visual acuity

Visual acuity (VA) is a measure of the patient's ability to resolve fine detail. It is the most commonly used measurement of visual function made by clinicians. VA is used to assess the adequacy of spectacle corrections and as a key indicator of ocular health. VA is also used to assess a person's fitness to drive or enter into some professions such as the police force and to enable registration as a partially sighted or blind person. The need to measure VA accurately is obvious.

There are three principal measures of VA:

1. Unaided VA, often called vision.

2. Habitual VA, with the patient's own spectacles.

3. Optimal VA, with the best refractive correction, i.e. after subjective refraction.

VA with the retinoscope result is also often recorded. Either vision and/or habitual VA should be measured immediately after the case history for legal reasons, to document the VA level prior to your examination. Habitual and optimal distance VA are routine measurements. Measuring distance unaided VA (vision) is optional, and should be measured with patients who:

- Do not wear spectacles

- Have lost/broken their spectacles so that you cannot measure habitual VA

- Do not wear spectacles for some distance viewing tasks (this information must therefore be obtained in the case history)

- Require the information for a report

- Wear their spectacles all the time for distance and yet you suspect they may not need to do so (does the young low hyperope need to wear the spectacles for distance tasks?).

3.2.2 Advantages and disadvantages

LogMAR visual acuity charts (Fig. 3.1) are widely recognised as providing the most reliable and discriminative VA measurements (Lovie-Kitchin 1988) and are standard for clinical research or clinical trials of ophthalmic devices or drugs (Ferris & Bailey 1996). Visual acuity measurements using a logMAR chart have been shown to be twice as repeatable as those from a Snellen chart (Lovie-Kitchin 1988) and over three times more sensitive to inter-ocular differences in VA and therefore substantially more sensitive to amblyopic changes, for example (McGraw et al. 2000). The Bailey–Lovie or ETDRS charts are the most commonly used logMAR charts for adults (Ferris & Bailey 1996) and the Glasgow Acuity Cards (commercially available as the Keeler crowded logMAR charts) have been designed specifically for children (McGraw et al. 2000). The major disadvantage of logMAR charts is that although they are available in printed, projector and computer-based chart form, they are not as widely available as Snellen charts. However, this is slowly changing. In particular, logMAR VA measurements are being promoted on computer-based visual assessment systems. The new generation of flat panel displays appear especially useful as they are light (easy to wall mount), have excellent resolution, luminance and contrast and are flicker-free. VA measurements on these systems have the advantage of allowing randomisation of letters, calculation of VA scores and conversion of VA into different notations. One practical disadvantage of printed panel logMAR charts is that patients may not be able to see the 'bottom line' of the chart (-0.3 logMAR, 6/3, 20/20). If they have been used to having their VA measured on a truncated VA chart and being able to see the bottom line, this may upset some patients. You should explain that the new chart includes lines with smaller text than the old one ('this new bottom line is just for superman/superwoman') and indicate, or even highlight, the 6/6 (20/20) line.

3.2.3 Procedure

1. Ensure the chart is at the appropriate distance and is calibrated correctly.

2. Leave the room lights on and illuminate the chart. The luminance of the chart should be between 80 and 320 cd/m^2. Seat the patient comfortably with an unobstructed view of the test chart. You should sit in front and to one side of the patient in order to monitor facial expressions and reactions.

3. If you are going to measure both vision and habitual VA, measure vision first to avoid memorisation. To measure vision, ask the patient to remove any spectacles. To measure habitual visual acuity, ask the patient to put their distance vision spectacles on.

4. Measure the visual acuity of the 'poorer' eye first, if a poorer eye is known from previous records or from the case history (to avoid a patient memorising the letters seen with the better eye and giving a false visual acuity with the poorer eye). Otherwise, measure VA in the right eye first.

5. Explain what measurement you are about to take. This can be as simple as 'now we shall find out what you can see in the distance'.

6. Instruct the patient: 'Please cover up your left/right eye with the palm of your hand/this occluder'. If using the patient's hand, make sure that the palm is being used as otherwise the patient may be able to peek

through their fingers. Some clinicians prefer to hold the occluder over the patient's eye themselves to ensure it is properly occluded.

7. Ask the patient: 'Please read the smallest line that you can see on the chart' or similar.

8. Continually monitor the patient's facial expressions and head position. Do not permit the patient to screw their eyes up or look around the occluder or through their fingers. A hyperopic shift is common in older patients and some PAL or varifocal wearers adapt to this change by habitually raising their chin to improve distance vision by viewing through the additional plus power in the intermediate section of the lens. This can be seen when assessing habitual VA as these varifocal wearers will raise their chin during measurements to improve VA. VAs should be measured through the distance portion of the lens. You should make a mental note that these patients will likely require additional plus (or less minus) power in their distance correction.

9. Once the patient has reached what they believe are the smallest letters they can see, they should be pushed to determine whether they can see any more. Use prompts such as 'Can you see any letters on the next line?' or 'Have a guess. It doesn't matter if you get any wrong'. Some patients are more cautious than others and only indicate those letters that they can see easily and clearly. Unless you push patients to guess, you could obtain different VA results depending on how cautious your patient is. Ideally, you should stop pushing patients to read more if they make four or more mistakes on a line of five letters (Carkeet 2001).

10. If the patient cannot see the largest letters on the chart, ask them to move closer to the letter until two or three lines can be seen (or use a printed panel chart at a reduced distance). The distance at which this occurs should be noted. This is a more accurate assessment than determining the position that the patient can 'count fingers' (Schulze-Bonsel et al. 2006). If the patient cannot see the letters even at the closest test distance,

use the following test sequence. Stop at the level at which the patient can accurately respond.

   a) Hand Movements (HM) @ Y cm: The patient can see a hand moving from a certain distance. Some computerised VA tests can provide accurate measurements down to the hand movements level (Schulze-Bonsel et al. 2006) and these should be used when available.

   b) Light Projection (Lproj.): The patient can report which direction light is coming from when you hold a penlight about 50 cm away. Ask the patient to point to the light and note the areas of the field in which the patient has light perception.

   c) Light Perception (LP): The patient can see the light but not where it is coming from. If they cannot see light, the vision is recorded as no light perception or NLP.

11. Record Vision/VA.

12. Repeat measurements for the other eye and binocularly.

3.2.4 Alternative procedures to assess VA in children

Amblyopia can be missed if single letters are used rather than a letter chart because of the lack of contour interaction. Ideally logMAR-based charts with contour bars at the end of lines, such as the logMAR crowded charts (McGraw & Winn 1993) should be used when measuring VA in children. The logMAR crowded charts have been shown to be over three times more sensitive to inter-ocular differences in VA than single letter Snellen charts and therefore substantially more sensitive to amblyopic changes (McGraw et al. 2000). Crowded and standard LogMAR charts can even be used in children who do not know their letters by providing them with a key card that includes a selection of the letters from the chart. You then point to a letter on the chart and ask the child to identify the letter on their key card. For children who are unable to use a key card, charts are now available in logMAR format that include pictures rather than letters, such as the Kay crowded picture test, which has been shown to provide comparable results to the logMAR crowded charts (Jones et al. 2003).

3.2.5 Recording

VA measurements can be scored in logMAR notation, using the Visual Acuity Rating (VAR) score or converting scores to an equivalent Snellen value. LogMAR or VAR could be used on your own record cards. However, equivalent Snellen values should generally be provided when writing referral letters and reports, as Snellen notation is universally understood, whereas logMAR is not at present. In all cases, it is preferable to score using a by-letter system rather than measuring the lowest line at which the majority of letters were correctly read. Comparisons of various logMAR scores with Snellen and other recording notations are shown in Table 3.1.

MAR is taken as the angle subtended by the gap between the limbs of a letter, which is one fifth of the vertical angle subtended by the letter. As a 6/6 (20/20) letter subtends 5 minutes of arc vertically, the MAR is 1 minute and the logMAR ($\log_{10}1$) is 0. Therefore 6/6 (20/20) is equivalent to a logMAR of 0. Letters smaller than 6/6 have a negative logMAR (the log of numbers less than 1 being negative). As there are five letters on each row of a logMAR chart and a step of 0.1 between rows, each letter is assigned a value of 0.02 (0.10/5). The logMAR score for a patient is the sum of all the letters correctly read. For example, if a patient reads all the letters down to the 0.00 row but none on the row below, their score is 0.00. If they get one letter wrong on the 0.00 row, their score is 0.02, two letters wrong 0.04, three 0.06, etc. If they read all of the letters on the 0.00 row and one letter on the row below, their score is −0.02, two letters on the line below −0.04, etc. Using a scoring method that gives credit for every letter read provides more repeatable and discriminative measurements than scoring per line (Bailey et al. 1991).

Adding units of 0.02 can be confusing and the fact that logMAR VAs better than 6/6 or 20/20 are negative is counterintuitive. The VAR score provides a simpler method for scoring logMAR charts. VAR = 100 − 50 logMAR. Therefore 0.00 logMAR = 100 VAR and each letter has a score of 1. For example, if a patient reads all the letters down to the 100 row and gets one letter wrong on this row, their score is 99, two letters wrong 98, etc. If they read all

Table 3.1 Distance visual acuity conversion table.

MAR*	LogMAR	VAR	Snellen (metric)	Snellen (imperial)	Decimal*
0.50	−0.30	115	6/3	20/10	2.0
0.63	−0.20	110	6/3.8	20/12.5	1.60
0.80	−0.10	105	6/4.8	20/16	1.25
1.00	0.00	100	6/6	20/20	1.00
1.25	0.10	95	6/7.5	20/25	0.80
1.60	0.20	90	6/9.5	20/32	0.63
2.0	0.30	85	6/12	20/40	0.50
2.5	0.40	80	6/15	20/50	0.40
3.2	0.50	75	6/19	20/63	0.32
4.0	0.60	70	6/24	20/80	0.25
5.0	0.70	65	6/30	20/100	0.20
6.3	0.80	60	6/38	20/125	0.16
8.0	0.90	55	6/48	20/160	0.125
10.0	1.00	50	6/60	20/200	0.10
20	1.30	35	6/120	20/400	0.05
40	1.60	20	6/240	20/800	0.025
100	2.00	0	6/600	20/2000	0.01

*Numbers rounded to simplify sequences.
MAR, minimum angle of resolution; VAR, visual acuity rating.

the letters on the 100 row and one letter on the row below, their score is 101, two letters on the line below 102, etc. A disadvantage of the VAR score is that it suggests that 100 (6/6) is normal VA, which is far from true for many patients with healthy eyes.

Vision or 'VA s̄ Rx' or VAsc or Vsc all mean visual acuity measured without a correction. VA c̄ Rx or VAcc or Vcc all mean visual acuity measured with a correction and generally refer to the VA with the patient's spectacles. VA measured with the patient's contact lenses would typically be recorded as VA c̄ CLs or similar. VAs are recorded for the right eye (RE or OD), left eye (LE or OS) and binocular (BE or OU).

Examples:

Vision. RE: 0.78, LE: 1.20 (logMAR)

VA sc. OD: 24, OS: 36 (VAR)

VA c Rx. RE: −0.18 (6/4), LE: −0.22 (6/4^{+2}), BE: −0.26 (6/4^{-2})

VAcc. RE: 118, LE: 114, BE: 122 (VAR)

Vcc. OD: −0.20, OS: −0.18, OU: −0.24 (logMAR)

3.2.6 Interpretation

Any deviation from normal age-matched results, as shown in Table 3.2, should be noted. Note that the

average VA for patients under 50 is about −0.14 logMAR (6/4.5, 20/15) and that 6/6 or 20/20 represents reduced VA for the vast majority of patients. 6/6 or 20/20 only becomes the average VA for patients over 70 years of age with healthy eyes. You must also check whether there has been any change in VA from the previous examination. In patients with normal or near normal VA, a significant change in VA is more than 0.1 logMAR or one line (e.g. Bailey 2006, McGraw et al. 2000). Also note any inter-ocular asymmetry of a line or more (McGraw et al. 2000), or a binocular result that is worse than the monocular response.

For low myopic refractive errors, a degradation of one line of vision corresponds to approximately −0.25 D of refractive error, e.g. a −1.00 D myope with an optimal VA of 6/4 should have vision of 6/9 or 6/12. Near horizontal and vertical astigmatic errors have a similar effect to the equivalent best mean sphere, so that a −1.00 uncorrected cylinder would have a similar effect to a −0.50 DS, which is a two-line drop in VA. Cylinders at oblique axes tend to give a slightly greater degradation in vision.

Because changes in astigmatism with age are negligible over the typical 1–4 year period between eye examinations, habitual VA reductions in spectacle-wearing myopes and myopic astigmats

Table 3.2 Normal age-matched visual acuity data for various notations (from Elliott et al. 1995). The average is shown with 95% confidence limits in brackets.

Age (years)	LogMAR	VAR	Snellen (metric)*	Snellen (imperial)*	Decimal
20–49	−0.14 (−0.02 to −0.26)	107 (101 to 113)	6/4.5 (6/6 to 6/3)	20/15 (20/20 to 20/10)	1.4 (1.0 to 1.8)
50–59	−0.10 (0.00 to −0.20)	105 (100 to 110)	6/5 (6/6 to 6/4)	20/15 (20/20 to 20/12)	1.25 (1.0 to 1.6)
60–69	−0.06 (0.04 to −0.16)	103 (98 to 108)	6/5⁻ (6/6⁻ to 6/4)	20/15⁻ (20/20⁻ to 20/12)	1.15 (0.9 to 1.45)
70+	−0.02 (0.08 to −0.12)	101 (96 to 106)	6/6 (6/7.5 to 6/4.5)	20/20 (20/25 to 20/15)	1.0 (0.8 to 1.3)

*Numbers rounded for simplification.

indicate the increase in spherical power required. For example, a myope of −1.00/−1.00 × 175 with a habitual VA of 6/12 (20/40) is likely to need an additional −1.00 DS (4 lines of VA lost at −0.25 DS per line) and a new refractive correction of approximately −2.00/−1.00 × 175. This rule can be used to check the accuracy of a subjective refraction result in myopes (and older hyperopes with no accommodation). By comparing habitual and optimal VA and using the one line of VA is equivalent to −0.25 DS rule, an estimate of the change in spherical Rx from the spectacles is gained. If this estimate is widely different from the actual subjective result, an error may be suspected and the subjective (and/or spectacle power) rechecked. If significant differences are found between the astigmatism in the spectacles and subjective refraction, an error in the determination of the refractive correction in the spectacles or subjective refraction or a pathological change in astigmatism (due to disorders such as keratoconus, cortical cataract or chalazion) may be suspected.

3.2.7 Most common errors

1. Allowing cautious patients to decide their acuity (i.e. not pushing them to guess).

2. Permitting the patient to screw their eyes up and improve their VA.

3. Permitting the patient to look around the occluder or through their fingers and view binocularly when measuring monocular VA.

4. Taking distance VAs in a PAL or varifocal wearer when they are not looking through the distance vision section of the lens.

5. Using an incorrect working distance.

6. Not recording the result immediately and guessing the result at the end of the examination.

3.3 DISTANCE VISUAL ACUITY USING SNELLEN CHARTS

Snellen charts were devised by the German ophthalmologist Hermann Snellen in 1862 and have been widely used ever since. There is not a standard Snellen chart and the letter size sequences, number of letters, varieties of letters, etc. vary from manufacturer to manufacturer. They typically contain one letter at a VA level of 6/60 (20/200; 0.1 logMAR) and increasing numbers of letters at smaller letter sizes with a typical bottom line of about 6/5 or 20/15 (≈ −0.1 logMAR).

3.3.1 Distance visual acuity

See section 3.2.1.

3.3.2 Advantages and disadvantages

Snellen charts have a major advantage at present in that they are widely available and Snellen notation of VA is universally understood. From a practical viewpoint, these charts can generally be produced in a smaller format as considerably fewer large letters are presented and this allows easier display on projector systems and the easy addition of other targets such as a duochrome and spotlight, etc. to wall charts. The charts provide a good target for refraction of patients with good VA as the number of lines between approximately 20/15 to 20/40 (6/5 to 6/12) is similar to logMAR charts and these lines typically have as many, if not more, letters than logMAR charts. Although the truncation of Snellen charts (to, say, 6/5 or 20/15 when some patients can see 6/3 or 20/10) can be a disadvantage, it can speed up the measurement and allows most patients to read your 'bottom line'.

However, Snellen chart VAs are much less repeatable than VA measured using logMAR charts (Lovie-Kitchin 1988) and over three times less sensitive to inter-ocular differences in VA (McGraw et al. 2000) and thus much less sensitive to amblyopia and other uniocular VA loss. Its main disadvantages occur at large (>6/12) and small letter sizes (<6/6). The majority of Snellen charts have one 6/60 letter, two 6/36 and three 6/24 letters, whereas logMAR charts have five letters on each of these lines and additional lines of letters at 6/48 and 6/30. Many Snellen charts do not contain lines of small letters and are truncated to 6/4, 6/4.5, 6/5 or even 6/6. This takes the approach of measuring 'distance vision adequacy' (i.e. determining whether distance VA is adequate for a patient's daily needs, similar to the approach used for near VA) rather than distance VA (a threshold measurement). This makes the detection of slightly reduced VA due to eye disease or uncorrected refractive error in patients with good VA impossible. For example, if your chart is truncated to 6/5 or 20/15, you will not be able to detect a VA loss from 6/3 (or 6/4) to 6/5 or from 20/10 to 20/15.

3.3.3 Procedure

1. Ensure the chart is at the appropriate distance and is calibrated correctly.

2. Leave the room lights on and illuminate the chart. The luminance of the chart should be between 80 and 320 cd/m². When using projector charts, the lights above the chart may need to be dimmed if the veiling luminance produced significantly reduces the contrast of the letters on the chart.

3. Seat the patient comfortably with an unobstructed view of the test chart. You should sit in front and to one side of the patient in order to monitor facial expressions and reactions.

4. If you are going to measure both vision and habitual VA, measure vision first to avoid memorisation. To measure vision, ask the patient to remove any spectacles. To measure habitual visual acuity, ask the patient to put their distance vision spectacles on.

5. Measure the visual acuity of the 'poorer' eye first, if a poorer eye is known from previous records or from the case history (to avoid a patient memorising the letters with the better eye and giving a false visual acuity with the poorer eye). Otherwise, measure VA in the right eye first.

6. Explain what measurement you are about to take. This can be as simple as 'now we shall find out what you can see in the distance'.

7. Instruct the patient: 'Please cover up your left/right eye with the palm of your hand/this occluder'. If using the patient's hand, make sure that the palm is being used as otherwise the patient may be able to peek through their fingers. Some clinicians prefer to hold the occluder over the patient's eye themselves to ensure it is properly occluded.

8. Ask the patient: 'Please read the smallest line that you can see on the chart'.

9. Continually monitor the patient's facial expressions and head position. Do not permit the patient to screw their eyes up or look around the occluder or through their fingers. A hyperopic shift is common in older patients and some varifocal wearers adapt to this change by habitually raising their chin to improve distance vision by viewing through the additional plus power in the intermediate section of the lens. This can be seen when assessing habitual VA as these varifocal wearers will raise their chin

during measurements to improve VA. VAs should be measured through the distance portion of the lens. You should make a mental note that these patients will likely require additional plus (or less minus) power in their distance correction.

10. Once the patient has reached what they believe are the smallest letters they can see, they should be pushed to determine whether they can see any more. Use prompts such as 'Can you see any letters on the next line?' or 'Have a guess. It doesn't matter if you get any wrong'. Some patients are more cautious than others and only indicate those letters that they can see easily and clearly. Unless you push patients to guess, you could obtain different VA results depending on how cautious your patient is.

11. If the patient cannot see the largest letters on the chart, ask them to move closer to the chart until two or three lines can be seen. Alternatively, a copy of a 6/60 letter on the back of your clipboard can be useful as it can be moved towards the patient until they can just see it. The distance at which this occurs should be noted. This is a more accurate assessment than determining the position that the patient can 'count fingers'. If the patient cannot see a 6/60 letter even at 1 m, use the following test sequence. Stop at the level at which the patient can accurately respond.
    a) Hand Movements: The patient can see a hand moving from a certain distance.
    b) Light Projection (Lproj.): The patient can report which direction light is coming from when you hold a penlight about 50 cm away. Ask the patient to point to the light and note the areas of the field in which the patient has light perception.
    c) Light Perception (LP): The patient can see the light but not where it is coming from. If they cannot see light, the vision is recorded as no light perception or NLP.

12. Record Vision/VA.

13. Repeat measurements for the other eye and binocularly.

3.3.4 Alternative procedures to assess VA in children

Keeler crowded logMAR charts (McGraw & Winn 1993) or the Kay crowded picture test should be used to measure VA in children as they are significantly more repeatable than Snellen charts (section 3.2.4) and substantially more sensitive to amblyopic changes (McGraw et al. 2000). Amblyopia can be missed if single letters are used rather than a letter chart because VA is better in amblyopia without contour interaction, so that charts with contour bars at the end of lines should be used. Standard Snellen charts can still be used even in children who do not know their letters by providing them with a key card that includes a selection of the letters from the chart. You then point to a letter on the chart (this is easy with wall charts used with a mirror as the chart is above the patient. With a projector chart you may need to get a clinical assistant to point to various letters) and ask the child to identify the letter on their key card. This is similar to the Sheridan-Gardner chart, which similarly uses a key card but the chart presents single letters on each page of a spiral bound booklet. For children who are unable to use the key card, charts that use targets of familiar objects, such as the Lea symbols of a box, apple, house and ball, can be used. Alternatively, a tumbling E or Llandolt C chart can be used, with children being asked to identify the legs of the E or the bite in the doughnut.

3.3.5 Recording

The Snellen fraction is defined as:
    Test Distance/Distance at which the letters subtend 5 min of arc.

1. Test distance can be provided in metres (metric) or feet (imperial).

2. Snellen VA can be labelled in either decimal or conventional Snellen notation (see Table 3.1 for comparison).

Vision or visual acuity is recorded as the smallest line in which the majority of the letters are seen, irrespective of subjective blur. Errors are recorded by appending a minus one, two or three to the Snellen fraction or decimal notation. If additional letters are seen on the following line, the Snellen fraction or decimal notation can be appended by a plus (usually up to no more than 3). If the patient could not see the 6/60 letter at 6 m, but could at 2 m, record 2/60. Similarly if the patient could not see the 20/200 letter at 20 feet, but could see the 20/120 letter at 5 feet, record 5/120.

Vision or 'VA s̄ Rx' or VAsc or Vsc all mean visual acuity measured without a correction. VA c̄ Rx or VAcc or Vcc all mean visual acuity measured with a correction and generally refer to the VA with the patient's spectacles. VA measured with the patient's contact lenses would typically be recorded as VA c̄ CLs or similar. VAs are recorded for the right eye (RE or OD), left eye (LE or OS) and binocular (BE or OU).

Examples:

Vision. RE: $6/36^{+1}$, LE: 2/60
VA sc. OD: $20/80^{-1}$, OS: 5/200
VA c̄ Rx. RE: $6/5^{-2}$, LE: 6/5, BE: 6/5
Vcc. OD: $20/15^{-1}$, OS: $20/20^{+2}$, OU: 20/15
VAcc. RE: 1.25^{-1}, LE: 1.00^{+3}, BE: 1.25

This last example is given in decimal format, which is commonly used in parts of Europe. It should not be confused with logMAR.

3.3.6 Interpretation

The following text is repeated from section 3.2.6 for convenience. Any deviation from normal age-matched results, as shown in Table 3.2, should be noted. An optimal VA of 6/6 (20/20) is often considered to be normal. It is, but only for the average patient over 70 years of age. The vast majority of young patients (and many older ones) have an optimal visual acuity better than 6/6 (20/20), and many young patients have VAs of 6/4 (20/25) and even 6/3 (20/10; see Table 3.2). It is important to use Snellen charts which measure down to 6/3 (20/10), otherwise a slight drop in VA (from 6/3 or 6/4 to 6/5 or 6/6; 20/10 to 20/15 or 20/20), which could indicate early ocular pathology or uncorrected refractive error, could be missed. If you have a chart with a bottom line of 6/5 or 6/6 (20/15 or 20/20), be aware that a young patient could have 6/3 (20/10) VA in one or both eyes, and complain of reduced vision even though they can see your 'bottom line'. You must also check whether there has been any change in VA from the previous examination and note any inter-ocular asymmetry

or a binocular result that is worse than the monocular response. Snellen chart measurements are less sensitive than logMAR charts to these VA differences due to the truncation at good VA levels and scarcity of lines and letters at poor VA levels.

For low myopic refractive errors, a degradation of one line of vision corresponds to approximately −0.25 D of refractive error, e.g. a −1.00 D myope with an optimal VA of 6/4 should have vision of 6/9 or 6/12. Near horizontal and vertical astigmatic errors have a similar effect to the equivalent best mean sphere, so that a −1.00 uncorrected cylinder would have a similar effect to a −0.50 DS, which is a two-line drop in VA. Cylinders at oblique axes tend to give a slightly greater degradation in vision.

Because changes in astigmatism with age are negligible over the typical 1–4 year period between eye examinations, habitual VA reductions in spectacle-wearing myopes and myopic astigmats provide a good estimate of the increase in spherical power required. For example, a myope of −1.00/ −1.00 × 175 with a habitual VA of 6/12 (20/40) is likely to need an additional 1.00 DS (4 lines of VA lost at −0.25 DS per line) and a new refractive correction of approximately −2.00/−1.00 × 175. This rule can be used to check the accuracy of a subjective refraction result in myopes (and older hyperopes with no accommodation). By comparing habitual and optimal VA and using the one line of VA is equivalent to −0.25 DS rule, an estimate of the change in spherical Rx from the spectacles is gained. If this estimate is widely different from the actual subjective result, an error may be suspected and the subjective refraction (and/or measurement of spectacle correction) rechecked. If significant differences are found between the astigmatism in the spectacles and subjective refraction, an error in the measurement of spectacle correction or subjective refraction or a pathological change in astigmatism (due to disorders such as keratoconus, chalazion and cataract) may be suspected.

3.3.7 Most common errors

1. Forgetting that patients could have VA better than your bottom line of typically 6/5 or 20/15.

2. Allowing 'cautious' patients to decide their acuity (i.e. not 'pushing' them to guess).

3. Permitting the patient to screw their eyes up and improve their VA.

4. Permitting the patient to look around the occluder or through their fingers and view binocularly when measuring monocular VA.

5. Taking VAs in a PAL or varifocal wearer when they are not looking through the distance vision section of the lens.

6. Using a chart with low illumination or contrast.

7. Using an incorrect working distance.

8. Not recording the result immediately and guessing the result at the end of the examination.

3.4 NEAR VISION ADEQUACY USING N- OR M-NOTATION NEAR CARDS

N- or M-notation near cards are used to determine whether near vision is adequate for the majority of near tasks and particularly reading. These cards therefore typically present sentences or paragraphs of words rather than isolated letters and often incorporate examples of near vision tasks such as sheet music, technical drawings and telephone directories (Fig. 3.2).

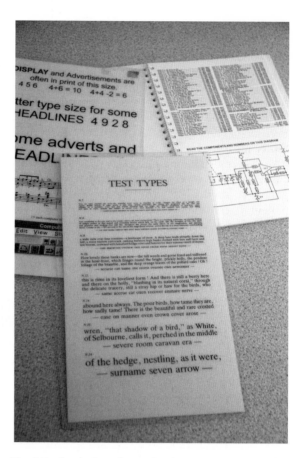

Fig. 3.2   A selection of near visual acuity charts.

3.4.1 Near visual acuity

In primary eye care examinations, 'near visual acuity' is rarely measured as it is unusual for a threshold to be measured. Most reading charts are truncated as the smallest print sizes are equivalent to distance VAs of about 6/9 (N5) and 20/20 (0.4 M) when used at 40 cm. Many patients could read sentences of text smaller than this if given the chance, so that a threshold is not measured. Thus 'near vision adequacy' is a more appropriate description of the measurements than near visual acuity. Near vision adequacy measurements have the added advantage that the measurement is quicker than a threshold measurement and most patients will be able to see the 'bottom line' of text. It is left to distance VA measurements, with their many advantages in this regard (fixed measurement distance,

same letter format, letters of similar legibility, etc.) to provide an accurate measurement of a patient's resolution.

There are three principal measures of near vision adequacy:

1. Unaided near VA or near vision.

2. Habitual near VA, with the patient's own spectacles.

3. Optimal near VA, with the best refractive correction.

Habitual and optimal near VA are routine measurements in presbyopes and on all patients who complain of near vision problems. Measuring near vision is optional, and should be measured with presbyopic patients who do not wear spectacles for all or certain near viewing tasks (this information must therefore be obtained in the case history) or if it is required for a report. A reading distance should always accompany a near VA as N8 (1.0 M) at 40 cm (2.5 MAR, equivalent to 6/15) is a totally different near VA to N8 (1.0 M) at 10 cm (10 MAR, 6/60).

3.4.2 Advantages and disadvantages

There are five main types of notations used to measure near VA: Equivalent Snellen, Jaeger, logMAR, M-scale and N-point. Cards using Jaeger notation should be thrown away as there is no standardisation of what J1 or J5, etc. means and different charts can give totally different sizes of print with the same J-value. Equivalent Snellen notation is a confusing notation, especially when near VAs are not measured at the standard 16″: What does 20/20 near VA at 8″ mean? In addition, near vision adequacy should indicate what patients can see at their own near working distance, not an arbitrary standard of 16″ (working distances for reading in patients with normal vision range from 10″ to 20″; Millodot & Millodot 1989). M-units are widely used in North America and indicate the distance in metres at which the height of a lower case 'x' subtends 5 minutes of arc. A 1.0 M letter 'x' is therefore 1.45 mm high. N-print uses the Times New Roman font and is the standard test in the UK and Australia. It is based on the 'point size' used by printers and word processing packages on modern computers, in which 1 point = 1/72 inch ($\approx$ 0.353 mm). This can be a useful aid when indicating to a patient the level of vision that would be provided for computer use by new lenses. N8 is approximately equal to 1.0 M and this 8 times conversion holds for all print sizes. Near logMAR charts have all the advantages of their distance chart compatriot, but these are minimal given that what is being measured is near vision adequacy rather than near visual acuity.

3.4.3 Procedure

1. Sit in front and to one side of the patient in order to monitor facial expressions and reactions.

2. Keep the room lights on. DO NOT routinely use additional lighting. Although this is commonly advocated in textbooks, you want to measure the patient's habitual near VA and patients often read without an additional anglepoise or goose-neck light. In addition, given that N5 at 40 cm is far from a threshold measurement (see Interpretation), increasing the illumination makes the test even easier. Higher illumination can also increase the depth of focus and artificially increase near VA in presbyopic patients. It is better to restrict the use of additional lighting to patients who indicate that they commonly use such lighting when performing near tasks and any patient who cannot easily read N5 (or 0.4 M) in their optimal near refractive correction without additional lighting. These latter patients must be encouraged to obtain additional light for near tasks in their home.

3. Instruct the patient to place the near vision card at their normal near working distance. Measure and record this distance (the Mallett near unit has a useful measuring device for this purpose).

4. Measure the near VA of the 'poorer' eye first, if a poorer eye is known from previous records or from the case history. Otherwise, measure the right eye first. Use an occluder or the patient's palm of their hand to cover the other eye. If using the patient's hand, make sure that the palm is being used as otherwise the patient may be able to peek through their fingers.

5. Explain to the patient what measurement you are about to take. This may be a simple 'Now we shall find out what you can see at close distances'.

6. Instruct the patient to read the smallest paragraph they can.

7. Unless the patient can see the smallest print, push them to determine whether they can see any more. Prompts such as 'Try and make out some of the words on the smaller paragraph' may be useful. Some patients are more cautious than others and only indicate those letters that they can see easily and clearly. Unless you push patients to guess, you could therefore obtain different near VA results depending on how cautious your patient is.

8. Repeat measurements for the left eye and binocularly.

3.4.4 Adaptation to the standard technique

Some patients with out-of-date reading spectacles change their working distance from their preferred distance to allow better near vision. This is most commonly a longer working distance than preferred because they now require a more positive near correction than that provided by their spectacles. This change in their near working distance will typically be identified in the case history. When measuring habitual near VA in such patients, it should be measured at their preferred working distance (which will identify a reduced near VA) rather than the adapted habitual distance. Measurement of the adapted distance may help indicate what change in correction is required. For example, if the patient has a preferred working distance of 40 cm, but adapts to a longer working distance of 50 cm to gain better vision at near, an additional +0.50 DS to the near refractive correction is suggested.

3.4.5 Recording

Note the working distance and then record the smallest paragraph size seen by the right and left eyes and binocularly. For approximate equivalents to other notations see Table 3.3. Some clinicians do not note the working distance unless it is different from the

'norm'. However, even patients with good vision present a wide range of normal working distances (22 cm to 50 cm for reading; Millodot & Millodot 1989; and further away for computer use), and as stated earlier a reading acuity is meaningless without a working distance. It can also be useful to record the working distance(s) used to determine near VA with the patient's own spectacles to allow a comparison with the one used to determine the reading add. This can also be useful for comparison if patients return to your practice dissatisfied with the near vision in any new spectacles. These cases are often due to problems with working distance determination rather than an incorrect refraction.

Near vision or 'NVA s̄ Rx' or NVAsc or NVsc all mean near visual acuity measured without a correction. NVA c̄ Rx or NVAcc or NVcc all mean near visual acuity measured with a correction and generally refer to the VA with the patient's spectacles. Near VA measured with the patient's contact lenses would typically be recorded as NVA c̄ CLs or similar. Near VAs are recorded for the right eye (RE or OD), left eye (LE or OS) and binocular (BE or OU) and should include the near working distance in centimetres or inches. If the patient can only read a paragraph slowly or with difficulty, include this information.

Examples:
Near vision. RE: N14, LE: N12 @ 40 cm
NVA sc. OD: 20/80, OS: 20/60 @ 16"
NVA c̄ Rx. RE: N5, LE: N5 (slowly), BE: N5 @ 35 cm

Table 3.3 Near visual acuity conversion table.

N-scale	M-units	Equivalent Snellen (imperial)	Equivalent Snellen (metric)	Common usage
2.5	0.32	20/16	6/5	
3	0.40	20/20	6/6	Medicine bottle labels
4	0.50	20/25	6/7.5	Medicine bottle labels
5	0.60	20/30	6/9	Footnotes, bibles
6	0.75	20/40	6/12	Telephone directories
8	1.0	20/50	6/15	Newspaper print
10	1.2	20/60	6/18	Magazines, books
12	1.6	20/80	6/24	Books
16	2.0	20/100	6/30	Children's books
20	2.5	20/125	6/36	Large print books
25	3.2	20/160	6/48	Large print books
32	4.0	20/200	6/60	Sub-headlines
40	5.0	20/250	6/75	Sub-headlines

Numbers rounded to simplify sequences.

NVA*cc*. RE: 0.4 M, LE: 0.4 M, BE: 0.4 M @
38 cm
NV*cc*. OD: 20/20 (diff.), OS: 20/20, OU: 20/15
@ 16″

3.4.6 Interpretation

When determining a reading addition, do not assume you have the correct add just because a patient can see the smallest text on your near chart such as N5, 0.4 M or 20/20. At 40 cm, 0.4 M is equivalent to about 20/20 or 6/6 distance VA and N5 is equivalent to 6/9 or 20/30. Therefore, a patient could have reduced distance VA and still read N5, 0.4 M or 20/20 at near. Apart from this truncation effect, near VA can be expected to be similar to distance VA in most cases provided that the eye is accommodating normally or that the reading addition is correct. Notable exceptions include patients with posterior sub-capsular cataract, where the near VA can be less than distance VA due to the effects of pupil constriction with convergence around the typically central cataract. Patients with some eye disorders, such as amblyopia, ARM and macular oedema can have significantly worse reading VA than distance VA (and isolated-letter near VA).

Finally, although near VA levels can be associated with a range of near tasks (Table 3.3), note that the poorer near VAs are threshold measurements (measurements of N5, 0.4 M and 20/20 may be truncated and not thresholds as discussed earlier) so that patients would not be able to read print of that size comfortably for any length of time. For example, to allow somebody to read newspaper print comfortably requires a near VA better than N8 or 1.0 M which is the typical size of newspaper print (Table 3.3) and a 'reading reserve' is needed. This should be between N4 (0.5 M) and N6 (0.75 M).

3.4.7 Most common errors

1. Not measuring or recording the test distance.

2. Not watching the patient to see if they are screwing their eyes up or looking at the chart with both eyes.

3. Measuring near VA with an additional light rather than the light levels typically used by the patient in their home or at work.

4. Measuring near VA at a standard fixed distance (16″ or 40 cm) rather than the near working distance typically used by the patient.

5. Using a dirty near vision chart.

6. Using a reading test on an illiterate patient.

3.5 SUPER PINHOLE VISUAL ACUITY TEST

The 'super' pinhole test (Hofeldt & Weiss 1998, Melki et al. 1999) is a pinhole visual acuity test (section 4.9.3) that incorporates adaptations to overcome the loss of light when a VA chart is viewed though a pinhole and cataract. It attempts to predict the visual acuity 'behind' cataract and thus the likely visual acuity after cataract surgery.

3.5.1 Potential vision assessment

Potential vision assessments predict the visual function of the neural system behind cataracts or other media opacities and thus predict the potential vision after cataract or other media opacity surgery. The most common cause of poor visual outcome after cataract surgery is ocular comorbidity and, particularly, age-related macular degeneration (ARMD). This has led to many patients with cataract and ARMD not being offered surgery and there are many low vision patients who have cataract as a secondary diagnosis (Elliott et al. 1997a). It is likely that some (many?) of these patients could benefit from cataract surgery (e.g. Ambrecht et al. 2003), although it should also be noted that cataract surgery may lead to the development of exudative macular degeneration in some patients with pre-operative macular changes (Wang et al. 2003, Klein et al. 2004). Potential vision testing can contribute to the decision of whether surgical intervention is appropriate. Potential vision testing can also be used in the decision of which eye should be operated on with a patient with bilateral cataract and to provide valuable prognostic information to the patient about the likely outcome of surgery.

3.5.2 Advantages and disadvantages

Although fundus biomicroscopy provides a much clearer view of the retina behind media opacity than direct ophthalmoscopy, subtle maculopathies can still provide inconclusive funduscopic findings. Schein et al. (1994) reported that 63% of patients who were predicted by an ophthalmic examination to have visual acuity of 6/12 (20/40, 0.5) or worse after surgery (the level at which cataract surgery is typically deemed 'unsuccessful') actually attained a visual acuity of 6/9 or better. This suggests that potential vision tests are required in addition to standard clinical tests such as case history information, dilated fundus examination and the swinging flashlight test. Unfortunately, a review of the currently available tests suggested that none of them are particularly useful (AHCPR 1993). The most commonly used tests, the potential acuity meter (PAM) and the various interferometers, cannot penetrate dense cataracts and suggest that potential vision is poor in these cases regardless of the state of the neural system (AHCPR 1993, Vianya-Estopa et al. 2006). In addition, the interferometers in particular can predict good postoperative vision in patients with certain retinal diseases that is not obtainable (AHCPR 1993). The 'super' pinhole test (Hofeldt & Weiss 1998, Melki et al. 1999) is a very simple potential vision test that has provided encouragingly accurate results, superior to the previous standard tests of the PAM and interferometers (Vianya-Estopa et al. 2006). This is simply a pinhole visual acuity test that incorporates adaptations to overcome the loss of light when a VA chart is viewed though a pinhole and cataract.

3.5.3 Procedure

1. Measure the potential visual acuity of the 'poorer' eye first to avoid a patient memorising the letters seen with the better eye and giving a false visual acuity with the poorer eye. Otherwise, measure VA in the right eye first.

2. Ensure that the patient is wearing their near correction.

3. Explain what measurement you are about to take. For example, 'this test will help us to estimate the vision you are likely to obtain after cataract surgery'.

4. Instruct the patient: 'Please cover up your left/right eye with the palm of your hand/this occluder'. If using the patient's

hand, make sure that the palm is being used as otherwise the patient may be able to peek through their fingers. Some clinicians prefer to hold the occluder over the patient's eye themselves to ensure it is properly occluded.

5. Hold a near VA card at an appropriate distance from the patient and illuminate it with a transilluminator or other bright light source (the Retinal Acuity Meter is a commercially available version of the super pinhole test and provides a brightly transilluminated near card with a multiple pinhole occluder).

6. Give the patient a multiple pinhole occluder and ask them to move it around until they obtain the best view possible of the near card through one of the pinholes.

7. Ask the patient to read the smallest line (or paragraph) that you can see on the chart.

8. Move the transilluminator to illuminate the text that the patient is reading or attempting to read.

9. Once the patient has reached what they believe are the smallest letters they can see, they should be pushed to determine whether they can see any more. Use prompts such as 'Can you see any letters on the next line?' or 'Have a guess. It doesn't matter if you get any wrong'. Also allow the patient to move the multiple pinhole occluder around to see if they can see further down the chart with the pinhole in a different position.

10. Repeat measurements for the other eye.

3.5.4 Recording

Record the near VA obtained with the super pinhole test:
    Super PH: RE: N14, LE: N12
    Super PH: OD: 0.4 M, OS: 0.4 M
    Super PH: OD: 20/20, OS: 20/30.

3.5.5 Interpretation

The near VA obtained with the super pinhole VA gives an indication of the possible near VA after uncomplicated cataract surgery. The test cannot bypass dense cataracts so that in such cases the super pinhole result is likely to be worse than the postoperative VA (Vianya-Estopa et al. 2006) and just represents the minimum VA that is likely to be obtained after surgery. Other results and assessments should be taken into account when considering the likely visual outcome after cataract surgery and these include the patient's age, indications from the case history and results from a dilated fundus examination and swinging flashlight test. Visual acuity in the pseudophakic eye is another useful indicator for patients undergoing second eye surgery.

3.5.6 Most common error

Not allowing the patient an opportunity to move the multiple pinhole occluder around to get the best possible potential visual acuity reading.

3.6 10-2 CENTRAL VISUAL FIELD ANALYSIS

The recommended approach to testing the macula region is to use a 10 degree, central threshold program with a spatial resolution of at least 2°. Examples include the Oculus 10-2, Humphrey Field Analyser 10-2 program, Medmont M700 Macula 10 and Octopus program 08.

3.6.1 Central visual function

The most common assessment of central visual function is visual acuity measurement. However, this provides just one assessment of central vision and offers little help in differential diagnosis. In addition, some ocular abnormalities can produce little or no reduction in visual acuity, but can produce other changes to central vision, such as centrocaecal scotomas, metamorphopsia (distorted vision) and changes in colour vision. The central visual field should be examined regularly in patients with age-related maculopathy, those taking certain medications such as hydroxychloroquine that are known to occasionally cause maculopathy, and in fixation-threatening scotomas in glaucoma.

3.6.2 Advantages and disadvantages

Standard automated perimetry has been shown to be much more sensitive, specific, reliable and valid for detecting central visual field changes than Amsler charts (Achard et al. 1995, Schuchard 1993). Standard Amsler charts are high contrast and, even threshold adaptations of the chart (using cross-polarising filters), are poor at detecting scotomas smaller than 6° (Schuchard 1993). Schuchard also found that more than half of the distortion reported in Amsler grids was at retinal locations that corresponded to the location of scotoma. Amsler charts rely heavily on subjective interpretation and may also be compromised by the 'completion phenomena', which perceptually fills small gaps in line stimuli (Achard et al. 1995).

3.6.3 Procedure

The same as central visual field analysis but replace program 30-2 with program 10-2 (section 3.15.3).

3.6.4 Recording

If no test locations are highlighted on the Total and Pattern Deviation probability plots then record 'SITA-Standard 10-2: WNL (within normal limits) R and L'. Print the fields for both eyes and attach to the record card. If a defect is evident then consider a confirmatory field. The single field analysis printout illustrates the data as an interpolated greyscale, raw data in decibels, and Total and Pattern deviation plots. It also summarises the field using global indices, reliability indices, and Gaze Tracking plots.

3.6.5 Interpretation

10° central visual field programs provide higher spatial resolution in the central 10° than the standard 25–30° visual field programs. Their interpretation is as discussed for 30-2 programs (section 3.15.5).

3.6.6 Most common errors

See section 3.12.6.

3.7 AMSLER CHARTS

The Amsler Grid is a rapid, qualitative technique designed to test the central 10° of the visual field, using a standard chart with a grid of white lines on a black background. Each square of the grid is 5 mm, subtending approximately 1° at 30 cm. The patient is requested to describe lines that are missing or distorted.

3.7.1 Macular testing

The Amsler Grid is an alternative to 10° central visual field analysis (section 3.6) if a quick assessment of macular function is required. It is particularly useful in cases with metamorphopsia or visual distortion. The central visual field should be examined regularly in patients with age-related maculopathy, and those taking certain medications such as hydroxychloroquine, that are associated with occasional maculopathy.

3.7.2 Advantages and disadvantages

Amsler charts measure the central 10° visual field and have the advantage that they provide quick and easy measurements and are portable, so can be used for home visits. The recording sheets can be used for home monitoring, although compliance has been shown to be poor (Fine et al. 1986) and it is likely that the white-on-black Amsler charts are more sensitive to macular changes than the black-on-white recording sheets (Roper-Hall 2006). Standard perimetry has been shown to be more sensitive, specific, reliable and valid for central visual field changes than Amsler charts (Achard et al. 1995, Schuchard 1993). Standard Amsler charts are high contrast and even threshold adaptations of the chart (using cross-polarising filters) are poor at detecting scotomas smaller than 6° (Schuchard 1993). Schuchard also found that more than half of the distortion reported in Amsler grids was at the retinal area that corresponded to the scotoma area, not a non-scotoma retinal area. Amsler charts rely heavily on subjective interpretation and may also be compromised by the 'completion phenomena', which perceptually fills small gaps in line stimuli (Achard et al. 1995).

3.7.3 Procedure

1. Seat the patient comfortably in the examining chair with the appropriate near correction. As the working distance for the test is 30 cm, ideally a 3.25 D near add should be used for absolute presbyopes. However, the patient's own spectacles are usually satisfactory given sufficient depth of focus. Use single vision glasses or trial lenses, but avoid multifocal lenses.

2. Position yourself so as to be able to occlude the non-viewing eye and measure the working distance. Get the patient to hold the chart at 30 cm.

3. Keep the room lights on. The method is qualitative and critical light levels are not essential; however, it is useful to be able to reproduce approximate ambient luminance levels.

4. Select the chart for testing:
   a) Chart 1: the standard chart used in every case. Consists of a 5 mm square, white grid with each square subtending approximately 1° from 30 cm, on a black background with a central, white fixation target.
   b) Chart 2: similar to Chart 1 but with two diagonal white lines to assist steady fixation in patients with a central scotoma.
   c) Chart 3: similar to Chart 1 but with a red grid. It has been reported to be useful in the toxic amblyopias and optic neuritis, but is also capable of testing the malingerer when used in conjunction with red and green filters.
   d) Chart 4: consists of scattered white dots with a central, white fixation target. It appears no more sensitive than the standard chart for relative scotomas and cannot detect metamorphopsia.
   e) Chart 5: consists of white parallel lines only and a central, white fixation point. The chart can be rotated to change the orientation of the lines and is used to investigate metamorphopsia along specific meridians.

f) Chart 6: similar to Chart 5 but has black lines on a white card with additional lines at 0.5° above and below fixation.

g) Chart 7: similar to Chart 1 but with additional 0.5° squares in the central 8°. This chart is used for detection of subtle macular disease.

5. Instruct the patient to view Chart 1 monocularly.

6. Ask the patient if they can see the central white dot. This is intended to determine whether the patient has a central relative (the dot looks blurred) or absolute scotoma. However, many patients with a central scotoma fixate eccentrically.

7. Ask the patient to keep looking at the central dot for the remainder of the test. They should be aware of the rest of the grid out of 'the corner of their eyes'.

8. Ask the patient if they can see all four sides and all four corners of the large square. This is intended to determine large scotomas, such as that produced by glaucoma.

9. Ask the patient if any of the small squares within the grid are missing or blurred.

10. Ask the patient if any of the lines that make up the grid appears wavy or distorted. This step is very important as it detects any metamorphopsia, which is usually caused by macular oedema.

11. Repeat steps 6 to 10 with any additional chart as deemed appropriate.

12. Record any defects or disturbances on an Amsler recording sheet. It is sometimes useful to have the patient draw the defects on a recording chart (Fig. 3.3).

3.7.4 Recording

Record defects or disturbances on an Amsler recording sheet. Always record the eye tested, the date of examination and the patient's name. Ensure that if no defects are detected, this is recorded clearly in the patient's file, e.g. Amsler charts: central fields full R and L (OD & OS).

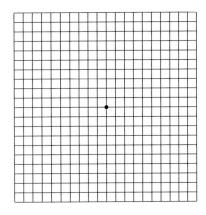

Fig. 3.3   The record sheet for the Amsler chart.

3.7.5 Interpretation

Metamorphopsia may indicate macular oedema. Although this can be advantageous clinically, great care must be taken when choosing the suitability of a patient for home monitoring with the test, as it can point out otherwise unnoticed problems that subsequently greatly annoy patients. For other patients, compliance can be poor (Fine et al. 1986). The step in the Amsler chart manual that suggests that you ask the patient to look for movement of lines, shining, or colours (entoptic phenomena) has been omitted as it can produce many artefacts.

3.7.6 Most common errors

1. Not ensuring that the patient views the central fixation target throughout the test.

2. Using an incorrect working distance.

3. Using an inappropriate near correction.

4. Using the patient's bifocals with a small reading area.

5. Performing the test binocularly.

3.8 PHOTOSTRESS RECOVERY TIME

Photostress recovery time (PSRT) is the time taken for visual acuity to return to normal levels after the retina has been bleached by a bright light source. It is a test of retinal function and is independent of ocular disease that affects other parts of the visual system.

3.8.1 Macular function

Long lasting after-images (longer than 15 seconds) produced by relatively brief flashes of light are due to photochemical changes in the receptors. Light absorption by rhodopsin (it is assumed that cone photopigments work in a similar fashion, although slightly faster) leads to the separation of the retinal chromophore from opsin. This process is called bleaching as it results in the loss of rhodopsin's purple colour. While the photopigment is being regenerated, the patient will see an after-image. Photostress recovery time determines the speed at which the photopigment regenerates.

3.8.2 Advantages and disadvantages

Photostress recovery time is solely dependent on the speed of regeneration of the photopigment and is therefore a test of retinal function. It should be independent of other disease within the visual pathway and to some extent will be independent of mild cataract as long as sufficient bleaching light can reach the retina. It is particularly useful when diagnosis of the cause of vision loss is difficult: is the vision loss caused by subtle macular changes or is there an underlying optic nerve or other visual pathway problem or amblyopia? Only macular disease will cause a prolonged photostress recovery time. The main disadvantage of the test is that there is no standardisation of the procedure. Recovery times are primarily dependent on the brightness of the light and the length of time used (Margrain & Thomson 2002), and it is best to obtain your own normal values with your own particular technique and instrumentation.

3.8.3 Procedure

1. Measure distance visual acuity of both eyes (section 3.2 or 3.3).

2. Ask the patient to remove their spectacles, but keep them in their lap so that they can be quickly put back on again.

3. Occlude the 'bad' eye. Hold your direct ophthalmoscope or other bright light source about 2–3 cm away from the patient's 'good' eye. Turn on the light and ask the patient to look directly at the light for exactly 10 s.

4. After 10 s, remove the ophthalmoscope, ask the patient to put his or her glasses back on and point to the letters one line larger than the patient's original visual acuity. Ask the patient to read those letters as quickly as he or she can after the after-image has disappeared.

5. Time how long it takes after removal of the bleaching light for the patient to read at least 2/3 of the letters on the line indicated.

6. Repeat the measurement for the 'bad' eye.

3.8.4 Recording

Record the time taken in seconds to recover to within one line of pre-bleached visual acuity.
    Examples:
        PSRT: RE 35, LE 40
        PSRT: OD 45, OS 105.

3.8.5 Interpretation

When used with patients with unilateral visual acuity loss, the results are compared between the 'good' and the 'bad' eye. If the recovery times are similar in the two eyes, then the cause of the poor visual acuity in the 'bad' eye is likely to be an optic nerve lesion. If the PSRT is much longer in the bad eye compared to the other eye, then the cause of the poor visual acuity is likely to be retinal. It is generally suggested that any PSRT longer than 50 s is abnormal, and suggests a macular disease rather than optic nerve abnormality. Of course, recovery times are primarily dependent on the brightness of the light and the length of time used (Margrain & Thomson 2002), and it is best to obtain your own normal values with your own particular technique and instrumentation.

3.8.6 Most common errors

1. Allowing the patient to lose fixation of the bleaching light.

2. Using a direct ophthalmoscope with batteries that are not fully charged.

3. Having the patient wait until the letters are clearly visible rather than just visible.

4. Timing inaccurately.

3.9 SIMPLE PENLIGHT GLARE TEST

The simple penlight glare test involves remeasuring distance visual acuity under glare conditions using a penlight at a fixed angle and distance from the eye.

3.9.1 Disability glare

Disability glare tests measure the reduction in a patient's vision due to a peripheral glare source. Light from the glare source is scattered within the patient's eye and forward light scatter produces a veiling luminance on the retina that reduces the contrast of the retinal image. In the following clinical conditions in which disability glare can be a problem, the site of increase in light scatter is indicated: corneal oedema (corneal epithelium especially) and opacity, post-refractive surgery (corneal epithelium), cataract (particularly posterior subcapsular cataract), post-cataract surgery (capsular remnants) and retinitis pigmentosa and other retinal disorders leaving a large reflective area on the retina. Light scatter within the retina may also be increased in conditions such as macular oedema.

3.9.2 Advantages and disadvantages

For routine optometric practice, disability glare is mainly used to help determine functional vision loss in patients with cataract. In these situations, the amount of intraocular light scatter is large and disability glare is probably best determined by remeasuring visual acuity while directing a glare source, such as a penlight or ophthalmoscope, into the eye. The disadvantage of this technique is the lack of standardisation of the amount of glare light reaching the eye. This can be remedied by using a standardised glare source such as the Brightness Acuity Tester (BAT) (Elliott & Bullimore 1993), although this is a relatively expensive instrument for what it provides. For more specialised practices, more sensitive measures of disability glare can be obtained using a low contrast visual acuity chart or the Pelli-Robson chart with a BAT. This can be useful when assessing disability glare in patients with relatively minor intraocular light scatter, such as in contact lens wearers or post-refractive surgery. Measurements of high and low contrast visual acuity or Pelli-Robson CS with a BAT glare source provide measurements of disability glare that are more repeatable than more complicated sine-wave grating based charts (Elliott & Bullimore 1993).

3.9.3 Procedure

1. Take the measurements with the patient wearing their own distance vision spectacles or contact lenses. It is difficult to measure disability glare with a trial frame/phoropter because the reduced aperture stops some of the glare light getting into the eye. You should check whether the spectacles or contact lenses are badly scratched as this could cause some disability glare.

2. Perform the test without dilating the pupils, so that the normal pupillary constriction from bright light will occur.

3. Occlude the eye not being tested.

4. Direct the penlight into the patient's eye from about 30 cm and at an angle of 30° from the eye. Alternatively, the slit-lamp illumination system can be used if it is in an appropriate position relative to the visual acuity chart. This helps to standardise the glare angle and distance of the glare source from the eye.

5. Re-measure visual acuity under these glare conditions.

3.9.4 Recording

Record as visual acuity with glare. For example:
VA with glare. RE: 6/24 LE: 6/18
VA with glare. OD: 20/80 OS: 20/60.

3.9.5 Interpretation

The amount of glare loss will differ depending on the test conditions such as the glare illumination and glare angle (disability glare is inversely proportional to the glare angle) and you should attempt to keep these constant and develop your own mean data for healthy eyes. Typically, most patients will show no change in visual acuity. A decrease in visual acuity of one line or less is normal. Some cataract patients can lose four lines of visual acuity and more. This test gives the patient's visual acuity under bright light conditions, which can be reduced with media opacification: corneal scars, post-refractive surgery, cataracts, posterior capsular opacification or central vitreous floaters. A poor visual acuity in glare conditions can provide justification for early referral of patients with cataract or posterior capsular opacification who have good visual acuity in normal light conditions.

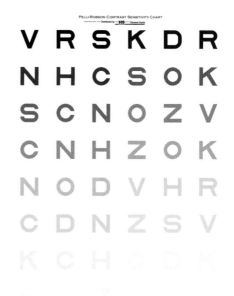

Fig. 3.4   The Pelli–Robson contrast sensitivity chart. (Reproduced with kind permission from Pelli et al. 1988).

3.9.6 Most common errors

1. Lack of standardisation of the glare source and its distance and angle from the eye.

2. Not directing the glare light into the eye.

3. As for visual acuity testing.

3.10 PELLI–ROBSON CONTRAST SENSITIVITY

The Pelli–Robson contrast sensitivity chart (Fig. 3.4) is an 86 × 63 cm chart that consists of 16 triplets of 4.9 cm (2.8° at 1 m) letters, and it assesses contrast sensitivity (CS) at a spatial frequency of about 0.50 to 1 cycle/degree. Within each triplet, the letters have the same contrast, and the contrast in each successive triplet decreases by a factor of 0.15 log units. Similar 'large letter' contrast sensitivity charts, such as the MARS test (Haymes et al. 2006) are available from other manufacturers.

3.10.1 Contrast sensitivity

Numerous studies have shown that contrast sensitivity (CS) provides useful information about functional or real-world vision that is not provided by visual acuity, including the likelihood of falling, control of balance, driving, motor vehicle crash involvement, reading, activities of daily living and perceived visual disability (reviewed in Elliott 2006). It is clear that CS should be included with visual acuity and visual fields in definitions of visual impairment and visual disability and for legal definitions of blindness (Leat et al. 1999). Thus, using CS in combination with visual acuity (and visual field assessment, when necessary) gives the clinician a better idea of how well a patient actually functions visually. In addition, CS can provide more sensitive measurements of subtle vision loss than visual acuity. There are many clinical situations in which CS can be reduced while VA remains at normal levels, including after refractive surgery, with minimal capsular opacification, with oxidative damage due to heavy smoking, in patients with optic neuritis and multiple sclerosis and in diabetics with little or no background retinopathy. For these reasons, CS measurements have become standard for most clinical trials of ophthalmic interventions, and they have been widely used in the assessment of refractive surgery, new intraocular implants, anticataract drug trials and potential treatments for age-related macular degeneration and optic neuritis. CS can therefore be used to help screen for visual pathway disorders and to explain symptoms of poor vision in a patient with good visual acuity. Patients with reduced visual acuity could have normal or reduced CS at low frequencies. Patients with reduced CS will have a poorer quality of vision than those with normal CS, despite the same acuity. When used in combination with visual acuity in this way, CS can be used to help explain symptoms of poor or deteriorating vision and to help justify referral of a cataract patient with reasonable visual acuity. Reduced CS can also explain a poor response to an optical aid by a low vision patient and suggest the need for a contrast enhancing CCTV. Binocular CS that is better than best monocular can also suggest the desirability of a binocular low vision aid over a monocular one.

3.10.2 Advantages and disadvantages

Pelli–Robson CS is quickly and simply measured and provides a reliable measurement of low spatial frequency CS (0.5–1 cycles/degree) when measured at the standard 1 m. It provides significantly more repeatable measures than sine-wave grating charts such as the Vistech or FACT charts (Elliott & Bullimore 1993, Pesudovs et al. 2004). If high contrast visual acuity is used to assess the high spatial frequency end of the CS curve, then a combination of Pelli–Robson CS and standard VA provides an indication of the whole CS curve. For example, a patient with low frequency CS loss only would have reduced Pelli–Robson CS and normal VA; a patient with high frequency CS loss only would have normal Pelli–Robson CS and reduced VA and a patient with CS loss at all frequencies would have reduced Pelli–Robson CS and reduced VA. The Pelli–Robson chart is ideal when determining functional vision loss in patients with low vision and moderate and dense cataract, when screening for low spatial frequency loss in patients with optic neuritis, multiple sclerosis or visual pathway lesions and when examining diabetics with little or no background retinopathy and patients with Parkinson's or Alzheimer's disease. The Pelli–Robson chart can be used at longer working distances such as 3 m, so that higher spatial frequencies are assessed and it becomes more sensitive to conditions such as early cataract. One disadvantage of the chart is that a variable endpoint can be gained depending on how long the patient is left to stare at the letters near threshold.

3.10.3 Procedure

1. Illuminate the chart (Fig. 3.4) to between 60 and 120 cd/m^2. If room lighting is inadequate, ensure the additional lighting provides a uniform luminance over the chart, and avoids specular reflections from the surface.

2. Sit/stand the patient 1 m from the chart, with the middle of the chart at eye level. Longer distances can be used if required.

3. Patients can wear their own distance spectacles as measurements are relatively immune to moderate dioptric blur.

4. Occlude one eye.

5. Ask the patient to read the lowest letters that they can see, and encourage the patient to guess. Once the patient states that they cannot see any further, indicate where the next lower contrast triplet is on the chart and ask the patient to keep looking at this point for at least 20 seconds. Generally, if given sufficient time, at least one more triplet of letters will become visible in this manner.

6. Count the reading of the letter C as an O as a correct response to further balance the legibility of the letters (Elliott 2006).

7. Score 0.05 log CS for every letter read correctly (the first triplet should be ignored as it has a log CS value of 0.00). This 'by-letter' scoring provides a more repeatable and sensitive measurement than the manufacturer's recommended scoring of the lowest line at which the patient can read two of the three letters (Elliott 2006).

8. Repeat the measurements in the other eye and binocularly as required.

3.10.4 Recording

Record the CS score in log units.
   Examples:
      Pelli–Robson. RE: 1.70 log CS, LE: 1.75 log CS, BE: 1.85 log CS

Pelli–Robson. OD: 1.70 log CS, OS: 1.25 log CS, OU: 1.65 log CS.

3.10.5 Interpretation

For patients between 20 and 50 years old, monocular CS should be 1.80 log units and above; for patients less than 20 years old and older than 50 years, monocular CS should be 1.65 log units and above. It is best to obtain your own norm values. If the monocular scores are equal, the binocular score should be 0.15 log units higher (binocular summation). With increasingly unequal monocular CS, the binocular summation will reduce and, in some patients, the best monocular score can be better than the binocular (binocular inhibition).

3.10.6 Most common errors

1. Not allowing the patient at least 20 seconds for the letters to become visible when the patient is near threshold.

2. Not pushing the patient to guess.

3. Inappropriate use of the occluder so that the patient can see the chart binocularly when monocular measurements are being made.

4. Inappropriate illumination (generally too low or not uniform).

3.10.7 Useful additional techniques: small letter CS and low contrast VA

Small letter CS is more sensitive than traditional VA to several clinical conditions, such as early cataract and contact lens oedema and should be ideal when attempting to measure subtle losses of vision such as after refractive surgery (Rabin & Wicks 1996). CS of very small letters, such as 20/30, correlates very highly with VA (Elliott & Situ 1998) and the ideal size for a small letter test may be about 20/50 (Rabin et al. 2004). 20/50 letters measure CS at about 7–10 cycles/degree. The measurement procedure is very similar to that for the Pelli–Robson chart.

Low contrast VA charts measure the smallest letter that can be resolved at a fixed contrast and do not measure CS. It is difficult to state which spatial frequencies the low contrast letter charts are measuring, because this depends on the VA threshold. If only the large letters at the top of the chart can be seen, the score gives an indication of CS at intermediate spatial frequencies. If a patient can see the small letters at the bottom of the chart, the score gives an indication of higher spatial frequencies. Low contrast VA scores are believed to indicate the slope of the high frequency end of the CSF. It has been suggested that they can be used to indicate the CSF when used in combination with a low frequency or peak CS measure such as the Pelli–Robson chart and a high contrast VA measurement. The lower the contrast of the acuity charts, the more sensitive they become to subtle vision loss. For example, for detecting subtle vision losses in aviators or subtle changes after refractive surgery, 5–10% charts should be used. For greater losses in vision, such as cataract, even the large letters on these very low contrast charts cannot be seen by some patients, and a higher contrast chart at about 25% is necessary. As with high contrast VA measurements, charts that follow the Bailey–Lovie (logMAR) design principles should be used (section 3.2). The measurement procedure is the same as for high contrast visual acuity and depends on whether the chart uses a logMAR (section 3.2) or Snellen (section 3.3) chart design.

3.11 FREQUENCY DOUBLING PERIMETRY

Frequency doubling perimetry (FDP) is based upon the frequency doubling illusion that occurs when a low spatial frequency grating (<1 cycle per degree) is flickered in counterphase at a high temporal frequency (>15 Hz), resulting in the perception of a doubled spatial frequency (Kelly 1981). The illusion was developed into a clinically viable technique using a grating of 0.25 cycles/degree and temporal frequency of 25 Hz, and incorporated into two central visual field instruments by Welch Allyn (FDP and Matrix perimeter; Delgado et al. 2002, Johnson & Samuels 1997). It was initially thought that the illusion was due to selective stimulation of the non-linear My cells, a type of magnocellular projecting retinal ganglion cells (Anderson & Johnson 2002).

This is now considered unlikely as there is no evidence for such cells in humans. The clinically developed stimulus is used as a flicker contrast threshold task, rather than being a true frequency doubling task. As such the stimulus is likely to still preferentially stimulate the magnocellular system (Quaid et al. 2004).

The suggested screening program is the N-30–5. The test uses four 10° square targets in each quadrant, a central 5° circle and two additional 10° targets in the nasal field. The −5 in the program title indicates that there is a 5% chance of a positive test being from a patient with a normal visual field. Two additional probability levels are also highlighted, 2% and 1%, in order to better delineate abnormality and assist in the clinical diagnosis. There is also a N-30–1 program that sets the probability of a positive test being from a patient with a normal visual field at 1%. This may be considered more appropriate in a population screening environment to avoid high numbers of false positives (section 1.2.2).

3.11.1 Central visual field screening

Perimetry enables the assessment of visual function throughout the visual field, the detection and analysis of damage along the visual pathway, and the monitoring of disease progression. Central visual field analysis can be a lengthy procedure and quicker and simpler techniques can be used for screening the central visual field. Central visual field screening can be considered for asymptomatic and risk free patients. For patients exhibiting significant risk factors for glaucoma, neurological disease, certain types of retinal disease or symptomatic patients, it is more appropriate to perform a central visual field analysis rather than use a screening technique. The FDP N-30–5 screening program, for example, may miss some small paracentral defects, likely due to the large stimulus size. If defects are suspected following screening (repeated twice) then central visual field analysis should be performed. Visual field screening should never be used to monitor disease progression.

3.11.2 Advantages and disadvantages

FDP provides a high level of sensitivity (≈85%) and specificity (≈90%) for early glaucoma (<6 dB mean deviation) (Delgado et al. 2002) for a rapid, 1–2 minute test. In addition, because the stimulus is relatively unaffected by optical blur, pupil size and ambient illumination, the test can be used in a pre-screening environment with normal room lighting, natural pupils and the patient's own spectacles, including multifocals. Patients tend to prefer performing FDP testing, especially when compared to standard automated perimetry. There is evidence to suggest that even in screening mode the FDP will identify some glaucoma defects prior to standard automated perimetry (Delgado et al. 2002).

The disadvantages include that the large targets sometimes miss small, early defects, particularly in the paracentral region. In a small number of patients there will be an artifactual, diffusely abnormal result in the second, generally left, eye tested. This is thought to be due to binocular rivalry. This phenomenon can be overcome by repeating the second eye test with the first eye occluded, or by ensuring that the second eye remains light adapted during the testing of the first eye. It is necessary always to test the right eye first.

3.11.3 Procedure

1. Turn on the instrument and allow to calibrate. The screening programs described are available on the original FDP and the newer Matrix instrument. The procedure described is for the FDP but is very similar for the Matrix.

2. Explain the test and the reasons for performing the assessment to the patient.

3. The FDP can be conducted with or without correction within about a 6 D range. If the patient's spectacles are worn ensure that the frame does not obscure the full view of the monitor. Do not use glasses that are tinted. Bifocals and progressive lenses *can* be used. Contact lens wearers should perform the test in their lenses and this is particularly useful for aphakes and high ametropes.

4. Seat the patient at the instrument and adjust the height of the instrument to ensure patient comfort.

5. Remove the calibration cap from the eyepiece.

6. Select Run Patient Tests.

7. Enter patient age.

8. Slide the patient visor to the right eye. It is important that the right eye is tested first (see Interpretation).

9. Give the patient the response button and ask them to place their forehead on the rest. Ensure that they can see all four corners of the monitor and the black fixation dot.

10. Explain the test to the patient: 'Can you see the black dot in the centre and the entire lit video screen? You need to stare at the black dot in the centre of the screen during the entire test. During the test you will see patterns of flickering black and white vertical bars that will appear briefly in different parts of the screen. The patterns will sometimes be very faint and you are not expected to see the bar patterns all the time. Each time you see the flickering black and white vertical bars, please press the response button once.'

11. If the patient is naïve to the test then run the demonstration program. Repeat until you are convinced the patient understands the procedure.

12. Select Run Screening N-30–5.

13. Following completion of the right eye test, slide the patient visor to the left eye position and repeat the test.

14. Print results or transfer to the Viewfinder program for further analysis, storage and printing.

15. At the end of a session replace the calibration cap.

3.11.4 Recording

If no errors are made at the 19 target locations, then record 'FDP: WNL (Within Normal Limits) R and L'. If there is a field defect, repeat the test, print and store both fields of both eyes and attach to the record card. If the original field defect is repeatable and if the patient is going to be referred to the secondary eye care system, then best practice would be to

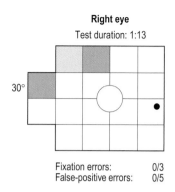

Right eye

Test duration: 1:13

| Fixation errors: | 0/3 |
| False-positive errors: | 0/5 |

Fig. 3.5 Printout from the FDP strategy N-30–5.

perform central visual field analysis (section 3.15) and include the single field analysis (section 3.15.5, Fig. 3.6) with the referral letter. Results are recorded as a non-interpolated greyscale illustrating the 19 target locations (Fig. 3.5). If clear or white the location is considered to be within normal limits for the patient's age, and there is a 5% chance that the negative finding is incorrect. The three levels of grey represent when the target was missed at 5% but seen at the 2% probability level; missed at 2% but seen at the 1% probability level; and missed at the 1% probability level. The test duration and rudimentary reliability indices (false positive and false negative catch trials and fixation losses) are also provided.

3.11.5 Interpretation

Note that following the collection of normal values that define the test, a systematic difference was found between the first and second eye tested. This difference has been incorporated into the test by designating the left eye as being the second eye tested. A repeatable cluster of two or more points at the <5% probability level, or a single repeatable point at the <1% probability level should be considered abnormal and the patient scheduled for central visual field analysis, and relevant ocular health assessment. Rudimentary reliability indices are provided (see section 3.15.5 for a full description of reliability indices). If there is more than one of three fixation losses and/or one of three false positives then the reliability of the result should be questioned and consideration given to repeating the examination.

3.11.6 Most common errors

1. Using a screening program incorrectly, such as to monitor a patient with a visual field defect.

2. Providing poor patient instruction: It is worth investing time to ensure that the naïve patient understands what is expected of them. If necessary, repeat the test until you are satisfied that the patient has performed adequately.

3. Examining the left eye first.

4. Failing to encourage and communicate with the patient.

5. Misinterpreting an initial field defect: It is important to be aware of the possible causes of artefact in cases where it would appear that a new defect has been detected, particularly in a patient with no previous experience of visual field screening or no history of field loss. A new defect is *not* a defect until it is repeated; 'if in doubt always repeat'. The effect of learning and fatigue can be dramatic.

6. Misinterpreting a generalised reduction in sensitivity in the left eye: One of the major problems encountered with FDP is that there is a sub-group of patients who encounter problems when testing the second eye. They experience a rivalry phenomenon, which results in a generalised defect in the second eye tested. The problem is overcome by retesting the left eye with a patch positioned over the right eye, or by ensuring that the left eye remains light adapted whilst the right eye is being tested.

3.12 FAST CENTRAL VISUAL FIELD ANALYSIS

The Humphrey Field Analyser (HFA) II, SITAFast, Central 24-2 tests 58 locations over the central 25° in a 6° grid pattern that straddles the horizontal and vertical midlines, i.e. targets are located 3° either side of the midlines. In addition, there are targets located on the nasal field between 25° and 30°. The SITAFast, 24-2 program rarely takes more than 3.5 minutes in a

normal patient, and can be as quick as 2.5 minutes. SITA employs methods of most likelihood to reduce testing time (Bengtsson & Heijl 1998). The Medmont M-700 uses a similar approach (Vingrys & Helfrich 1990). The Octopus Tendency Oriented Perimetry (TOP) uses another approach based upon the principle that neighbouring target locations will have similar levels of sensitivity (Chaglasian 2001). The Oculus perimeters (Easyfield Centerfield and Twinfield) and the Henson Pro also have the option of a fast, staircase based, threshold estimation strategy. These strategies are useful for screening, but *not* for monitoring of disease. The Matrix perimeter uses frequency doubling technology to evaluate the central visual field using 5° targets in a 24-2 pattern. It uses a 4-step, modified ZEST procedure (for review of the various threshold estimation techniques see McKendrick 2005) to rapidly estimate threshold ($\approx$4 minutes per eye).

3.12.1 Fast central visual field analysis

In spite of SITAfast and the other related techniques, designed to rapidly estimate threshold, they should be considered as screening techniques, to be used when a defect is not suspected. They take approximately the same time to test the visual field as traditional screening methods (sections 3.13 and 3.14). Fast central visual field screening can be considered part of a routine eye examination for asymptomatic and risk free patients. For patients exhibiting significant risk factors for glaucoma, neurological disease, certain types of retinal disease or symptomatic patients, it is more appropriate to perform a more accurate central visual field analysis. If defects are suspected following the fast threshold technique then central visual field analysis should be performed. Fast central visual field analysis should never be used to monitor disease progression.

3.12.2 Advantages and disadvantages

Fast thresholding strategies can produce an estimation of visual field sensitivity in a time (2.5–4 minutes per eye) similar to single stimulus, suprathreshold screeners. Humphrey's SITAFast (Swedish Interactive Thresholding Algorithm) is a strategy that provides similar accuracy to the old Fastpac strategy, but takes half the time (Bengtsson & Heijl 1998). All of the fast central field analysis techniques have the advantage over suprathreshold screening techniques in that they are better able to detect early visual field defects, and can give an idea of defect depth and area. They have the disadvantage of taking longer than some suprathreshold techniques. When compared to techniques for full central field analysis, they are quicker but less precise and with worse test–retest characteristics.

3.12.3 Procedure

The example used is the Humphrey Field Analyser, SITAFast, 24-2.

1. Explain the test and the reasons for performing the assessment to the patient.

2. When performing visual field screening, pupils should be 3 mm or greater, whenever possible. It is considered acceptable to perform visual field testing whilst a pupil is dilating, provided the pupil is at least 3 mm at the start of the test.

3. Reduce ambient illumination and turn on the instrument.

4. For most visual field screeners: Contact lens wearers should perform the visual field test in their lenses. This is particularly useful for aphakes and high ametropes. Full aperture trial case lenses should otherwise always be used for all necessary near vision correction. Reduced aperture lenses and masked cylindrical lenses (i.e. those with opaque masks running along the direction of the axis) can result in visual field artefacts. Similarly, bifocal and progressive addition spectacles and small aperture spectacles should be avoided. Best sphere should be used for any cylinder less than 1.50 D. If the cylinder is greater than 1.50 D then place the appropriate spherical lens in the back cell of the lens holder and the cylindrical lens in the cell immediately in front of the sphere. You should use a translucent occluder if the patient has latent nystagmus.

5. Seat the patient at the instrument and adjust the height of the instrument to ensure patient comfort.

6. Select 'Central 24-2' and then subsequently select 'Change Parameters' and 'Test Strategy' to ensure 'SITAFast' is used.

7. Select the eye to be tested first, and unless otherwise indicated select 'Right'.

8. Enter the patient ID. Let the patient adapt to the bowl luminance while entering the data. This is a very important, but frequently overlooked, procedure, as it ensures a consistent level of retinal adaptation over the duration of the test. Enter as much patient data as possible but always include patient name using the surname first, date of birth (this is often formatted as month-day-year) and patient file number if appropriate. It is often useful to enter the prescription lenses used and pupil size. It is also possible to enter a diagnostic code, VA, IOP and cup-to-disc ratio.

9. Occlude the left eye and give the patient the response button.

10. Place the patient's head in the headrest. Explain the test to the patient: 'I want you to keep looking at the yellow light in the middle of the bowl. When you see a light flashing off to the side of the yellow light, please press this button. There will be times during the test when you will not be able to see any lights flashing and this is normal. Remember to keep looking at the yellow light in the middle of the bowl all the time'.

11. Align the patient using the video eye monitor.

12. Ensure that the vertex distance of the trial lens is adjusted appropriately and the trial lens is centred in front of the eye.

13. Select 'Demo' for a naïve patient. Repeat until you are happy that the patient understands the procedure.

14. Select 'Start'.

15. Some models will have a Gaze Monitoring feature. Once initialised, select 'Start'.

16. Monitor fixation and encourage the patient throughout the test.

17. Never leave the patient unattended.

18. When the test is completed, store the result on disk then select 'Test Other Eye'. Occlude the patient's right eye and align the left eye with the appropriate correction having been placed in the lens holder.

19. When the left eye is completed, store the results on disk and print the results if required.

3.12.4 Recording

If no test locations are highlighted on the Total and Pattern Deviation probability plots then record 'SITAFast: WNL (Within Normal Limits) R and L'. If there is a field defect, repeat the test, print and store both fields of both eyes and attach to the record card. SITAStandard (or equivalent) could be used instead of SITAFast for the repeated field. The single field analysis of the repeated field should accompany any referral to the secondary eye care system. The single field analysis printout illustrates the data as an interpolated greyscale, raw data in decibels, and Total and Pattern deviation plots. It also summarises the field using the glaucoma hemifield test, global indices, reliability indices, and Gaze Tracking plots (section 3.15.5 and Fig. 3.6).

3.12.5 Interpretation

These are interpreted in exactly the same way as the strategies for full central field analysis (see section 3.15.5).

3.12.6 Most common errors

1. Using an inappropriate spectacle or lens type: Only use full aperture lenses in order to reduce the possibility of lens rim artefact. Do not use multifocal or varifocal lenses as these will frequently result in an artefactual reduction of sensitivity in the lower visual field. Frames with a small eye size should also be avoided as they may result in a mid-peripheral lens rim artefact.

2. Poorly aligning the patient: Great care needs to be taken when initially aligning the patient. Ensure the instrument height is appropriate for the patient, relative to the height of the chair. The patient should be sat comfortably throughout the test, with their back supported. Over-extension of the neck and a bent back with hunched shoulders and neck should both be avoided. If supplementary lenses are being used, ensure the patient's eye is centred within the lens when viewing through the video monitor. Throughout the examination, check that the patient's forehead has remained touching the rest.

3. Misinterpreting an initial field defect: It is important to be aware of the possible causes of artefact in cases where it would appear that a new defect has been detected, particularly in a patient with no previous experience of visual field screening or no history of field loss. A new defect is *not* a defect until it is repeated; 'if in doubt always repeat'. The effect of learning and fatigue can be dramatic (Hudson et al. 1994).

4. Using visual field screeners incorrectly, such as using a screening technique to monitor a patient with a visual field defect.

5. Providing poor patient instruction: It is worth investing time to ensure that the naïve patient understands what is expected of them. If necessary, repeat the test until you are satisfied that the patient has performed adequately.

6. Failing to encourage and communicate with the patient: It is essential that the patient is encouraged and coerced throughout the examination period, e.g. informing of the time remaining, using phrases such as 'you are doing well' or 'keep looking straight ahead'. It has been shown that such human contact and encouragement is the most effective way to achieve the best result.

7. Examining the right eye with a left eye program.

8. Misinterpreting an upper field defect: The effect of blepharoptosis or dermatochalasis should always be carefully considered. Always note the position of the upper lid

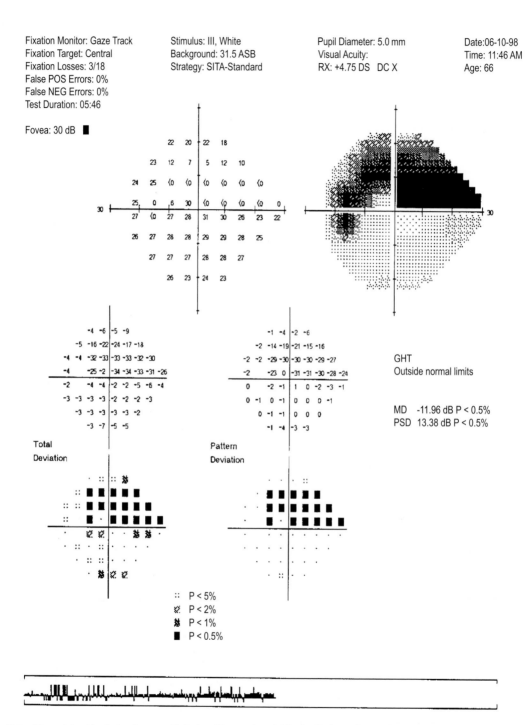

Fig. 3.6 The printout includes the sensitivity level for each point in decibels; an interpolated greyscale display; the total deviation in decibels and probability of each point being normal in a non-interpolated greyscale; the pattern deviation in decibels and probability of each point being normal in a non-interpolated greyscale; the glaucoma hemifield test; the gaze track plot; and global indices.

and consider taping if it is obstructing the field of view.

9. Using an incorrect vertex distance for the trial lenses. Use the rear cell of the trial lens holder for the spherical correction. Use the cell immediately in front for the cylindrical correction should one be required ($\geq$1.50 DC). Keep the vertex distance to a minimum so as to reduce the possibility of lens rim artefact.

10. Misinterpreting a generalised reduction in sensitivity. When the glaucoma hemifield test classifies the field as having a 'general reduction of sensitivity', the Mean Defect/Deviation is abnormal and/or the Total Deviation probability plot shows a majority of test locations as being outside normal limits; care should be taken when interpreting the results. There is usually an obvious clinical reason for such a result, with the most likely association being with cataracts or small pupils. Occasionally, such a result can be associated with an inappropriate refractive correction or poor visual acuity. Remember, 'if in doubt always repeat'.

3.13 MULTIPLE STIMULUS SUPRATHRESHOLD STRATEGY

The Henson multiple stimulus suprathreshold program tests 26 points within the central 25° visual field using eight presentations of between two and four points. A threshold value is first determined (the level at which the light can just be detected) at several mid-peripheral points 10° from fixation, and the expected threshold values for the entire visual field are extrapolated. All target locations are then tested at 5 dB brighter than these values (5 dB suprathreshold). If any point is repeatedly missed, the program can be extended to screen 68 or 136 points in the central field. Typical test duration is between 2 and 4 minutes.

3.13.1 Central visual field screening

Perimetry enables the assessment of visual function throughout the visual field, the detection and analysis of damage along the visual pathway, and the monitoring of disease progression. Central visual field analysis can be a lengthy procedure and quicker and simpler techniques are used for screening the central visual field. Central visual field screening can be considered part of a routine eye examination for asymptomatic and risk free patients. For patients exhibiting significant risk factors for glaucoma, neurological disease, certain types of retinal disease or symptomatic patients, it can be more appropriate to perform a central visual field analysis rather than use a screening technique. Suprathreshold screening, like Henson multiple stimulus, can miss shallow or small scotomas. If defects are suspected following screening then central visual field analysis should be performed. Visual field screening should never be used to monitor the progression of a disease.

3.13.2 Advantages and disadvantages

The Henson Pro includes a new threshold algorithm (HEART), which improves test–retest variability (Henson & Artes 2002) and an automatic measurement of patient response times. Henson & Artes (2002) showed that a large percentage of false positive responses can be detected by comparing their latencies to the average response time of a patient. The procedure takes longer than the FDP screening program, and can take as long as fast thresholding strategies. It is likely to miss some early, small and/or shallow defects and there is no information provided with respect to patient reliability.

3.13.3 Procedure

1. Explain the test and the reasons for performing the assessment to the patient.

2. When performing visual field screening, pupils should be 3 mm or more whenever possible. It is considered acceptable to perform visual field testing whilst a pupil is dilating, provided the pupil is at least 3 mm at the start of the test.

3. Reduce ambient illumination and turn on the instrument.

4. Contact lens wearers should perform the visual field test in their lenses. This is

particularly useful for aphakes and high ametropes. Full aperture trial case lenses should otherwise always be used for all necessary near vision correction. Reduced aperture lenses and masked cylindrical lenses (i.e. those with opaque masks running along the direction of the axis) can result in visual field artefacts. Similarly, bifocal and progressive addition spectacles and small aperture spectacles should be avoided. Best sphere should be used for any cylinder less than 1.50 D. If the cylinder is greater than 1.50 D then place the appropriate spherical lens in the back cell of the lens holder and the cylindrical lens in the cell immediately in front of the sphere. You should use a translucent occluder if the patient has latent nystagmus.

5. Seat the patient at the instrument and adjust the height of the instrument to ensure patient comfort.

6. Select F1: 'Multiple stimulus suprathreshold' from the main menu.

7. Occlude the left eye and adjust the chin rest for the right eye, and place the patient's head in the rest.

8. Ensure that the vertex distance of the trial lens is adjusted appropriately.

9. Explain the test to the patient: 'I would like you to keep looking at the central red light throughout the test. Some lights will flash on the screen and you will see them "out of the corner of your eyes". Please tell me how many flashing lights you see'.

10. The computer screen provides instructions to guide you through the rest of the examination. First, you must estimate the patient's threshold. The target presentations are set at a bright level and subsequently lowered until none can be seen. One step above this level is taken as threshold. Press the PRESENT button and ask the patient how many flashes of light they saw. If the patient saw none, press the up-arrow button; if one or more, press the down-arrow button. The computer will repeat this procedure until there have been two 'none' responses (and two up-arrow button presses).

11. The program will then set the targets at 5 dB above this threshold level in order to screen for a field defect at a suprathreshold level.

12. The program presents eight stimuli of between two and four points. Press the PRESENT button. If the patient correctly determines the number of targets presented, press the right-arrow button to proceed to the next presentation and press the PRESENT button once again. Continue in this way for all eight presentations or until a target is missed.

13. If a target is missed, present again. If the patient incorrectly identifies the number of targets for a second time, ask the patient to describe the position of the seen targets. They are best described using the positions of the hours on a clock.

14. The targets will be described on the computer screen as A, B, C or D. Press the button that describes the target(s) missed. Then press the PRESENT button again and repeat the procedure.

15. If the same target(s) were missed again, then the computer suggests that you extend the screening program. Press F2 (EXTEND). This extends the screening program to 68 points. The computer screen now also contains a dial that indicates whether the field is normal, suspect or defective.

16. Once you have completed screening the 68 points, reassess any points missed at higher suprathreshold values. Return to the presentation where a target or targets were missed using the right-arrow button and increase the intensity of the presentation to 8 dB above threshold by pressing the up-arrow button. Present the target at this intensity level. If it is missed at this level, increase the intensity to 12 dB above threshold by again pressing the up-arrow button, and present again.

17. If the screening program indicates that the field is suspect or defective, then press F3 (PRINT/SAVE). You will then be asked to input the patient's details and can save the field information on disk and/or request a printout.

3.13.4 Recording

If no errors are made on the eight initial presentations or if the Henson indicates the field is normal on the extended program, then record 'Henson suprathreshold: All points seen (suprathreshold level)'. For example, Henson suprathreshold: all points seen @ 2.6 R and L. If there is a field defect, then repeat the test, print the fields of both tests and both eyes and attach to the record card. Figure 3.7 shows the printout of a field result. If the original field defect is repeatable and if the patient is going to be referred to the secondary eye care system, then best practice would be to perform central visual field analysis (section 3.15) and include the single field analysis (section 3.15.5, Fig. 3.6) or similar with the referral letter.

3.13.5 Interpretation

The program indicates whether the visual field is normal, suspicious or has a field defect. It considers the number, depth and clustering properties of any missed targets when interpreting any field defect. The printout of the visual field indicates whether a

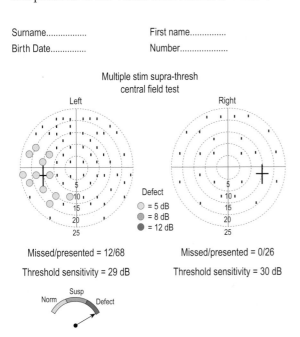

Surname................. First name...............
Birth Date.............. Number....................

Multiple stim supra-thresh central field test

Left   Right

Defect
○ = 5 dB
◔ = 8 dB
● = 12 dB

Missed/presented = 12/68   Missed/presented = 0/26

Threshold sensitivity = 29 dB   Threshold sensitivity = 30 dB

Norm Susp Defect

Fig. 3.7 The printout of a field result using the Henson multiple-stimulus suprathreshold screening strategy.

point was seen at the 5 dB suprathreshold level or was missed at the 5 dB, 8 dB or 12 dB suprathreshold level.

It is likely that a proportion of early glaucomatous defects detected using central field analysis will be missed using a screening technique of this type. The program does not present any reliability indices such as the number of fixation losses and the percentage of false positive and false negative errors, as this information cannot be obtained when using multiple stimulus presentations. It is left to the clinical judgement of the operator as to whether a field defect could be due to unreliable responses from the patient. Reliability indices are provided with the full threshold strategy, and the reliability of the patient's responses can be quantified using this secondary assessment.

3.13.6 Most common errors

See section 3.12.6.

3.14 SINGLE POINT SUPRA-THRESHOLD SCREENING

Single point, suprathreshold central screening is designed to determine whether the sensitivity of the visual field is greater than a specific, pre-determined level. It can provide an estimate of the size and location of moderate to severe defects, but will not quantify the depth of the defect. There are several alternate approaches that either estimate a suprathreshold screening level relative to age matched normal values (recommended technique) or relative to initially tested seed points (Anderson & Patella 1999, Weijland et al. 2004). These are then tested in a 2 or 3 level/zone strategy. The 3 zone strategy, the recommended technique, will test once (Octopus 2-LT) or twice (HFA 3 zone, Oculus 3 zone) at the screening level, and if missed will test again with the brightest stimulus level. If seen at the initial screening level, usually 4 dB to 6 dB brighter than the expected threshold, the location is recorded as being within normal limits. If missed at the initial screening level but seen at the maximum brightness then it is recorded as a relative defect. If missed at both screening levels the location will be designated an absolute defect. The Oculus and Humphrey perimeters offer an additional 'quantify defects' screening strategy, whereby the locations missed twice at the initial screening level are quantified using a full threshold, staircase strategy.

3.14.1 Central visual field screening

Central visual field analysis can be a lengthy procedure and quicker and simpler techniques are used for screening the central visual field. Central visual field screening can be considered for asymptomatic and risk free patients. Suprathreshold screening is likely to miss shallow defects <5 dB. For patients exhibiting significant risk factors for glaucoma, neurological disease, certain types of retinal disease or symptomatic patients, it is more appropriate to perform a central visual field analysis rather than use a screening technique. If defects are suspected following screening then central visual field analysis should ideally be performed. Single point, suprathreshold central screening should never be used to monitor disease progression.

3.14.2 Advantages and disadvantages

Single point suprathreshold screening techniques of the central visual field have become largely redundant following the introduction of fast threshold estimation techniques (section 3.12). They frequently take as long to perform, and can take longer if a defect is present. The sensitivity and specificity for early glaucoma is not as good as that reported for the FDP screening technique (section 3.11). Single point screening is likely to miss early, shallow defects (<5 dB). However, they are still occasionally used for full field screening, particularly for suspected neurological defects (section 3.16).

3.14.3 Procedure

The example used is the Humphrey Field Analyser, 3 zone, 24-2.

1. Follow steps 1 to 5 of 'Fast central visual field analysis' (section 3.12.3).

2. Select 'Screening' test type from the 'Main Menu'.

3. Select 'Central 24-2'.

4. Select 'Change Parameters'.

5. Select 'Three Zone' test strategy.

6. Select 'Age Reference Level' test mode.

7. Follow steps 7 to 20 of 'Fast central visual field analysis' (section 3.12.3).

3.14.4 Recording

If no test locations are highlighted on the printout then record '24-2, 3 zone: WNL (Within Normal Limits) R and L'. The printout illustrates the data with symbols that designate the location as 'within normal limits', 'relative defect' and 'absolute defect'. There is usually some indication of patient reliability, e.g. test time, catch trials and fixation losses. If there is a field defect, repeat the test, print and store both fields of both eyes and attach to the record card. If the original field defect is repeatable and if the patient is going to be referred to the secondary eye care system, then best practice would be to perform central visual field analysis (section 3.15) and include the single field analysis (section 3.15.5, Fig. 3.6) with the referral letter.

3.14.5 Interpretation

Identify any clusters of relative or absolute defect. Repeatable isolated absolute defects should be investigated further, as should any repeatable cluster of three or more relative defects. As with all visual field analysis, the position and shape of a defect, along with additional clinical findings, will dictate the management of the patient.

3.14.6 Most common errors

See section 3.12.6.

3.15 30-2 AND 24-2 CENTRAL VISUAL FIELD ANALYSIS

The most commonly used perimeter and programs for central visual field analysis is the Humphrey

Field Analyser (HFA), programs 30-2 and 24-2. The 30-2 program tests 76 locations over the central 30° in a 6° grid pattern that straddles the horizontal and vertical midlines, i.e. targets are located 3° either side of the midlines (Anderson & Patella 1999, Lalle 2001). Equivalent programs can be found on most perimeters, such as the Henson Pro (Henson 2000), Medmont M700 (Vingrys & Helfrich 1990), Octopus 1-2-3, 101 or 301 (Chaglasian 2001, Weijland et al. 2004), Matrix and Oculus Easyfield, Centerfield and Twinfield perimeters. The 24-2 program examines the central 25°, with the addition of more peripheral targets in the nasal step region, and consequently testing time is reduced by up to 20% compared to the 30-2 strategy. It is often used in follow-up assessments and to lessen the likelihood of any fatigue effect.

3.15.1 Central visual field analysis

Standard threshold automated perimetry is the standard of care for the diagnosis and management of many ocular and neurological diseases. In particular it plays an invaluable role in the diagnosis and management of the glaucomas. Analysis of the central visual field should be performed on all patients with:

- Risk factors for glaucoma

- Abnormal screening test (e.g. positive automated screening test, frequency doubling test, confrontation or Amsler)

- Symptoms consistent with neurological disease (for example, headache including migraine, dizziness, tingling of limbs) or neuro-ophthalmic disease

- Symptoms consistent with central field loss, e.g. non-refractive reduced vision, positive scotoma, scintillating scotoma.

In addition, threshold fields are always required when monitoring a known defect, and they should always be included in protocols for the management of glaucoma. Typical screening strategies are suprathreshold with stimuli presented 5 to 6 dB above threshold, so that subtle field defects may be missed.

3.15.2 Advantages and disadvantages

The instrument should be capable of monitoring fixation, providing full threshold fields in less than 10 minutes, providing reliability indices and analysing the results. A rapid threshold estimation algorithm, such as the HFA's SITAStandard or the Octopus Dynamic Strategy, is recommended. These strategies take approximately 7 to 9 minutes per eye, without compromising the accuracy or repeatability of the result (Wild et al. 1999). The use of faster, less repeatable, thresholding strategies (e.g. HFA SITAFast and Octopus TOPs; section 3.12) may be considered as an alternative for some patients with a demonstrated history of fatigue, although the number of such patients has reduced considerably with the advent of the 8 minute threshold test. There has been discussion that SITA should not be used in patients suspected of conditions other than glaucoma as they are optimised specifically for glaucoma. However, clinically the advantage of the reduced test time makes such a compromise worthy of consideration, and no evidence has been presented that suggests a reduction in diagnostic capability for non-glaucomatous defects. The Matrix offers a new alternative, employing the frequency doubling illusion. In response to concerns over the ability of the original FDP screening instrument, with its large targets, to detect subtle, early defects, a second generation machine was recently launched, the FDT Matrix, which uses smaller 5 degree targets and measures with a standard 24-2 pattern. An adapted ZEST-type, fixed 4 step strategy is used to estimate the sensitivity and ensure a standardised test time (<4 minutes), regardless of defect.

3.15.3 Procedure

The following procedure, although specific to the HFAII, can be considered a template for most modern perimeters.

1. Reduce ambient room illumination and turn on the instrument. When performing visual field assessment, pupils should be 3 mm or more whenever possible. Below 2.5 mm the results will be diffraction limited and will demonstrate a generalised reduction in sensitivity. Very large pupils will blur the

stimuli due to increased aberrations. However, the effect is usually minimal when examining a standard 30 degree field size and it is considered acceptable to perform visual field testing whilst a pupil is dilating, provided the pupil is at least 3 mm at the start of the test.

2. Seat the patient at the perimeter and adjust the height of the instrument and the chin rest to ensure the patient is comfortable.

3. At the 'Main Menu' select 'Central 30-2' (or 'central 24-2').

4. Select the eye to be tested first, and unless otherwise indicated select 'Right'.

5. Enter the patient ID. Let the patient adapt to the bowl luminance while entering the data. This is a very important, but frequently overlooked, procedure, as it ensures a consistent level of retinal adaptation over the duration of the test. Enter as much patient data as possible but always include patient name using the surname first, date of birth (nb: this is often formatted as month-day-year) and patient file number if appropriate. It is often useful to enter the prescription lenses used and pupil size. It is also possible to enter a diagnostic code, VA, IOP and cup-to-disc ratio.

6. Select 'Change Parameters', followed by 'Test Strategy' and ensure 'SITAStandard' is selected. If a full threshold strategy is considered appropriate, select 'Full Threshold'.

7. Occlude the left eye, give the patient the response button and place any appropriate correction into the lens holder positioned before the right eye. Contact lens wearers should perform the visual field test in their lenses. This is particularly useful for aphakes and high ametropes. Full aperture trial case lenses should otherwise always be used for all necessary near vision correction. Reduced aperture lenses and masked cylindrical lenses (i.e. those with opaque masks running along the direction of the axis) can result in visual field artefacts. Similarly, bifocal and progressive addition spectacles and small aperture spectacles should be avoided. Best sphere should be used for any cylinder less than 1.50 D. If the cylinder is greater than 1.50 D then place the appropriate spherical lens in the back cell of the lens holder and the cylindrical lens in the cell immediately in front of the sphere. You should use a translucent occluder if the patient has latent nystagmus.

8. Place the patient's head in the headrest. Explain the test to the patient: 'I want you to keep looking at the yellow light in the middle of the bowl. When you see a light flashing off to the side of the yellow light, please press this button. There will be times during the test when you will not be able to see any lights flashing and this is normal. Remember to keep looking at the yellow light in the middle of the bowl all the time'.

9. Align the patient using the video eye monitor.

10. Ensure that the vertex distance of the trial lens is adjusted appropriately.

11. Select 'Demo' for a naïve patient. Repeat until you are happy that the patient understands the procedure. Use the diamond fixation target for patients who have poor central vision.

12. Select 'Start'.

13. Some models will have a Gaze Monitoring feature. Once initialised select 'Start'.

14. Monitor fixation and encourage the patient throughout the test.

15. Never leave the patient unattended. Patients often need constant encouragement.

16. If false negative catch trials are noted, advise the patient to rest by keeping the response button pressed down, which will pause the test.

17. If false positive catch trials are noted, pause the test and re-instruct the patient.

18. When the test is completed, store the result on disk then select 'Test Other Eye'. Occlude the patient's right eye and align the left eye with the appropriate correction having been placed in the lens holder.

19. When the left eye visual field is completed, store the results on disk and select 'Print' or the print icon.

20. Print all results and return to the 'Main Menu'.

3.15.4 Recording

If no test locations are highlighted on the Total and Pattern Deviation probability plots then record 'SITAStandard (30-2): WNL (Within Normal Limits) R and L'. Print the fields for both eyes and attach to the record card. If a new defect has been detected, particularly in a patient with no previous experience of perimetry or no history of field loss, then repeat the field measurement. Confirmation of visual field abnormalities is essential for distinguishing reproducible visual field loss from long-term variability (section 1.2.4). The single field analysis printout illustrates the data as an interpolated greyscale, raw data in decibels, and Total and Pattern deviation plots (Fig. 3.6). It also summarises the field using the glaucoma hemifield test, global indices, reliability indices, and Gaze Tracking plots. When monitoring glaucoma, the Glaucoma Progression Analysis (GPA), which is based upon the Early Manifest Glaucoma Trial (Leskea et al. 2004), is designed to identify true glaucoma progression.

3.15.5 Interpretation

Visual fields should be interpreted with respect to their reliability, as a single field and with respect to change over time.

Reliability indices

The reliability indices consist of the following (for a review see Lalle 2001):

Fixation losses. These are assessed by presenting suprathreshold targets in the blind spot (Heijl–Krakau technique). They are flagged if more than 20% occur, however this has been found to be too stringent and 30% is a more appropriate cut-off (Katz & Sommer 1988). If fixation losses are flagged, only discard the field if you feel that the patient was struggling to fixate, or if false negatives are also flagged.

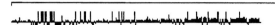

Fig. 3.8 Example of gaze tracking plots. Upward deflections indicate fixation losses and downward deflections are recorded when the position of the eye cannot be determined or there is a blink. The upper plot is typical of a patient with good fixation. The lower plot would indicate poor fixation throughout the test.

The HFAII also employs gaze tracking throughout the test, displayed as a bar chart on the monitor and the printout (Fig. 3.8). Upward deflections indicate eye movements and downward deflections are recorded when the position of the eye cannot be determined or there is a blink.

False positives. These errors indicate a 'trigger happy' patient who is responding to the sound of the perimeter when no target is presented. They should be less than 20%. Intervene immediately if false positives start to appear during the test and re-instruct the patient. If false positives are greater than 20%, the result should be discarded and the field repeated. For a repeat field, the test speed could be reduced.

False negatives. These errors accumulate when a patient fails to respond to a suprathreshold target at a given location; these are associated with fatigue and/or inattention. They should also be less than 20%. If you notice false negatives accumulating, particularly toward the end of an examination, give the patient a rest. This will often ensure that the false negative score does not reach significance. If the false negative rate does not improve, despite a rest, it can be better to continue on another day.

For strategies other than SITA there will also be an estimate of the intra-test variance called the short-term fluctuation, which should be within normal limits (not have a reported p-value).

Single field analysis

The single field analysis (Fig. 3.6, section 3.12.4) includes: the sensitivity level for each point in decibels;

an interpolated greyscale display; the total deviation in decibels and probability of each point being normal in a non-interpolated greyscale; the pattern deviation in decibels and probability of each point being normal in a non-interpolated greyscale and the glaucoma hemifield analysis. The Octopus and Oculus perimeters also include a defect curve.

- Total deviation (TD) compares the result to an age-matched normal population and states the probability of each point being abnormal on a point-by-point basis.

- Pattern deviation (PD) compares the result to an age-matched normal population corrected for the overall level of sensitivity for the individual. The probability of any point varying from this level is stated on a point-by-point basis. This enhances the ability to observe mappable scotomata within a generalised depression, which may be induced by small pupils or poor media.

- If there are no abnormal points on the TD and PD plots, then the patient can be considered as having a normal field.

- A generalised depression will be most easily appreciated by looking for a majority of abnormal points on the TD probability chart. Clusters of two or more non-edge points together on the PD chart (p < 0.05) should be considered suspicious. An isolated point within the central 10° (p < 0.05) should also be considered suspicious. If a cluster of abnormal points exists it should be interpreted with respect to its underlying anatomical correlate and subsequent clinical significance. Many artefacts show large jumps in sensitivity, from −1 to −28 dB, for example.

- The glaucoma hemifield test analyses the relative symmetry of five pre-defined areas in the superior and inferior field, as well as judging the overall level of sensitivity compared to age-matched normal values. The visual field is then classified as being 'within normal limits', 'outside normal limits', 'borderline', 'abnormally high sensitivity', or to have a 'general reduction of sensitivity'. Note that some other visual

defects are not picked up by the glaucoma hemifield test, so it should not be relied upon to interpret all visual field losses. The defect curve ranks the test locations from most to least sensitive and plots relative to the 5% and 95% confidence interval for normal visual fields.

The global indices

The global indices are data reduction statistics designed to describe specific characteristics of the glaucomatous visual field (Heijl et al. 1987). In summary:

- Mean deviation (MD) is the mean difference in decibels between the 'normal' expected hill of vision and the patient's hill of vision. If the deviation is significantly outside the norms, a P value will be given. It is useful to monitor the overall change in the visual field (Fig. 3.9a).

- Pattern standard deviation (PSD) is a measure of the degree to which the shape of the patient's field deviates from age-matched normal. A low PSD indicates a smooth hill of vision, while a high PSD indicates an irregular hill. PSD characterises localised changes in the visual field (Fig. 3.9b). The value is expressed in decibels and any value of 2 dB or greater will have a P value next to it indicating the significance of the deviation. Note that it gets better as the field defect advances to more severe stages, as the field becomes more uniform once again.

- Short-term fluctuation (SF) is a measure of the intra-test variance. It has proven to be of little clinical value.

- Corrected pattern standard deviation (CPSD) is PSD corrected for the SF. These latter two indices are no longer provided on SITA fields.

The probability of the global indices being normal is stated on the printout.

Visual field progression

Change in the visual field of a single patient over time is best appreciated using the Overview printout. Caution is recommended when considering

(a)

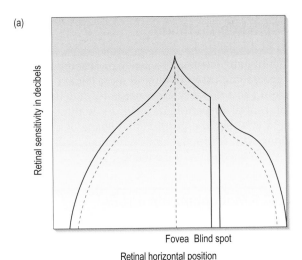

(b)

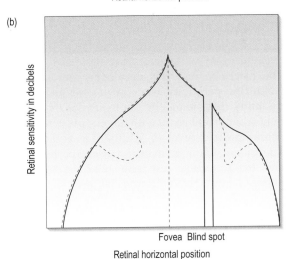

Fig. 3.9   The hill of vision, showing changes that would produce (a) a significant mean defect, MD and (b) a significant pattern standard deviation, PSD.

change in the visual field due to the high level of inter-test variability, particularly when a defect is present (Heijl et al. 1989). The mantra should be 'if in doubt always repeat'. If a glaucomatous defect is being followed, the Glaucoma Progression Analysis (GPA) can be considered. This is a refinement of the original Glaucoma Change Probability analysis and was developed for the Early Manifest Glaucoma Trial. GPA uses the pattern deviation database rather than the total deviation database, and is therefore more robust to the effects of cataract and reduced

pupil size. The analysis uses estimates of the inherent variability within glaucomatous visual fields. This is combined with the Early Manifest Glaucoma Trial criterion of three significantly deteriorating points repeated over three examinations. A minimum of two baseline and one follow-up examinations are required. Each exam is then compared to baseline and to the two prior visual fields. Abnormal points are highlighted, as are those that progress on two or three consecutive examinations.

It is also possible, but not recommended, in the Change Analysis printout, to monitor change in the global indices by linear regression analysis and overall change by means of a box-plot chart.

3.15.6 Most common errors

See section 3.12.6.

3.16 30 TO 60 DEGREE SUPRATHRESHOLD VISUAL FIELD SCREENING

The recommended approach to peripheral field testing is to first record a fast threshold central test (see section 3.12) followed by a peripheral suprathreshold screening program that tests between 30 and 60 degrees, e.g. Humphrey Field Analyser Peripheral 60 screening program and Medmont M700 Peripheral 30–50. Similar programs can be found on most modern bowl perimeters. Alternative methods would include a full field suprathreshold screening program such as that found on the Octopus (programs 07 and N1), Medmont M700 (Full 50 and Neurological 50), Humphrey Field Analyser (Full Field 120), Oculus and Henson Pro, or combining a fast threshold central test with a fast threshold peripheral test.

3.16.1 Screening the peripheral visual field

Peripheral testing should be considered in some neurological cases, occasional retinal (particular retinitis pigmentosa) and glaucoma cases, when patients report symptoms of poor peripheral vision and when assessing vision standards.

3.16.2 Advantages and disadvantages

Virtually all visual field defects, including those due to chiasmal or post- chiasmal lesions, are reflected within the central 30° visual field (e.g. Wellings 1989). This is simply due to the anatomy of the visual pathway. There is a systematic bias towards representation of the central visual field, with over 80% of the visual pathway dedicated to processing the central 30° of vision (Drasdo & Peaston 1980).

3.16.3 Procedure

The example used is the Humphrey Field Analyser, Three-zone, Peripheral 60.

1. Following completion of the 30-2 program select 'Screening' test type from the 'Main Menu'.

2. Select 'Peripheral 60'.

3. Select 'Right'.

4. Select 'Change Parameters'.

5. Select 'Three Zone' test strategy.

6. Select 'Age Reference Level' test mode.

7. Follow steps 7 to 20 of 'Fast central visual field analysis' (section 3.12.3).

8. Print results as a merged file with the central 30-degree threshold result, if possible.

3.16.4 Recording

If all test locations are labelled as being 'within normal limits' on the printout then record 'Peripheral 60, 3 zone: WNL (Within Normal Limits) R and L'. If there is a defect evident then print the fields for both eyes, attach to the record card and consider a confirmatory field. The printout illustrates the data with symbols that designate the location as 'within normal limits', 'relative defect' and 'absolute defect'. There is usually some indication of patient reliability, e.g. test time, catch trials and fixation losses. The combined printout will show the threshold 30-2 result as a greyscale, surrounded by the Peripheral 60 symbols.

3.16.5 Interpretation

Identify any clusters of relative or absolute defect. Repeatable clusters of three or more relative defects should be noted. Look for continuity of defect from the central to peripheral field. As with all visual field analysis, the position and shape of a defect, along with additional clinical findings, will dictate the management of the patient.

3.16.6 Most common errors

See section 3.12.6.

3.17 BINOCULAR ESTERMAN TEST

The Esterman test was developed for use with Goldmann perimetry as a way of assessing visual disability (Esterman 1982). It expresses the visual field as a percentage of seen targets, presented at a suprathreshold level of 10 dB (III3e equivalent). The monocular Esterman test uses 100 locations and the binocular test uses 120. The stimulus pattern favours the inferior visual field.

3.17.1 Visual field screening for driving requirements

The binocular Esterman test has proven increasingly popular as a method for evaluating the visual field for driving standards. The monocular Esterman test can be used for assessing visual disability.

3.17.2 Advantages and disadvantages

The binocular Esterman grid is now available on several of the automated perimeters, including the Humphrey Field Analyser, and gives an automated score. As such it has gained in popularity for the evaluation of visual impairment, visual disability and driving standards (Anderson & Patella 1999). It has not been validated for use with standard automated perimetry, but has become a standard of measurement in many circumstances, including the driving standard in several countries.

3.17.3 Procedure

The example used is the Humphrey Field Analyser binocular Esterman test. Other perimeters have similar testing procedures.

1. Reduce ambient illumination and turn on the instrument.

2. The patient should be seated at the perimeter and the height of the instrument and the position of the chin rest should be adjusted to ensure patient comfort.

3. At the 'Main Menu' select 'Specialty Test'.

4. Select 'Esterman Binocular'.

5. Enter the patient ID. Let the patient adapt to the bowl luminance while entering the data.

6. Move the chin rest to the extreme right position.

7. Position the patient's chin on the left chin rest.

8. Give the patient the response button. Use the habitual prescription used for driving, and do not attempt to use trial case lenses.

9. Explain the test to the patient: 'I want you to keep looking at the yellow light in the middle of the bowl. When you see a light flashing off to the side of the yellow light, please press this button. There will be times during the test when you will not be able to see any lights flashing and this is normal. Remember to keep looking at the yellow light in the middle of the bowl all the time'.

10. Select 'Start'.

11. Encourage the patient throughout the test and never leave the patient unattended. Note that there is no way of monitoring fixation.

12. If false positive catch trials appear, it can be useful to pause the screening and re-educate the patient before completing the test. If false positive catch trials get too high, the field screening will have to be repeated (see Interpretation).

13. When the test is completed store the result on disk and select 'Print' or the print icon.

14. Print the result and return to the 'Main Menu'.

3.17.4 Recording

The printout uses a non-interpolated greyscale to illustrate those grid locations that were seen (open circle) at the 10 dB screening level, and those that were missed (black box). The number of seen and missed points are also stated as a proportion of the total 120 grid locations and an efficiency score is expressed as the percentage seen. The efficiency score is then used to judge the patient's disability. At the end of the test, print the result and record the efficiency score as a percentage.

3.17.5 Interpretation

The results are interpreted as a percentage of visual function, giving an indication of visual disability. For driving standards it is often necessary to assess the extent of the horizontal binocular visual field. Several jurisdictions consider 120° or more of continuous horizontal field to be the required standard. The percentage rate of false positives is an important check of the reliability of the test, as some patients can try to improve their chances of 'passing' this driving standard test by pressing the response button when a light was not seen. Typically, a false positive score above 20% means that the visual fields are unreliable and not acceptable to a driving standards agency, so that the test must be repeated.

3.17.6 Most common errors

These are the same as for visual field screening (section 3.12.6), plus:

1. Not using the patient's habitual prescription.

2. Selecting the monocular test and testing binocularly, or vice versa.

3.18 CONFRONTATION FIELD TESTING

Confrontation field testing provides a gross assessment of the patient's visual field using a comparison of the patient's visual field with the examiner's field using simple targets such as a 15 mm diameter red or 4 mm white bead at the end of a stick or the examiner's fingers.

3.18.1 Gross visual field screening

A variety of very simple visual field tests are available and include confrontation fields, kinetic boundary testing, colour comparison fields and oculo-kinetic perimetry (OKP). The confrontation test can be used in primary eye care patients with very gross field defects to provide an assessment of their functional visual field.

3.18.2 Advantages and disadvantages

The prime use of confrontation tests as visual field screeners is during home (domiciliary) visits, which are outside the scope of this text. Their only advantages are that they are portable and inexpensive. The most sensitive method appears to be examination of the central visual field with a red target(s) (Elliott et al. 1997b, Pandit et al. 2001). From a visual field screening point of view, all of these tests have been shown to be insensitive to all but gross field defects such as homonymous hemianopias when compared to automated perimetry (Elliott et al. 1997b, Pandit et al. 2001). It is advisable for general medical practitioners who suspect a patient may have a visual field defect to refer such patients for automated field testing rather than relying on the results of a confrontation test.

3.18.3 Procedure

1. Explain to the patients that you are going to measure the area over which they can see rather than how well they can see detail.

2. Keep the room lights on. The absolute level is irrelevant as the technique involves a comparison of the patient's and examiner's visual fields.

3. Sit between 66 cm and 1 m away from, and directly facing, the patient. You should be at approximately the same height as the patient.

4. Ask the patient to remove any glasses and occlude their left eye using the palm of their hand (not fingers).

5. You should similarly occlude your right eye.

6. Ask the patient to fixate your open eye (left) with their open eye (right). Some patients may feel uncomfortable if asked to stare into your eye directly, and you can suggest they look at the middle of your lower lid.

7. Show the patient the bead-on-a-stick and explain that you are going to move it inwards from outside the field of view and you want the patient to indicate when they can first see the target. Explain that you will continue to move the target into the centre of their vision and you want them to indicate if it disappears or fades at any point.

8. Hold the bead-on-a-stick in a plane equidistant between you and the patient and outside your field of view along one of the eight principal radial meridians. Slowly move the bead inwards until the patient reports it is just seen. Compare this point to the point when you first saw the target. Then slowly move the target towards fixation and ask the patient to indicate if it disappears or becomes less distinct.

9. Repeat this procedure for all eight radial meridians. At all times watch that the patient does not lose fixation of your eye to look towards the target. If this occurs, repeat the measurement.

10. Repeat for the other eye.

3.18.4 Recording

Record the type of confrontation target used and whether there were any significant differences between your own visual field and the patient's visual field. A normal result could be recorded as 'Fields grossly full to confrontation, 15 mm Red'.

3.18.5 Interpretation

Confrontation testing involves a comparison of your visual field with the patient's visual field. Providing there is no obvious abnormality in your field, the patient's field is considered within normal limits if it matches your own. It is useful in the detection and monitoring of large absolute defects, e.g. quadrantanopsia and homonymous, heteronymous or altitudinal hemianopsia.

3.18.6 Most common errors

1. Using too cluttered a background to the visual field (loud tie or blouse, wall picture, bookcase).
2. Moving the target too fast.
3. Allowing the patient to lose fixation.
4. Believing that other visual field assessments are not necessary if confrontation does not show a defect.

3.19 FARNSWORTH–MUNSELL D-15

The Farnsworth–Munsell D-15 test consists of 16 caps that each contain a paper of a different colour (Fig. 3.10). The differences between the colours are relatively large and the test was designed to separate patients into those with a mild colour defect who pass the test and those with a moderate to severe defect who fail the test.

3.19.1 Acquired colour vision testing

Acquired colour defects are normally monocular or unequal in the two eyes, found about equally in males and females, can progress (or regress) and most often involve a loss of blue sensitivity leading to blue–green and yellow–violet discrimination loss accompanied by decreased vision. Acquired

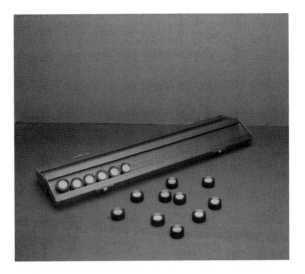

Fig. 3.10   The Farnsworth D-15 colour vision test.

defects may be due to the presence of an anomaly involving the ocular media, retina or the visual pathways. The causes of the anomalies can be due to ocular or systemic diseases and disorders, drugs or toxic substances. In patients with acquired colour deficiencies, their colour problems can get ignored because other aspects of vision, such as visual acuity, contrast sensitivity or visual fields, are reduced and take precedence. Although these latter tests may be more routinely measured in patients with ocular abnormality and may be more important from a diagnostic perspective, colour vision is an important part of the assessment of a patient's functional vision. Depending on the prognosis for the condition, young patients with an acquired colour defect should be counselled that their condition reduces their chances of joining certain occupations, as discussed in section 3.21.1. Relatively common causes of acquired colour defects in the working population include diabetes and glaucoma. Note that diabetes can cause blue–yellow defects even prior to the appearance of ophthalmoscopically visible retinopathy (e.g. Ismail & Whitaker 1998). Patients who acquire a colour vision problem who have already started a career that requires good colour vision should be warned of possible problems. For example, general medical practitioners should be warned of the difficulties in identifying the presence and extent of various coloured clinical signs such as body colour changes, skin rashes, blood in urine, faeces, sputum and vomit and test strips for blood and urine (Cole 2004). A tritan-type defect occurs with increasing age due to the yellowing of the lens and receptor changes and cataract (particularly nuclear cataract) and age-related maculopathy in particular can lead to more severe colour defects in the elderly population. Hobbies that may be affected by colour defects include art, photography, interior decorating and electronics. The famous impressionist artist, Claude Monet (1840–1926) had great trouble with acquired colour defects due to cataract in his later life. Finally, elderly individuals with colour defects should be warned against differentiating tablets based purely on their perceived colour.

3.19.2 Advantages and disadvantages

Because the Ishihara test is relatively poor at grading the severity of congenital and acquired colour defects and monitoring acquired colour defects, and cannot detect blue–yellow defects, an additional colour vision test is required. The Farnsworth–Munsell D-15 test can grade the severity of colour vision problems and can test for blue–yellow and red–green defects, so that it can be used to detect and monitor all patients with acquired colour deficiency. It is more sensitive to protan loss than the City University test (section 3.20) (Oliphant & Hovis 1998). However, the D-15 is not as sensitive to subtle colour vision defects as the Ishihara test and patients with a mild red–green defect could pass the D-15 and yet fail the Ishihara. Therefore, the D-15 must never be used as a screening test, particularly given that passing the more stringent Ishihara test is a common requirement for some professions (section 3.21.1). The usefulness of any colour vision test is influenced by whether it is used as part of the entrance requirements to certain professions in the region where you are working.

3.19.3 Procedure

1. You must use the proper quantity and quality of illumination, as the colour temperature of the illuminant will affect the colours of the test. Colour vision testing is normally performed under a standard daylight source,

such as one of the Gretag Macbeth Sol-Source daylight desk lamps. This simulates natural daylight conditions provided by direct sunlight and a clear sky. As these desk lamps are expensive, alternative sources are also used. For example, you can use high colour rendering fluorescent lights (>5000 K) or a Kodak Wratten number 78AA filter (found in camera shops) placed in front of the patient's eye in conjunction with a 100 watt incandescent light source. Natural daylight is not recommended due to its variability in both the quality and quantity of light, although even this is preferable to tungsten lighting.

2. If grading the severity of a congenital colour vision defect detected using the Ishihara test, measure colour vision binocularly. Explain to the patient that you are going to assess the extent of their colour vision difficulty.

3. If screening for an acquired defect, measure colour vision monocularly. Explain to the patient that you are going to test their colour vision.

4. Ask the patient to use their near vision correction and avoid tinted spectacles or contact lenses.

5. Arrange the loose colour caps in a random order in front of the patient near to the box that contains the pilot colour cap.

6. Ask the patient to place the test cap that most closely resembles the colour of the pilot cap next to it in the box. This then becomes the reference cap for the next test cap, and so on (Fig. 3.10) until all caps are in place. Allow the patient time to review the ordering and make any necessary adjustments.

7. Close the box, turn it over and open it again to determine the order in which the caps have been arranged.

8. If the caps have been arranged in the correct order, or with just one or two transpositions of adjacent caps, record the result as normal.

9. If mistakes have been made in the arrangement of the caps, record the arrangement order on the D-15 score sheet

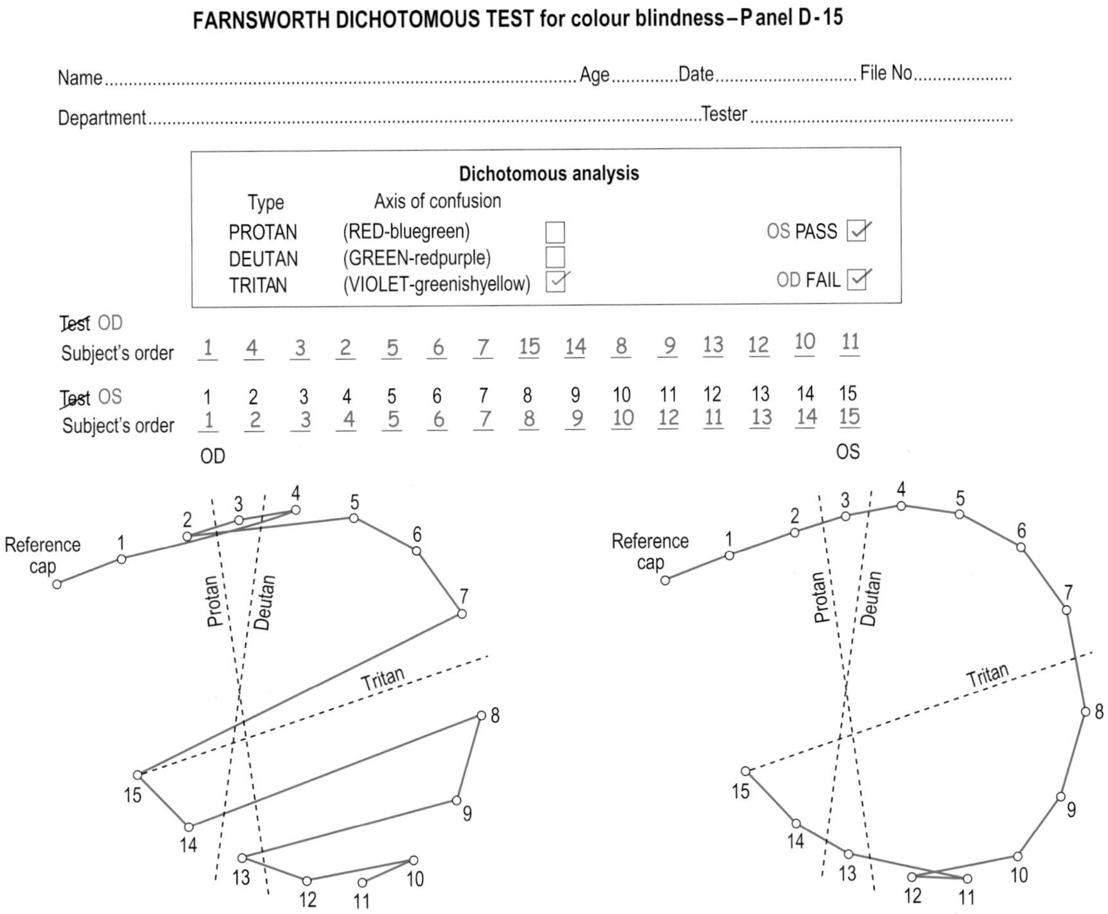

FARNSWORTH DICHOTOMOUS TEST for colour blindness – Panel D-15

Name.. Age.............Date..............................File No....................

Department..Tester...

Dichotomous analysis

Type	Axis of confusion		
PROTAN	(RED-bluegreen)	☐	OS PASS ☑
DEUTAN	(GREEN-redpurple)	☐	
TRITAN	(VIOLET-greenishyellow)	☑	OD FAIL ☑

Test OD
Subject's order: 1 4 3 2 5 6 7 15 14 8 9 13 12 10 11

Test OS
Subject's order: 1 2 3 4 5 6 7 8 9 10 11 12 13 14 15

OD   OS

Fig. 3.11   A D-15 scoring sheet showing a tritan defect in the right eye and a passed test in the left eye.

(Fig. 3.11). Draw lines from the numbers on the score sheet according to the patient's arrangement of the caps. Repeat the test and plot your retest results on a different score sheet (indicate which score relates to which test).

10. Any patients who are diagnosed as colour defective should be counselled regarding the effects of the modified colour vision on (as appropriate) jobs, hobbies and future career restrictions.

who make errors. It is also important to record any advice given to the patient and their family.
Examples:
Ishihara failed; D-15 no errors: Mild R/G defect. patient advised re. effect & future career restrictions
Ishihara failed; D-15 failed/see attached: mod./severe R/G defect. patient advised re. effect & future career restrictions
See attached sheet (Fig. 3.11): D-15. OD: Acquired tritan defect. OS: No errors. Fail: patient advised re. possible effect on job as interior decorator.

3.19.4 Recording

Patients with normal colour vision should make no errors and this can be recorded. The D-15 score sheet should be plotted and retained for patients

3.19.5 Interpretation

Patients with normal colour vision should make no errors. Patients with mild colour vision defects may make minor errors, such as reversals of adjacent caps or one crossing of the D-15 score sheet. These errors still constitute a pass for this test. A failure, as specified by Farnsworth, is two or more crossings of the D-15 score sheet (Fig. 3.11). These crossings should parallel one of the protan, deutan or tritan axes marked on the score sheets.

3.19.6 Most common errors

1. Using an inappropriate light source.
2. Believing that a pass on the D-15 test means that the patient has normal colour vision.

3.20 THE CITY UNIVERSITY TEST

The City University test (Birch 1997a) contains 10 plates that each displays a central coloured dot surrounded by four coloured dots derived from the Farnsworth–Munsell D-15 test. The patient's task is to select the peripheral coloured dot that looks most similar in colour to the central dot. Three of the peripheral colours are chosen as typical isochromatic confusion colours for patients with a protan, deutan or tritan deficiency respectively. The fourth colour is very similar to the central coloured dot and is the one chosen by patients with normal colour vision.

3.20.1 Acquired colour vision testing

See section 3.19.1.

3.20.2 Advantages and disadvantages

Because the Ishihara test is relatively poor at grading the severity of congenital and acquired colour defects and monitoring acquired colour defects, and cannot detect blue–yellow defects, an additional colour vision test is required. The second edition of the TCU (City University test) (Birch 1997a) is preferred as the third edition has not been independently evaluated and it is substantially different from the second edition. It can grade the severity of colour vision problems and can test for

blue–yellow and red–green defects so that it can be used to detect and monitor all patients with acquired colour deficiency. However, the second edition TCU is not as sensitive to subtle colour vision defects as the Ishihara and patients with a mild red–green defect could pass TCU and yet fail the Ishihara. Therefore the TCU should never be used on its own as a screening test, particularly given that passing the more stringent Ishihara test is a common requirement for some professions (section 3.21.1). TCU is less sensitive to protan loss than the Farnsworth D-15 (section 3.19; Oliphant & Hovis 1998). The usefulness of any colour vision test is influenced by whether it is used as part of the entrance requirements to certain professions in the region where you are working.

3.20.3 Procedure

1. You must use the proper quantity and quality of illumination as described in 3.19.3 or 3.21.3.

2. If grading the severity of a congenital colour vision defect detected using the Ishihara test, measure colour vision binocularly. Explain to the patient that you are going to assess the extent of their colour vision difficulty.

3. If screening for an acquired defect, measure colour vision monocularly. Explain to the patient that you are going to test their colour vision.

4. Ask the patient to use their near vision correction and avoid tinted spectacles or contact lenses.

5. Hold the test in your hand or place it on the table in front of the patient, about 35 cm away with the pages at right angles to the patient's line of sight. The cap colours can become soiled with time and some practitioners use white cotton gloves (photographer's) for themselves and/or the patient.

6. Show the demonstration plate A to the patient and describe the test: 'Here are four coloured spots surrounding one in the middle. Please tell me which of the four spots is nearest in colour to the one in the middle. Either point or tell me whether it is

the top, bottom, left or right, but please don't touch the pages.'

7. Show the test plates 1 to 10 in turn. Allow about 3 seconds per page, with a slightly longer time for the first few pages while the patient becomes familiar with the task.

8. Record the patient's choices in the appropriate column on the record card (either right, left or both eyes).

9. Any patients who are diagnosed as colour defective should be counselled regarding the effects of the modified colour vision on

(as appropriate) jobs, hobbies and future career restrictions.

3.20.4 Recording

Patients with normal colour vision should make no errors and this can be recorded. The TCU record form (Fig. 3.12) indicates the most likely of the four spots which will be identified as most similar to the middle by colour normals, protans, deutans and tritans. This can be used to categorise a colour defect in a patient who makes some mistakes. Score

Fig. 3.12 The TCU record form. (Reproduced with the permission of Keeler Ltd.)

City University colour vision test

Address .... Patient ....

Examiner .... Male/Female   Date .... / .... / 200 ....

Spectacles worn? Yes/No   RE/LE/BE

Illumination ('Daylight')   Type .... Level ....

FORMULA: Here are four colour spots surrounding one in the centre. Tell me which spot looks most near in *colour* to the one in the centre. Use the words 'TOP', 'BOTTOM', 'RIGHT' or 'LEFT'. Please do not touch the pages.

Page (A is for demonstration)	Subject's choice of match R | L | Both	Normal	Diagnosis Protan	Diagnosis Deutan	Diagnosis Tritan
1		B ⬇	R	L	T
2		R ▷	B	L	T
3		L ◁	R	T	B
4		R ▷	L	B	T
5		L ◁	T	B	R
6		B ⬇	L	T	R
7		L ◁	T	R	B
8		R ▷	L	B	T
9		B ⬇	L	T	R
10		T ⬆	B	L	R

(Rows 1–6: 'Chroma four'; Rows 7–10: 'Chroma two')

SCORE		Normal	Protan	Deutan	Tritan
	At chroma four	/6	/6	/6	/6
	At chroma two	/4	/4	/4	/4
	Overall	/10	/10	/10	/10

Probable type of Daltonism   P; PA, EPA mixed
D, DA, EDA
Tritan

the patient's responses out of 10. The number of mistakes in the normal column indicates the severity of the colour defect. Record if the patient was unusually slow and record any advice given to the patient and their family.

Examples:

Ishihara failed; TCU no errors: Mild R/G defect. patient advised re. effect & future career restrictions

Ishihara failed; TCU 4/10 deutan: Moderate deutan. patient advised re. effect & future career restrictions

TCU. RE: no errors, but slow; OS: 8/10 tritan: Severe acquired tritan defect. patient advised re. possible effect on job as interior decorator.

3.20.5 Interpretation

Cut-off points can be changed to vary the sensitivity and specificity of a test. The cut-off points given below are the ones typically used. A patient 'fails' the test if they make more than two mistakes. A patient who makes one or two mistakes is 'borderline' and may require retesting or testing with a more extensive battery of tests. The TCU grades the severity and classifies the colour deficiency (Birch 1997a). Patients who fail the Ishihara and then pass the TCU have a mild red–green defect, and are unlikely to have trouble with most occupations.

3.20.6 Most common errors

1. Using an inappropriate light source.

2. Allowing the patient too long to look at the figures.

3. Suggesting to the patient which spot might be correct.

3.21 THE ISHIHARA COLOUR VISION TEST

The Ishihara test is the most commonly used pseudoisochromatic plate test for colour vision defects. The Ishihara test is made up of several plates that present various numbers made up of coloured dots of varying size embedded in a background of different coloured dots (Fig. 3.13). The colours of the number and background dots are chosen so that they are confused by patients with red–green colour defects (i.e. they appear isochromatic to those with colour defects) but discriminated by patients with normal colour vision. Plate 1 is a demonstration plate that should be read by all literate patients and can be used to indicate malingerers. Different designs of pseudoisochromatic plates follow, and include transformation (plates 2–9), vanishing (10–17) and hidden digit (18–21) plates. Normal trichromats can see numbers on all but the hidden digit plates. Patients with red–green colour deficiency do not see a number on the vanishing plates, see a different number than normals on the transformation plates and *can* see a number on the hidden digit plates. Classification plates, which attempt to differentiate protans and deutans, are found on plates 22–25. Two numbers are shown on each plate. The right-hand number (blue–purple) is not seen or seen less well by deutans, and the left-hand number (red–purple) is not seen or less well seen by protans. The rest of the plates contain pseudoisochromatic pathways and are used for

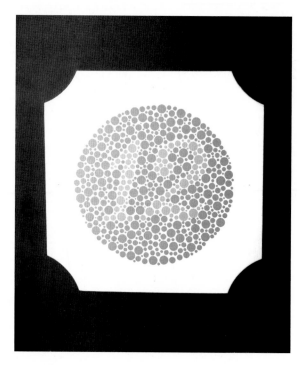

Fig. 3.13   The demonstration plate of the Ishihara pseudoisochromatic plates.

patients who cannot read letters, such as young children. The patient's task is to trace the pathway.

3.21.1 Congenital colour vision testing

Congenital colour deficiency is found in both eyes equally and does not change over time. It is virtually always a red–green deficiency and is far more common in males than females as it is an X-linked disorder. Approximately 8% (1 in 12) of the male and 0.5% of the female population are red–green deficient. Dichromats, with only two of the three cone photopigments, have the most severe type of colour vision anomaly. Deuteranopes (1%) lack the 'green-catching' chlorolabe, and protanopes (1%) lack the 'red-catching' erythrolabe and both confuse all colours from red, through orange and yellow to green. Anomalous trichromats have all three photopigments, but either the red or green photopigments provide less discriminative colour vision than normal. The level of colour vision anomaly can range from near normal to near dichromat levels. Protanomalous trichromats (1%) and deuteranomalous trichromats (5%) confuse colours such as red and brown, green and brown, yellow and orange, pink and grey, purple-red and grey. These colours are more likely to be confused if they are pale or dull or made in dim lighting. In addition, all protans are relatively insensitive to red light. These confusions of colour create difficulties in a variety of everyday situations (Cole 2004), including:

- Matching coloured objects such as clothes, paints and materials used in crafts and hobbies

- Differentiating differently coloured objects such as ripe and unripe fruit, school workbooks, features on maps

- Judging when meat is cooked

- Recognising skin rashes and sunburn.

Patients with colour deficiency will also have difficulty with road traffic signals, and protans, because of their relative insensitivity to red light, have difficulty seeing low intensity red lights such as car and bicycle retroreflectors. Colour vision defects also reduce the chances of being accepted for certain jobs within the armed forces, police force, fire brigade,

aviation and railway industry, etc. For example, at the present time in the UK, a patient with a colour deficiency who fails the Ishihara test cannot become a pilot, air traffic control officer, flight engineer or flight navigator in the armed forces or with the civil aviation authority and is unable to become a firefighter, train driver or railway signaller. In addition to exclusion from these occupations, the presence of a colour deficiency results in greater difficulty in pursuing a career that stresses the ability to discriminate colour. Such careers include histology, photography, the paint and textiles industries, interior decorating and electronics. Medical practitioners have been shown to have difficulties in identifying the presence and extent of coloured clinical signs (e.g. body colour changes, skin rashes, blood in urine, faeces, sputum and vomit, test strips for blood and urine, etc., Cole 2004) and should be aware of their colour deficiency and its effects. Optometrists with colour deficiency report difficulties identifying disc pallor, the redness of inflamed eyes and skin rashes and differentiating retinal pigment and haemorrhage (Cole 2004).

Due to the increased use of colour as a teaching aid in schools, it is important to test the colour vision of children soon after the commencement of school. For any moderate to severe colour defectives, it can also be useful to inform the child's school of the condition and its implications (e.g. Box 3.1).

All hereditary colour defectives should be reassured about their condition: that it is not a disease and the condition will always remain but will not get worse. Young colour defectives and their parents should be counselled regarding the effects of the modified colour vision on their everyday life and on future career restrictions.

3.21.2 Advantages and disadvantages

The Ishihara test is a very efficient screening test for red–green colour deficiency (Birch 1997b) and provides quick and simple measurements. It is by far the most commonly used colour vision test and is a required entrance test for several professions throughout the world, including the armed forces, aviation and railway industries.

Disadvantages include the fact that the Ishihara plates do not assess tritan colour problems. In addition, it is designed as a screening test around the normal/abnormal boundary and is therefore less

Box 3.1   Information that could be conveyed to teachers of children with colour vision deficiencies (see colorvisiontesting.com)

Re: John Jones

John has protanopia, a relatively severe form of congenital colour vision deficiency. He sees colours, but sees them differently to other children and will confuse some colours, particularly reds, greens and browns, but also purples, oranges and yellows. These colours are more likely to be confused if they are pale or dull or viewed in dim lighting. Here are some suggestions that may help John and other pupils with colour vision problems:

- Colour deficient children may confuse coloured workbooks or colour-coded reading schemes and make errors when making or reading colour-coded bar charts and pie charts, etc.
- Crayons, coloured pencils, and pens can more easily be identified if labelled with the name of the colour. A colour deficient child may prefer to use their own set of labelled coloured pencils.
- Coloured chalk can be very difficult for a colour deficient child to see, particularly on green chalkboards. White chalk is much easier to see.
- Colour deficient students may appreciate help from a classmate when assignments require colour recognition, such as colour coding different countries on a world map or making colour-coded pie charts, etc.

Particularly for young children:

- Colour deficient children will have difficulty with colour-matching activities.
- Most colour deficient children can identify pure primary colours and it is typically just different shades that give them problems. It can help them to be taught 'all' the colours.
- Label a picture with words or symbols when the response requires colour recognition.
- Make sure a child's colour vision has been tested before they have to learn their colours or colour-enhanced instructional materials are used.
- If they cannot learn certain colours, let them know you understand some colours look the same to them and it is 'OK'.

useful for grading the severity of a defect or for monitoring an acquired colour deficiency (section 3.19.1). To grade the severity of a congenital or acquired colour deficiency, for monitoring acquired colour defects, and detecting blue–yellow defects, either the City University (section 3.20) or Farnsworth D-15 tests (section 3.19) or similar tests are recommended. Note that, after several years, the colours on the Ishihara plates can fade and the test loses its validity.

3.21.3 Procedure

1. You must use the proper quantity and quality of illumination, as the colour temperature of the illuminant will affect the colours of the test. Colour vision testing is normally performed under a standard daylight source, such as one of the Gretag Macbeth Sol-Source daylight desk lamps. This simulates natural daylight conditions provided by direct sunlight and a

clear sky. As these desk lamps are expensive, alternative sources are also used. For example, you can use high colour rendering fluorescent lights (>5000 K) or a Kodak Wratten number 78AA filter (found in camera shops) placed in front of the patient's eye in conjunction with a 100 watt incandescent light source. Natural daylight is not recommended due to its variability in both the quality and quantity of light, although even this is preferable to tungsten lighting.

2. Explain to the patient that you are going to test their colour vision.

3. If screening for a congenital defect, measure colour vision binocularly. If screening for an acquired defect, measure colour vision monocularly.

4. Ask the patient to use their near vision correction and hold the booklet at a typical reading distance. Tinted spectacles or contact lenses should be avoided.

Table 3.4 The Ishihara 24-plates edition scoring sheet.

Plate	Normal person	Person with red-green deficiency	Person with total colour blindness
1	12	12	12
2	8	3	X
3	29	70	X
4	5	2	X
5	3	5	X
6	15	17	X
7	74	21	X
8	6	X	X
9	45	X	X
10	5	X	X
11	7	X	X
12	16	X	X
13	73	X	X
14	X	5	X
15	X	45	X

Plate	Normal person	Protan		Deutan	
		Strong	Mild	Strong	Mild
16	26	6	(2)6	2	2(6)
17	42	2	(4)2	4	4(2)

X means that the plate cannot be read. Numbers in parentheses mean that the plate can be read but not as easily as the other numbers.

5. Ask the patient to read the numbers, starting at plate one. The patient should only be allowed about 3 seconds to view each plate.

6. Use the results sheet to keep a count of any errors. Allow patients another attempt if they make mistakes that are *not* the specific mistakes that red–green colour defectives make.

7. If a patient makes three or more errors, use the classification plates and attempt to categorise the colour defect. Two numbers are shown on each plate and if the patient only reads one number or one number is less visible than the other, the patient can be categorised as deutan (blue-purple letter is not seen or is less visible) or protan (red-purple letter is not seen or is less visible).

8. Any patient who is diagnosed as colour defective should be counselled regarding the effects of the modified colour vision on their everyday life and on future career restrictions.

3.21.4 Recording

Record the number of plates correctly determined from the number of plates attempted. Patients with normal colour vision will make few, if any, errors. If a patient fails the test, attempt to categorise the defect using the result from the classification plates. You should also record any advice given to the patient and their family.
Examples:
Ishihara 15/16 correct. Normal colour vision
Ishihara 8/16 correct. Deutan. patient advised re. effect & future career restrictions
Ishihara 2/16 correct. Protan. patient advised re. effect & future career restrictions.

3.21.5 Interpretation

Patients with red–green colour defects will make specific errors as indicated in Table 3.4. Generally, three or more errors constitutes a fail (Birch 1997b), although entrance requirements for some professions allow no errors. Some clinicians do not present the hidden-digit plates, which are not very sensitive to colour deficiency, and just present transformation and vanishing plates (Birch 1997b). Mistakes that are *not* the specific mistakes that red–green colour defectives make should be viewed with caution, as they are much less likely to indicate red–green colour deficiency.

3.21.6 Most common errors

1. Using an inappropriate light source.
2. Attempting to assess an acquired colour deficiency using only the Ishihara test.
3. Allowing the patient too long to look at the figures.
4. When screening a patient for a certain occupation or vocation, using the Ishihara test rather than the test(s) specified in the appropriate vocational standards.

3.21.7 Alternative procedure: Standard Pseudoisochromatic Plates Part 2

The SPP-2 is another very efficient screening test for red–green colour deficiency (Hovis et al. 1996) and has the advantage over the Ishihara in that it can also be used to screen for blue–yellow defects (Vu et al. 1999). Its major disadvantage is that it is not used as a standard entrance requirement for certain professions like the Ishihara test and therefore is less commonly used. Table 3.5 is a modified score sheet for the SPP-2. Place an 'X' through the figures on each plate that were missed and record the total number of blue–yellow, red–green and scotopic errors. Asking the patient to identify which number is more distinct when two figures are seen on each page may only be helpful when testing for subtle differences between the two eyes. If the only BY error was on plate 4, then repeat the plate to rule out the error being caused by the patient's expectation of seeing only one figure. When totalling the errors, ignore any mistakes of '2' on plate 3 and '3' on plate 6. The '2' is very difficult to discern and almost everyone misses it. The

Table 3.5   The SPP-2 scoring sheet.

Plate	Right eye or binocular		Left eye or binocular repeat	
3	2	4	2	4
	BY	BY	BY	BY
4	6	7	6	7
	BY	BY	BY	BY
5	3	2	3	2
	BY	RG	BY	RG
6	6	3	6	3
	BY		BY	
7	5	9	5	9
	BY	S	BY	S
8	9	8	9	8
	BY	RG	BY	RG
9	5	2	5	2
	BY	RG	BY	RG
10	2	6	2	6
	BY	RG	BY	RG
11	3	5	3	5
	BY	RG	BY	RG
12	4	3	4	3
	RG/BY	S	RG/BY	S

Number of BY errors ___.
Number of RG errors ___.
Number of scotopic errors ___.

'3' is a reference that can be used to compare the visibility of the two numbers on the page. A patient over 60 years of age fails the test if they make two or more errors, a patient less than 20 years of age fails the blue–yellow part of the test with two or more errors. The failure criteria for all other patients is one or more errors. Classifying an error based on a fail on plate 12 can be confusing because the figure can be missed by individuals with either a protan or tritan defect. In this case, errors on other plates should be considered. With other red–green errors, but not blue–yellow, classify the patient as a protan. With no other red–green errors, then the error should be classified as blue–yellow. With acquired defects, both red–green and blue–yellow errors can occur along with failing plate 12 and additional testing should be carried out with either the D-15 or TCU (sections 3.19 and 3.20).

3.22 BIBLIOGRAPHY AND FURTHER READING

Adams, A.J. and Haegerstrom-Portnoy, G. (1987) Colour deficiency. In: *Diagnosis and management of vision care* (ed. J.F. Amos). Boston: Butterworth-Heinemann.

Bailey, I.L. (2006) Visual acuity. In: *Borish's Clinical refraction*, 2nd edn (ed. W.J. Benjamin). St Louis: Butterworth-Heinemann.

Birch, J. (2001) *Diagnosis of defective colour vision*, 2nd edn. Boston: Butterworth-Heinemann.

Bullimore, M.A. (1997) Visual acuity. In: *The ocular examination: measurements and findings* (ed. K. Zadnik). Philadelphia: W.B. Saunders.

Elliott, D.B. (1997) Supplementary clinical tests of vision. In: *The ocular examination: measurement and findings* (ed. K. Zadnik). Philadelphia: W.B. Saunders.

Elliott, D.B. (2006) Contrast sensitivity and glare testing. In: *Borish's Clinical refraction*, 2nd edn (ed. W.J. Benjamin). St Louis: Butterworth-Heinemann.

Flanagan, J.G., Buys, Y. and Trope, G.E. (1996) *Automated perimetry: an interactive primer*. Waterloo, Canada: Lifelearn Eyecare.

3.23 REFERENCES

Achard, O.A., Safran, A.B., Duret, F.C. et al. (1995) Role of the completion phenomenon in the evaluation of Amsler grid results. *American Journal of Ophthalmology* **120**, 322–329.

AHCPR report: Cataract Management Guideline Panel (1993) *Cataract in adults: management of real world impairment*. Clinical Practice Guideline, Number **4**. Rockville, Maryland. US Department of Health and Human Services, Public Health Service, Agency for Health Care Policy and Research. AHCPR Pub. No. 93-0542, Feb. 1993.

Ambrecht, A.M., Findlay, C., Aspinall, P.A. et al. (2003) Cataract surgery in patients with age-related macular degeneration – one-year outcomes. *Journal of Cataract and Refractive Surgery* **29**, 686–693.

Anderson, A.J. and Johnson, C.A. (2002) Mechanisms isolated by frequency doubling technology perimetry. *Investigative Ophthalmology and Visual Science* **43**, 398–401.

Anderson, D.R. and Patella, V.M. (1999) *Automated static perimetry*. St Louis: Mosby.

Bailey, I.L. (2006) Visual acuity. In: *Borish's Clinical refraction*, 2nd edn (ed. W.J. Benjamin). St Louis: Butterworth-Heinemann.

Bailey, I.L. and Lovie, J.E. (1976) New design principles for visual acuity letter charts. *American Journal of Optometry and Physiological Optics* **53**, 740–745.

Bailey, I.L., Bullimore, M.A., Raasch, T.W. et al. (1991) Clinical grading and the effects of scaling. *Investigative Ophthalmology and Visual Science* **32**: 422–432.

Bengtsson, B. and Heijl, A. (1998) SITA Fast, a new rapid perimetric threshold test. Description of methods and evaluation in patients with manifest and suspect glaucoma. *Acta Ophthalmologica Scandinavica* **76**, 431–437.

Birch, J. (1997a) Clinical use of the City University Test 2nd edition. *Ophthalmic and Physiological Optics* **17**, 466–472.

Birch, J. (1997b) Efficiency of the Ishihara test for identifying red-green colour deficiency. *Ophthalmic and Physiological Optics* **17**, 403–408.

Carkeet, A. (2001) Modeling logMAR visual acuity scores: effects of termination rules and alternative forced-choice options. *Optometry and Vision Science* **78**, 529–538.

Chaglasian, M.A. (2001) The Octopus perimeter. In: *Primary care of the glaucomas*, 2nd edn. (eds M. Fingeret and T. Lewis). New York: McGraw-Hill, pp. 255–270.

Cole, B.L. (2004) The handicap of abnormal colour vision. *Clinical and Experimental Optometry* **87**, 258–275.

Delgado, M.F., Nguyen, N.T., Cox, T.A. et al. (2002) Automated perimetry: a report by the American Academy of Ophthalmology. *Ophthalmology* **109**, 2362–2374.

Drasdo, N. and Peaston, W.C. (1980) Sampling systems for visual field assessment and computerised perimetry. *The British Journal of Ophthalmology* **64**, 705–712.

Elliott, D.B. (2006) Contrast sensitivity and glare testing. In: *Borish's Clinical refraction*, 2nd edn (ed. W.J. Benjamin). St Louis: Butterworth-Heinemann.

Elliott, D.B. and Bullimore, M.A. (1993) Assessing the reliability, discriminative ability, and validity of disability glare tests. *Investigative Ophthalmology and Visual Science* **34**, 108–119.

Elliott, D.B. and Situ, P. (1998) Visual acuity versus letter contrast sensitivity in early cataract.*Vision Research* **38**, 2047–2052.

Elliott, D.B., Yang, K.C. and Whitaker, D. (1995) Visual acuity changes throughout adulthood in normal, healthy eyes: seeing beyond 6/6. *Optometry and Vision Science* **72**, 186–191.

Elliott, D.B., Trukolo-Ilic, M., Strong, J.G. et al. (1997a) Demographic characteristics of the vision-disabled elderly. *Investigative Ophthalmology and Visual Science* **38**, 2566–2575.

Elliott, D.B., North, I. and Flanagan, J. (1997b) Confrontation visual field tests. *Ophthalmic and Physiological Optics* **17**, S17–S24.

Esterman, B. (1982) Functional scoring of the binocular field. *Ophthalmology* **89**, 1226–1234.

Ferris, F.L. and Bailey, I. (1996) Standardizing the measurement of visual acuity for clinical research studies: Guidelines from the Eye Care Technology Forum. *Ophthalmology* **103**, 181–182.

Fine, A.M., Elman, M.J., Ebert, J.E. et al. (1986) Earliest symptoms caused by neovascular membranes in the macula. *Archives of Ophthalmology* **104**, 513–514.

Haymes, S.A., Roberts, K.F., Cruess, A.F. et al. (2006) The letter contrast sensitivity test: clinical evaluation of a new design. *Investigative Ophthalmology and Visual Science* **47**, 2739–2745.

Heijl, A., Lindgren, G. and Olsson, J. (1987) A package for the statistical analysis of visual fields. *Documenta Ophthalmologica Proceedings Series* **49**, 153–168.

Heijl, A., Lindgren, A. and Lindgren, G. (1989) Test re-test variability in glaucomatous visual fields. *American Journal of Ophthalmology* **108**, 130–135.

Henson, D.B. (2000) *Visual fields*. Oxford, UK: Butterworth-Heinemann.

Henson, D.B. and Artes, P.H. (2002) New developments in supra-threshold perimetry. *Ophthalmic and Physiological Optics* **22**, 463–468.

Hofeldt, A.J. and Weiss, M.J. (1998) Illuminated near card assessment of potential acuity in eyes with cataract. *Ophthalmology* **105**, 1531–1536.

Hovis, J.K., Cawker, C.L. and Cranton, D. (1996) Comparison of the standard pseudoisochromatic plates – Parts 1 and 2 – as screening tests for congenital red-green color vision deficiencies. *Journal of the American Optometric Association* **67**, 320–326.

http://colorvisiontesting.com/color4.htm.

Hudson, C., Wild, J.M., O'Neill, E.C. (1994) Fatigue effects during a single session of automated static threshold perimetry. *Investigative Ophthalmology and Visual Science* **35**, 268–280.

Ismail, G.M. and Whitaker, D. (1998) Early detection of changes in visual function in diabetes mellitus. *Ophthalmic and Physiological Optics* **18**, 3–12.

Johnson, C.A. (1997) Perimetry and visual field testing. In: *The ocular examination: measurements and findings* (ed. K. Zadnik). Philadelphia: W.B. Saunders.

Johnson, C.A. and Samuels, S.J. (1997) Screening for glaucomatous visual field loss with frequency doubling perimetry. *Investigative Ophthalmology and Visual Science* **38**: 413–425.

Jones, D., Westall, C., Averbeck, K. et al. (2003) Visual acuity assessment: a comparison of two tests for measuring children's vision. *Ophthalmic and Physiological Optics* **23**, 541–546.

Katz, J. and Sommer, A. (1988) Reliability indices of automated perimetric tests. *Archives of Ophthalmology* **106**, 1252–1254.

Kelly, D.H. (1981) Non-linear visual responses to flickering sinusoidal gratings. *Journal of the Optical Society of America* **71**, 1051–1055.

Klein, R., Peto, T., Bird, A. et al. (2004) The epidemiology of age-related macular age-related degeneration. *American Journal of Ophthalmology* **137**, 486–495.

Lalle, P. (2001) The Humphrey visual field analyzer. In: *Primary care of the glaucomas*, 2nd edn (eds M. Fingeret and T. Lewis). New York: McGraw-Hill, pp. 213–253.

Leat, S.J., Legge, G.E. and Bullimore, M.A. (1999) What is low vision? A re-evaluation of definitions. *Optometry and Vision Science* **76**, 198–211.

Leskea, M.C., Heijl, A., Hyman, L. et al. (2004) Factors for progression and glaucoma treatment: the Early Manifest Glaucoma Trial. *Current Opinion in Ophthalmology* **15**, 102–106.

Lovie-Kitchin, J.E. (1988) Validity and reliability of visual acuity measurements. *Ophthalmic and Physiological Optics* **8**, 363–370.

McGraw, P.V. and Winn, B. (1993) Glasgow Acuity Cards: a new test for the measurement of letter acuity in children. *Ophthalmic and Physiological Optics* **13**, 400–404.

McGraw, P.V., Winn, B., Gray, L.S. et al. (2000) Improving the reliability of visual acuity measures in young children. *Ophthalmic and Physiological Optics* **20**, 173–184.

McKendrick, A.M. (2005) Recent developments in perimetry: test stimuli and procedures. *Clinical and Experimental Optometry* **88**, 73–80.

Margrain, T.H. and Thomson, D. (2002) Sources of variability in the clinical photostress test. *Ophthalmic and Physiological Optics* **22**, 61–67.

Melki, S.A., Safar, A., Martin, J. et al. (1999) Potential acuity pinhole – a simple method to measure potential visual acuity in patients with cataracts, comparison to potential acuity meter. *Ophthalmology* **106**, 1262–1267.

Millodot, M. and Millodot, S. (1989) Presbyopia correction and the accommodation in reserve. *Ophthalmic and Physiological Optics* **9**, 126–132.

Oliphant, D. and Hovis, J.K. (1998) Comparison of the D-15 and City University (second) color vision tests. *Vision Research* **38**, 3461–3465.

Pandit, R.J., Gales, K. and Griffiths, P.G. (2001) Effectiveness of testing visual fields by confrontation. *Lancet* **358** (9295), 1820.

Pelli, D.G., Robson, J.G. and Wilkins, A.J. (1988) The design of a new letter chart for measuring contrast sensitivity. *Clinical Vision Sciences* **2**, 187–199.

Pesudovs, K., Hazel, C.A., Doran, R.M. et al. (2004) The usefulness of Vistech and FACT contrast sensitivity charts for cataract and refractive surgery outcomes research. *The British Journal of Ophthalmology* **88**, 11–16.

Quaid, P.T., Simpson, T.L. and Flanagan, J.G. (2004) Frequency doubling illusion: detection versus resolution. *Optometry and Vision Science* **82**, 36–42.

Rabin, J. and Wicks, J. (1996) Measuring resolution in the contrast domain – the small letter contrast test. *Optometry and Vision Science* **73**, 398–403.

Rabin, J.C., Kim, L,. Leon, G. et al. (2004) Quantification of visual resolution in the contrast domain. *Investigative Ophthalmology and Visual Science* **45**, E-Abstract 4351.

Roper-Hall, M.J. (2006) The usefulness of the Amsler chart. *Eye* **20**, 508.

Schein, O.D., Steinberg, E.P., Javitt, J.C. et al. (1994) Variation in cataract surgery practice and clinical outcomes. *Ophthalmology* **101**, 1142–1152.

Schuchard, R.A. (1993) Validity and interpretation of Amsler grid reports. *Archives of Ophthalmology* **111**, 776–780.

Schulze-Bonsel, K., Feltgen, N., Burau, H. et al. (2006) Visual acuities 'hand motion' and 'counting fingers' can be quantified with the Freiburg visual acuity test. *Investigative Ophthalmology and Visual Science* **47**, 1236–1240.

Vianya-Estopa, M., Douthwaite, W.A., Noble, B.A. et al. (2006) Capabilities of potential vision test measurements: a clinical evaluation in the presence of cataract or macular disease. *Journal of Cataract and Refractive Surgery* **32**, 1151–1160.

Vingrys, A.J. and Helfrich, K.A. (1990) The Opticom M-600TM: a new LED automated perimeter. *Clinical and Experimental Optometry* **73**, 3–17.

Vu, B.L., Easterbrook, M. and Hovis, J.K. (1999) Detection of color vision defects in chloroquine retinopathy. *Ophthalmology* **106**, 1799–1803.

Wang, J.J., Klein, R., Smith, W. et al. (2003) Cataract surgery and the 5-year incidence of late-stage age-related maculopathy: pooled findings from the Beaver Dam and Blue Mountains eye studies. *Ophthalmology* **110**, 1960–1967.

Weijland, A., Fankhauser, F., Bebie, H. et al. (2004) *Automated perimetry visual field digest*, 5th edn. Bern, Switzerland: Haag-Streit International.

Wellings, P.C. (1989) Detection and recognition of visual field defects resulting from lesions involving the visual pathways. *Australian and New Zealand Journal of Ophthalmology* **17**, 331–335.

Wild, J.M., Pacey, I.E., O'Neill, E.C. et al. (1999) The SITA perimetric threshold algorithms in glaucoma. *Investigative Ophthalmology and Visual Science* **40**, 1998–2009.

DETERMINATION OF THE REFRACTIVE CORRECTION

DAVID B. ELLIOTT

4.1 RELEVANT CASE HISTORY INFORMATION

The case history can provide significant information about the need for a refractive correction or change in refractive correction and even the type of ametropia that might be present.

4.1.1 Symptoms

Symptoms of blurred vision or an inability to see well enough for certain tasks (reading the blackboard, schoolbooks or a newspaper, watching TV, driving, etc.) suggest undiagnosed ametropia or a change in ametropia in those already wearing spectacles. If these symptoms are due to ametropia, they usually have a gradual onset. Near vision blur with good distance vision suggests hyperopia or presbyopia depending on the patient's age. Distance vision blur with good near vision suggests myopia and blur at all distances can indicate significant astigmatism. You should ask whether the blurred vision is in one eye or both. Headaches and asthenopia can accompany uncorrected hyperopia and presbyopia. Myopes who squint to see can develop frontal headaches and uncorrected astigmatism can often lead to complaints of asthenopia.

4.1.2 Ocular history

If a patient already wears spectacles or contact lenses, the ocular history can suggest the type of ametropia. Knowledge of the age at which spectacles were first worn can also help to indicate the ametropia. For example, patients who first wore spectacles at age 8–12 are likely to be childhood-onset myopes and those who first wore spectacles at age 18–22 are likely to be adult-onset myopes.

Adult-onset myopes (often 1.00–3.00 D) are typically less myopic than childhood-onset myopes (often 3.00–6.00 D) (e.g. Grosvenor & Scott 1991). Patients who first wore spectacles at age 45–55 are presbyopes and are likely to be emmetropic or slightly hyperopic at distance. The earlier they needed reading glasses, the more likely they are to be hyperopic. Finally, the natural progression of the type of ametropia given the patient's age can indicate what change in refractive correction to suspect. For example, a childhood-onset myope who obtained their first spectacles at age 12 and is now 16 is likely to have increased myopia given the typical progression of myopia after onset.

Any mention of cataracts in the case history should lead to a careful investigation for increased myopia (nuclear cataract) or astigmatic change (cortical cataract) (Pesudovs & Elliott 2003).

4.1.3 Family ocular history

When examining children who do not wear spectacles, it is useful to ask whether any of the patient's family wear glasses or contact lenses. Mutti and colleagues (2002) reported that juvenile onset myopia was evident in 33% of the offspring of two myopic parents, compared with only 6% of the children of two non-myopic parents.

4.1.4 General health

Diabetes, either undiagnosed or poorly controlled, can lead to wide fluctuations in refractive error, with either hyperopic or myopic shifts. In addition, a variety of systemic medications can lead to refractive error shifts (Locke 1987).

4.2 RELEVANT VISUAL ACUITY INFORMATION

Visual acuity (VA) measurements can also provide significant information about the need for a refractive correction or change in refractive correction and the type of ametropia.

4.2.1 Distance vision vs. near vision (i.e. unaided measurements)

Reduced distance vision (unaided distance VA) with normal near vision (unaided near VA) indicates myopia, while normal distance vision with reduced near vision indicates moderate to severe hyperopia or presbyopia depending on the patient's age. Young hyperopes typically have no vision loss because they can accommodate to see well at both distance and near. As patients get older, accommodation is lost, so that reduced near vision becomes more likely. Reduced vision at both distance and near can indicate astigmatism, which could be combined with either hyperopia or myopia. The vision measurements should reflect the symptoms presented in the case history.

4.2.2 Distance vision (unaided distance VA)

Distance vision measurements can be used to predict the refractive corrections of myopes and older hyperopes (i.e. hyperopes over 60 years of age who do not have any accommodation). For low myopic refractive errors and hyperopic changes in absolute presbyopes, a degradation of one line of vision (on a logMAR chart) corresponds to approximately −0.25 D of refractive error, e.g. a −1.00 D myope with an optimal VA of 6/4.5 (20/15; typical of a 20-year-old patient) should have vision loss of about four lines and distance vision of 6/12 or 20/40. Similarly, an older +1.00 D hyperope with optimal VA of 6/6 or 20/20 should have a vision loss of about four lines and distance vision of 6/15 or 20/50. Near horizontal and vertical astigmatic errors have a similar effect to the equivalent best mean sphere, so that a −1.00 DC would have a similar effect to a −0.50 DS, a two-line drop in vision. Cylinders at oblique axes tend to give a slightly greater degradation in vision.

4.2.3 Habitual distance VA

For low myopic refractive changes (and hyperopic changes in an absolute presbyope), a degradation of one line of visual acuity (VA) on a logMAR chart corresponds to approximately −0.25 D of refractive error. Therefore, a myope of −1.00 DS with a habitual VA of 6/9 (three-line loss in VA from 6/4.5 or 20/15) is likely to need a change in refractive correction of about −0.75 DS and an updated prescription to approximately −1.75 DS. An older hyperope of +1.00 DS with a habitual VA of 6/9 (two-line loss in VA from 6/6 or 20/20) is likely to need a change in refractive correction of +0.50 DS and an updated prescription to approximately +1.50 DS. Astigmatism in adults changes with age from with-the-rule in young adults to against-the-rule in older patients. However, these changes in astigmatism are negligible over the typical 1–3-year period between eye examinations, so that habitual distance VA reductions in spectacle wearing myopic astigmats and older hyperopic astigmats indicate the increase in spherical power required. Therefore, a myope of −1.00/−0.50 × 180 with a habitual VA of 6/12 or 20/40 (four-line VA loss from 6/4.5 or 20/15) is likely to need a change in refractive correction of −1.00 DS and an updated prescription to approximately −2.00/−0.50 × 180. Similarly, an older hyperope of +1.50/−0.75 × 90 with a habitual VA of 6/12 or 20/40 (three-line loss from 6/6 or 20/20) is likely to need a change in refractive correction of +0.75 DS and an updated prescription to approximately +2.25/−0.75 × 90.

4.2.4 Near VA

An estimate of myopia can be determined from the patient's far point. Ask the patient to remove any spectacles and bring in the near VA card until they can just see it. The far point provides an estimate of the mean sphere refractive correction. For example, patients with far points of 33 cm, 25 cm and 20 cm have mean sphere refractive corrections of approximately −3.00 DS, −4.00 DS and −5.00 DS respectively.

4.3 KERATOMETRY

This is an optical instrument that measures the radius of curvature of the anterior corneal surface along the two principal meridians.

4.3.1 Corneal topography

The topography of the anterior corneal surface can be assessed using computerised videokeratoscopes and the curvature of the corneal cap can be estimated using keratometry. Videokeratoscopes illuminate the cornea with a Placido disc series of concentric rings and the reflections from the cornea are captured and analysed. The results are displayed as colour coded topographic maps, with areas with the same radius of curvature displayed in the same colour. Steep areas of the cornea are typically shown as red, average areas as yellow and green and flat areas as blue. Different shades of these colours are used to provide smaller step sizes. Keratoscopy is mainly used:

■ Before and after refractive surgery. Prior to surgery, it is used to screen for otherwise sub-clinical disorders such as early keratoconus. Postoperatively, it is used to determine the outcome of surgery, particularly in relation to the centration and symmetry of the ablation zone. When patients have postoperative irregular astigmatism or asymmetry, keratoscopy is an essential part of the 'refinement' process.

■ For the early detection and better management of keratoconus and other corneal disorders.

■ For fitting contact lenses, particularly to abnormal corneas, such as keratoconic and post-refractive surgery (although here it is working to low accuracy). The limited range of parameter variation (radius and diameter) of soft lenses means that the use of videokeratoscopes for the determination of fit of these lenses is an overkill.

■ To assess contact lens induced corneal change. Keratoscopes are more sensitive to such changes than keratometry because they assess most of the corneal surface whereas a keratometer only measures a single radius of curvature around 1.5 mm off the instrument axis.

■ In the management of patient post-penetrating keratoplasty.

■ As part of orthokeratology.

There are many different systems available that use different approaches and there is insufficient space to describe them in this text. Suffice to say that all of them require an accurately focused image before image acquisition by the computer. The algorithms for image analysis vary with the manufacturer and rely on assumptions that may or may not be valid. The main differences in the various instruments are associated with how an accurate focus is achieved and how the data are finally displayed.

The procedure that is much more commonly used to measure the anterior curvature of the cornea, keratometry, will be described. In contact lens fitting, keratometer measurements are used to indicate the corneal curvature, thus allowing an appropriate contact lens curvature to be deduced for the first trial contact lens. In contact lens aftercare, keratometer readings can be used to monitor lens-induced corneal surface changes. For example, distortion of the keratometer mires can indicate unwanted mechanical action of the lens on the cornea, and a steepening cornea can indicate oedema. The keratometer can also be used to measure the base curve of rigid contact lenses, and provide an indication of tear film quality. Non-invasive tear break-up time can be measured as the number of seconds between a blink and the first indication of distortion of the mire images (section 6.7). Keratometry can also be used to detect keratoconus and other disorders of the cornea that change its shape, but it is much less sensitive to these changes than videokeratoscopy.

4.3.2 Advantages and disadvantages

One-position variable doubling keratometers (Bausch and Lomb type) or two-position variable doubling keratometers or copies of them are widely used in optometric practice. The one-position instrument is said to be quicker to use since once aligned on one of the corneal principal meridians, both principal meridians can be measured without further adjustment, hence the 'one-position' name. Disadvantages include that the instrument design assumes that the principal meridians lie at exactly 90° to each other, which is not always the case, especially when the cornea has been subjected to contact lens wear. Also, since it is a one-position instrument, both the vertical and

horizontal mires are imaged at the same time and in higher degrees of corneal toricity this can mean the vertical mire is not in focus at the same focusing position as the horizontal mire. Of course, if required the keratometer can always be turned to the second principal meridian and the second reading taken in a 'two-position' style. Lastly, the Bausch and Lomb keratometer tends to use a shorter working distance than other instruments and this can lead to larger measurement errors.

Two position variable mire keratometers include the Javal Schiotz and copies. Measurements of corneal radii are achieved by the physical movement of the mires along an arc. The main criticism of this instrument is that unlike the variable doubling keratometer, where measurements are made on a linear scale, radii that fall at the extreme ends of the arc are non-linear and this can lead to measurement inaccuracy. Although two-position variable doubling instruments do require a second adjustment of the instrument to find and measure the second principal meridian, they tend to be more accurate because of a longer working distance. Perhaps the best instrument is the two-position variable doubling keratometer, especially if it is of telecentric design. The advantage of telecentricity is that focusing of the eyepiece of the telescope is not necessary and therefore there are no inaccuracies due to focusing errors. Unfortunately, these telecentric instruments can be expensive and are not commonly encountered.

4.3.3 Procedure (Bausch and Lomb one-position keratometer)

1. Seat the patient comfortably in front of the keratometer, and ask them to remove any spectacles. Sit opposite the patient, across the instrument table, and dim the room lighting.

2. Explain the procedure to the patient: 'I am going to measure the shape of the front of your eye/cornea'. You may add: '. . . so that I will know which contact lens to fit' or '. . . so that I can tell whether the contact lens is changing the shape of your cornea.'

3. Adjust the eyepiece of the instrument by directing the telescope to a distant object

(such as the cubicle wall), turning the eyepiece anti-clockwise as far as it will go and then turning the eyepiece clockwise until the black cross hair just comes into sharp focus.

4. Adjust the height of the patient's chair and the instrument to a comfortable position for both you and the patient. Ask the patient to lean forward and place their chin in the chin rest and forehead against the headrest. Occlude the eye not being tested by swinging the instrument's occluder into place. Then adjust the chin rest so that the outer canthus aligns with the headrest marker.

5. Ask the patient to look at the image of their own eye in the centre of the instrument and to open the eye wide after a full blink. If a high refractive error prevents the patient seeing their own eye, then ask them to look down the centre of the instrument. Make vertical adjustments of the instrument if the patient is unable to see into the centre.

6. Align the instrument so that the lower right mire image is centred on the crosshairs, and lock the instrument into place.

7. Adjust the focusing of the instrument by turning the focusing knob until the mires are clear and the lower right mire is no longer doubled.

8. If you cannot focus the mires, check to see that the patient's head is firmly against the headrest. If the patient is in the correct position, and the mires are still out of focus, adjust the position of the headrest forward or backward while continuing to focus until the mires are in focus.

9. Measure the principal meridian that is closest to the horizontal first. Rotate the instrument so that the plus signs are set 'in step' (Fig. 4.1b). This ensures that the instrument is aligned precisely on a principal meridian. Use one hand to adjust the focusing knob to ensure a single, clear

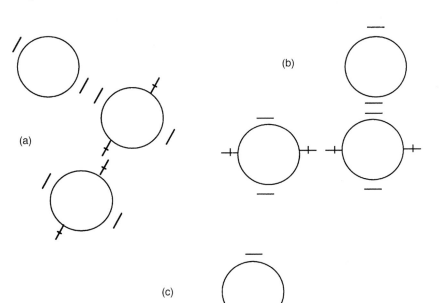

Fig. 4.1 Alignment of the mires on a Bausch and Lomb keratometer. (a) The view when the mires are off the principal meridians. (b) The view when the mires are on the principal meridians. (c) The view when the plus and minus signs are overlapping to measure the 'horizontal' and 'vertical' radii of curvature.

Fig. 4.2 The mire images as seen on the Javal Schiotz keratometer. (a) Aligned mire images along the horizontal. (b) Mires from (a) touching with no overlap. (c) Non-aligned mire images. (d) Mire images from (c) brought into alignment along an oblique meridian. (e) Mires from (d) touching with no overlap.

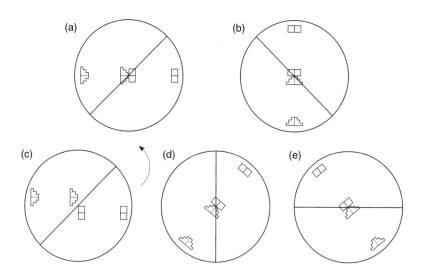

plus sign, and adjust the horizontal alignment wheel to superimpose the two plus signs with the other hand (Fig. 4.1c). Note that you will need to constantly adjust the instrument position to maintain image focus, so keratometric measurements are always a two-handed operation. Note the radius of curvature (or dioptric power) and orientation of this meridian.

10. Measure the second principal meridian, which is theoretically 90° to the primary one. Adjust the focusing knob to give the best focus for the minus signs and then adjust the vertical alignment wheel until the minus signs are superimposed (Fig. 4.1c). Note the radius of curvature (or dioptric power) and orientation of this meridian. On a toric cornea, the plus signs will be out of focus and not superimposed, but this does not matter as you have completed your measurement of the near horizontal principal meridian.

11. Repeat the measurements on the other eye.

4.3.4 Procedure for two-position variable doubling type keratometer

1. Set up the patient and the instrument as described in steps 1–8 above.

2. Move the telescope forward by adjusting the focusing knob appropriately. You may need to make minor adjustments both horizontally and vertically to centre the mire images and achieve a view as depicted in Figure 4.2. If the blocks and staircase are in step (Fig. 4.2a), then the orientation of the instrument arc is aligned to one of the two principal meridians and you can now proceed to step 4.

3. If the picture you see is similar to Figure 4.2c, where the blocks and staircase are out of step, then the angle of the instrument arc is not aligned along a principal meridian. Move the arc slowly until the staircase and block mires are in step and are able to be brought into contact by turning the knurled knob situated below the arc as in Figure 4.2d.

4. Ask the patient to blink and then keep their eyes as wide open as possible. Turn the knurled knob situated below the arc until the staircase and block mires are just touching. You must simultaneously adjust the instrument position to maintain focus of the mire images. If you turn the knob too much and the mires overlap, a white area of overlap will be seen. Adjust the position of the mires until they are just touching with no overlap. If the hair wire does not cross through the middle of the touching mires, make final horizontal and vertical adjustments to achieve this.

5. Read off the angle of the arc from the degree scale of the instrument and the radius of curvature along this meridian from the mm scale.

6. Turn the arc through 90° and make adjustments as in steps 4 and 5 to achieve a picture similar to 4.13b or 4.13e. Note the reading off the scales. This is the corneal radius along the other meridian.

4.3.5 Recording

The results can be recorded with the radius of curvature of the horizontal meridian first followed by the vertical as follows:

R 7.75 @ 175 / 7.60 @ 85

L 7.70 @ 180 / 7.60 @ 90.

The @ nomenclature can be replaced by 'along'. A degree sign (°) should not be used after the axis direction. It is possible for the ° to be confused with a 0, so that 15 degrees could become 150 degrees. If the mires are distorted, this must be recorded.

Alternatively, the results can be recorded in dioptres, in which case the amount of corneal astigmatism is usually calculated and recorded. Note that this is the total corneal astigmatism due to the anterior and posterior corneal surfaces and is usually derived by assuming a corneal refractive index of 1.3375. The difference between the two powers equals the approximate total corneal astigmatism and the meridian with the lower power corresponds to the corneal cylinder axis.

OD: 42.00 @ 175 / 43.75 @ 85, −1.75 × 175, mires distorted

OS: 43.50 @ 180 / 44.25 @ 90, −0.75 × 180, mires clear.

4.3.6 Interpretation

The power of the anterior corneal surface (Fc) is estimated from the radii measurements (r) using the equation $Fc = (n - 1)/r$. A small radius means a steep corneal surface, which is more powerful and more myopic (or less hyperopic). Larger radii mean flatter surfaces, which are less powerful and more hyperopic (or less myopic). The refractive index (n) of the cornea is about 1.376, but most keratometers use a value for n of 1.3375. The lower value for n is intended to compensate for the negative power of the posterior corneal surface. It is assumed that the posterior surface reduces the overall corneal power by about 10%. This also assumes that the two surfaces have the same proportion of astigmatism. Other factors also lead to slight errors in keratometry readings: keratometers assume that the cornea is spherical (most are elliptical) and that the visual axis runs through the corneal apex, which it usually does not.

The anterior radii of curvature of the cornea are usually between 7.25 mm and 8.50 mm, with myopes having steeper (smaller) radii and hyperopes having flatter (larger) radii. Dioptric powers range between 46.50 D and 40.00 D, and the estimated corneal astigmatism is usually less than 2.00 D. It is most common to find the flattest corneal meridian lying near the horizontal (with-the-rule astigmatism, WTR) in younger patients. This is likely due to lid tension steepening the vertical meridian. Little change in curvature occurs between the mid-teens and the late 40s. Over the age of 40 there is a significant shift towards against-the-rule astigmatism (the flattest meridian is along the vertical, ATR), likely due to relaxed lid tension. The corneal astigmatism is called oblique when the principal meridians are between 30° and 60° and 120° and 150°. Unusually steep readings with irregular principal meridians can be indicative of keratoconus. Large changes in the degree of astigmatism within a short time can be indicative of keratoconus, lid neoplasms, pterygium, or a chalazion. Large changes in spectacle astigmatism without corneal astigmatic changes in the elderly are likely to be due to cortical cataract. Keratometer readings can also be used to help indicate whether ametropia is refractive or axial. For example, a patient with increasing myopia but no change in keratometry readings probably has axial myopia. An anisometrope with different keratometry readings probably has refractive anisometropia, while an anisometrope with similar keratometry readings probably has axial anisometropia.

The amount of corneal astigmatism determined using keratometry can be used to estimate spectacle astigmatism using certain formulae. The most commonly used formula is Javal's rule, which is:

Spectacle astigmatism = 1.25 (corneal cylinder)+ (−0.50 D × 90).

The 1.25 factor was proposed to account for the change in cylinder power due to the vertex distance of spectacles, and the 0.50 of against-the-rule astigmatism is used to account for the astigmatism believed to be from the lens. Note that the 1.25 factor is theoretically incorrect as, although it works for a −1.00 cylinder with a −8.00 sphere, a factor of 0.75 is required for a −1.00 cylinder with a +8.00 sphere. A modification to Javal's rule has been proposed (Grosvenor et al. 1988):

Spectacle astigmatism = 1.00 (corneal cylinder) + (−0.50 D × 90).

These estimates of astigmatism can be very inaccurate (by up to 2.00 DC) for some patients and are much less accurate than either retinoscopy or autorefraction (Elliott et al. 1994, Mote & Fry 1939). They are particularly inaccurate for small degrees of astigmatism and should only be used for patients with astigmatism greater than about 1.00 D (Elliott et al. 1994).

4.3.7 Most common errors

1. Not maintaining mire image focus when attempting superimposition of the mire image.

2. Not getting the patient to keep their head against the headrest.

3. Forgetting to focus the eyepieces.

4. Not centring the mire images.

5. Not getting the patient to fixate properly.

6. Not determining the correct axis.

7. Regularly estimating spectacle astigmatism from keratometry readings. This is usually only valuable for high astigmatism, when subjective responses and other objective assessments such as retinoscopy and autorefraction are unavailable or unreliable.

8. Forgetting to calibrate the instrument on a regular basis.

4.4 FOCIMETRY

Focimeters measure the vertex power, axis direction and optical centres of ophthalmic lenses. These devices are also referred to by trade names in some countries, including lensometer or lensmeter (America) and vertometer (Australia). Automatic focimeters are available that measure the lens characteristics mentioned above once the lens has been appropriately positioned and provide a printout of the results. These are very simple to use and the measurement procedure will not be explained. Their main disadvantage is that they break down more often than non-automated focimeters (Steele et al. 2006).

4.4.1 Spectacle lens identification

It is often important to determine the spectacle details. You may want to check that they have been made to the specifications you ordered, or you may wish to determine the parameters of the spectacles that a patient is wearing. It is important to know the spectacle prescription so that you can compare it with the optimal refractive correction that you will subsequently determine during refraction.

4.4.2 Advantages and disadvantages

Focimeters provide simple and accurate measurements of vertex power, axis direction and optical centres. Focimeters do not provide information about all the important features of spectacle lenses, however, and it is important to consider that changes in other spectacle characteristics could cause patients problems and need to be checked. These include base curve and lens form, segment style, height, size and inset, centre or edge thickness, optical and surface quality and the presence of a lens tint and/or surface coating (antireflection, anti-scratch).

4.4.3 Procedure

1. Explain the test to the patient: 'I am going to measure the power of your spectacles.'

2. Set the power of the focimeter to zero and focus the eyepiece (turn it as far anti-clockwise as possible, then slowly turn it clockwise until the target and graticule first come into sharp focus).

3. Measure the back surface power (BVP) by placing the spectacles on the focimeter with the back (ocular) surface away from you. Position the middle of the right lens against the lens stop.

4. Look into the focimeter and adjust the lens position vertically (using the lens table) and horizontally until the illuminated target is placed in the middle of the reticule. If the lens is high powered, you may need to turn the power wheel to bring the target into focus before it can be centred.

5. Fix the lens into position using the lens retainer.

6. To obtain the power of the sphere, turn the power wheel to bring the target into focus.
   a) If the entire target is focused at the same time (Fig. 4.3), the lens is a sphere and there is no cylindrical component. Record the sphere power for the right eye from the power wheel or the internal scale and go to step 8.
   b) If parts of the target are in focus at different powers and to record in the standard negative cylinder format, turn the power wheel until the meridian with the most plus power (or least minus power) is brought into focus.
   c) With focimeters using line targets, rotate the axis wheel until the sphere line (Fig. 4.3a) is in focus and the line is continuous without breaks. You may need to use the power wheel to gain best focus.
   d) Record the sphere power from the power wheel or internal scale.

7. To obtain the power and axis of the cylinder:
   a) Focus the image in the meridian at 90° from the first meridian by turning the power wheel towards the most minus (or least plus) power.
   b) Read off the power when this meridian is in focus. With focimeters using line targets, the cylinder lines will be in focus.

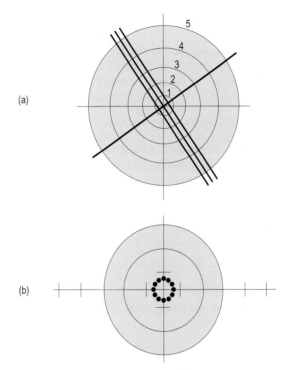

(a)

(b)

Fig. 4.3   The entire focimeter target is in focus at the same time, indicating a spherical lens. The graticule scale allows measurement of prism. (a) A focimeter that uses a cylindrical (3-line) and spherical (1-line) target. The graticule scale is numbered 1–5. (b) A focimeter that uses a circle-of-dots target. The graticule scale is indicated by the intersecting lines and runs from 1–5 horizontally and 1–3 vertically in both directions from the centre. With an astigmatic lens, the dots become lines orientated along the two principal meridians.

   c) Record the difference between the sphere power from step 6.d) and the new meridian power as the cylinder power.
   d) Record the orientation of the second meridian from the eyepiece protractor or the axis wheel as the cylinder axis. With focimeters using line targets, this will be the orientation of the cylinder lines (Fig. 4.3a).

8. Make sure the target is centred in the graticule and dot the right lens using the focimeter's marking device. This could be just one spot (the lens optical centre) or three dots (the middle is the lens optical centre, the other two indicate the horizontal line).

9. Release the lens retainer and repeat steps 4 to 7 for the left eye. Do not change the vertical position of the lenses between measurements of the right and left lenses as you need to determine if any vertical prism is incorporated in the spectacles.

10. Move the lens horizontally until the target is in the same vertical plane as the centre of the graticule and dot the left lens using the focimeter's marking device.

11. If the target is above or below the centre of the reticule, vertical prism is present and should be recorded to the nearest $0.5^\triangle$ using the graticule scale (Fig. 4.3).

12. Remove the spectacles from the focimeter and measure the distance between the right and left optical centres to calculate the distance between centres (DBC). Record the DBC in mm.

13. For front-surface solid multifocal lenses, the reading add must be measured using front vertex power (FVP). Turn the lens around so that the ocular surface faces you and reposition the spectacles in the focimeter. Measure the FVP along one meridian in the distance portion of the spectacles. Measure the FVP along the same meridian in the near portion of the spectacles. The difference between these powers is the reading addition. Repeat the measurement in the left lens. For low-powered lenses, the FVP approximately equals the BVP, and the BVP add can be measured.

14. For progressive addition lenses (PALs), the appropriate position on each lens to measure the distance and near prescription, optical centres and any prism must first be found (Fig. 4.4). A faint mark is etched into both the nasal and temporal sides of each lens, and this must be found and marked with a non-permanent marker. The mark may also indicate the PAL manufacturer and the power of the addition. Use the manufacturer's marking up card, to find the appropriate distance and near centres and measure the spherocylindrical power as previously described. Use the card to determine where to mark the optical

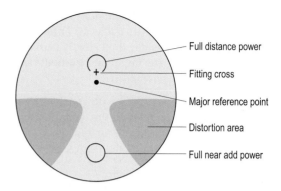

Fig. 4.4   An example of the important points and areas of a progressive addition lens.

centres and where to check for any prism (Fig. 4.4).

15. Compare the distance DBC and the patient's distance interpupillary distance (PD). If these distances are different, calculate the induced horizontal prism using Prentice's rule (induced prism = Fc, where F is the power of the lens along the horizontal meridian and c is the difference between the DBC and PD in cm). The direction of the prism also needs to be deduced.

4.4.4 Recording

Record the spherocylinder correction in minus cylinder form for both eyes and the reading addition power if a multifocal. Also record any prism, the type of lens, any tints or coatings etc. Use 'x' rather than the word 'axis'. Record the spherical and cylindrical power to the nearest 0.25 D, and the cylinder axis to the nearest 2.5°. The axis should be between 2.5° and 180°. Use 180 rather than 0 degrees. For example:

D28 segment bifocal, CR39, MAR coat

RE: $-2.00/-1.00 \times 35$

LE: -2.25 DS

Add: $+2.00$ DS

NV spectacles, CR39

OD: $+2.25/-0.75 \times 80$

OS: $+2.50/-0.50 \times 105$.

4.4.5 Interpretation

One of the most common errors in focimetry is an axis reading incorrect by 90° (Steele et al. 2006). Given that the cylindrical axes in the two eyes are often mirror images of each other (for example, both axes 90° or both axes 180°; right axis 175°, left 5°; right 20°, left 160°; right 45°, left 135°, etc.; Solsona 1975), if axes are 90° different to this (for example, 180° and 90°; 175° and 95°; 20° and 50°; both axes 45°; both axes 135°) then recheck the two cylindrical axes. Reading additions are typically the same in both eyes, so that if they are read as different, they should be rechecked.

4.4.6 Most common errors

1. Not focusing the focimeter eyepiece. This can lead to inaccuracies for high-powered lenses.
2. Not measuring the reading addition using FVP measurements for front-surface solid multifocals.
3. Reading one or both of the cylindrical axes incorrectly by 90°.
4. Ignoring the relative vertical position of the target between the right and left lens, thereby missing vertical prism.
5. Changing the vertical position of the lenses between measurements of the right and left lenses, thereby incorrectly reading vertical prism.

4.5 ANATOMICAL INTER-PUPILLARY DISTANCE

The interpupillary distance (PD) is the distance between the centres of the pupils of the eyes.

4.5.1 Interpupillary distance

The PD is measured for two reasons:

1. To place the optical centre of the phoropter/trial frame lenses in front of the patient's visual axes to control prism and avoid aberrations.

2. So that the optical centre of spectacle lenses can be placed in front of the patient's visual axis to avoid unwanted prism and aberrations or deliberately placed elsewhere to produce desired prism.

4.5.2 Advantages and disadvantages

Measurement of the anatomical PD is quick and convenient to use during an eye examination and it requires no instrumentation other than a simple millimetre ruler. The repeatability of anatomical binocular PD measurements is similar to that for a pupillometer (Holland & Siderov 1999, Osuobeni & Al-Fahdi 1994). A pupillometer could be considered when refracting or dispensing a patient with a large amount of ametropia, where slight discrepancies in PD could lead to induced prism, and for monocular measurements when dispensing progressive addition lenses.

4.5.3 Procedure

1. Keep the room lights on.

2. Explain the test to the patient: 'I am going to measure the distance between your eyes so that I can put your lenses in the correct position for your eyes.'

3. Face the patient directly at the distance desired for the near PD (usually about 40 cm).

4. Rest the PD ruler on the bridge of the patient's nose or on the forehead so that the millimetre scale is within the spectacle plane. Steady your hand with your fingers on the patient's temple to ensure that the ruler is held firmly in place.

Distance PD

5. Close your right eye and ask the patient to look at your left eye. (It is usually easiest to indicate with your finger the eye that you want the patient to fixate). To allow a patient with unilateral strabismus to fixate, you may need to cover the fellow eye.

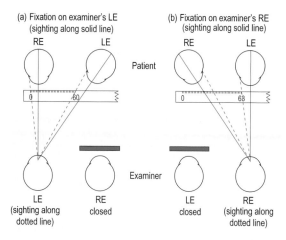

Fig. 4.5   (a) Measurement of near PD. (b) Measurement of distance PD.

6. Choose a point of reference on the patient's right eye. The temporal pupil margin is usually most convenient, although the centre of the pupil or the temporal limbus margin may also be used and the latter may be essential with patients with dark irides. Align the zero point on the ruler with this reference point.

7. Close your left eye, open your right and ask the patient to change fixation to your open right eye. Take care not to move the ruler or your head position. By sighting again to the appropriate reference point on the patient's left eye, you will obtain a reading for the distance PD (Fig. 4.5). This would be the left nasal pupil margin if you used the temporal pupil margin of the right eye.

Near PD

8. Move laterally to place your dominant eye opposite the patient's nose.

9. Ensure that you are still at a distance from the patient equal to their near working distance. Normally this is done at 40 cm but, if desired, the near PD can be measured for a closer or farther working distance.

10. Using your dominant eye only, choose a point of reference on the patient's right eye and align the zero point on the ruler with this reference point.

11. Look over to the patient's left eye and note the reading on the ruler that aligns with the corresponding reference point on the left eye (Fig. 4.5).

4.5.4 Alternative procedures

The near PD can also be measured during the distance PD measurement. During step 6, after aligning the zero mark on the ruler with the reference point, look over to the patient's left eye and note the reading on the ruler that aligns with the corresponding reference point on the left eye. The only difference to the procedure described above is that the target is not placed at the patient's midline. Any error is likely to be negligible.

When measuring monocular distance PDs you must use the middle of the patient's pupil as the reference point. The right monocular PD is measured from the middle of the patient's right pupil to the centre of the bridge of the nose. To determine the left monocular PD, you need to subtract the right monocular PD from the total distance PD. For example, if the total distance PD is 65 mm and the right monocular PD is 32 mm, the left monocular PD is 33 mm. It is not advisable to move the ruler to measure the left monocular PD (i.e. making the centre of the bridge of the nose the zero reference point) as this will lead to an additional error.

4.5.5 Recording

The values are normally recorded as distance PD/near PD (in mm). For example, PD: 63/60.

4.5.6 Interpretation

For women, the distance PD is most commonly in the range of 55–65 mm, and for men, 60–70 mm. Young children may have PDs as low as 45 mm. The distance PD value is usually 3–4 mm greater than the near PD at 40 cm. Inaccuracies in anatomical PD can occur due to parallax error when there is a large difference between your PD and the patient's PD. However, the error is slight, with an 8 mm difference in the examiner and patient's PDs leading to a 0.5 mm error in the measured patient PD (Brown

1991). The repeatability of anatomical PDs taken by an experienced practitioner is approximately ±1–2 mm (Holland & Siderov 1999, Osuobeni & Al-Fahdi 1994). Repeatability between practitioners is slightly poorer at about ±1.5−2 mm (Holland & Siderov 1999).

4.5.7 Most common errors

1. Moving the ruler during the measurement. Make sure it is held firmly and steadily in position. After taking the distance PD reading, it is a good idea to re-open your left eye, have the patient switch fixation back to it and check that the zero mark on the ruler is still aligned with the original reference point on the patient's right eye.

2. Using an inaccurate near test distance. Most commonly, unwittingly drifting in closer than 40 cm so the near PD turns out to be lower than it should be. The test distance should not affect the distance PD measurement.

3. Using a PD ruler that is not accurately calibrated, such as some give-away rulers provided by optical companies.

4.5.8 Alternative procedure: corneal reflection pupillometer

Pupillometers allow monocular PDs to be measured more accurately than an anatomical measurement (Holland & Siderov 1999). This is beneficial when ordering spectacles for high refractive errors or for progressive addition lenses where precise centration of each lens along the patient's visual axes is necessary. In addition, the procedure is quick and simple and could be performed by a clinical assistant and the examiner does not need to be binocular. The PD measured with a corneal reflection pupillometer will typically be 0.5–1 mm smaller than the anatomical PD (Holland & Siderov 1999, Osuobeni & Al-Fahdi 1994). This is because pupillometers measure the 'physiological PD', the distance between the two principal corneal reflexes, and locate the visual axes, whereas the anatomical PD locates the lines of sight or optical axes. Note that many pupillometers use a correction for the parallax error mentioned in the

anatomical PD section (Brown 1991). Inaccuracies can occur if the pupillometer sits higher or (usually) lower on the bridge than the intended spectacle frame and the nose is not straight, so that the monocular PDs can be shifted to one side.

4.6 PHOROPTER OR TRIAL FRAME?

A phoropter is a unit that is placed in front of the patient's head and contains all the equipment necessary to measure a patient's ametropia, heterophoria and accommodation. It can also be called a refractor, refractor head or refracting unit. A trial frame is an adjustable spectacle frame that includes cells into which all the various lenses required to measure a patient's ametropia, heterophoria and accommodation can be placed.

4.6.1 Advantages of a phoropter

The use of a phoropter (Fig. 4.6) is the preferred technique for distance vision refraction of the majority of patients. A video clip introduction to the phoropter is provided on the website 🖾. The main advantages of phoropters are:

- A quicker refraction: As the lenses are all contained within the phoropter, it is much quicker to change lens powers for both retinoscopy and subjective refraction than with a trial frame. This may also provide less back strain for the examiner.

- Comfort: The trial frame containing several lenses can become uncomfortably heavy, particularly for older patients.

- Jackson cross-cylinder alignment: On all modern phoropters, the Jackson cross-cylinder (JCC) is automatically aligned with the cylinder axis in the phoropter.

- No lens smear: Trial case lenses can become covered with fingerprints, and require regular cleaning. The trial frame should also be regularly cleaned.

- Risley prisms: These are standard on phoropters and make measurements of

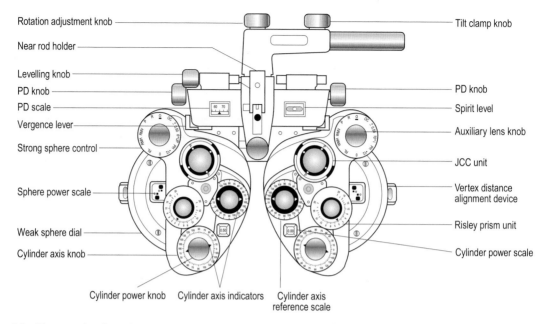

Fig. 4.6　Diagram of a phoropter.

subjective heterophoria and fusional reserves faster and easier and allow for easy use of the binocular prism dissociated accommodative balance technique.

- Computerisation: Computerised phoropters are available and can include data links to an automated focimeter (lensmeter) and/or autorefractor.

- High-tech: Some patients may prefer high-tech phoropters rather than the ancient-looking trial frame.

4.6.2 Advantages of a trial frame

A video clip introduction to the trial frame is provided on the website ⬛. In the routine refraction of presbyopic patients, the trial frame (Fig. 4.7) is preferred for the final determination of the near addition, as the test can be performed at the patient's preferred working distance and position, and the range of clear vision can be easily measured and compared to the near vision requirements of the patient. A trial frame is also useful to illustrate the improvement in distance vision in the 'real world' that a pair of spectacles could provide. For example, the new refractive correction can be placed into

the trial frame and the patient shown the improvement of their vision while looking through the window of the practice.

A trial frame is required for refractions during home (domiciliary) visits and is preferred when refracting:

- Patients who provide poor subjective responses: Some patients, despite normal or near normal visual acuity, provide poor subjective responses and cannot seem to discriminate between the view provided with and without a 0.25 DS lens or a ±0.25 Jackson cross-cylinder (JCC). Using larger dioptric changes in sphere (±0.50 or ±0.75 DS) and a higher-powered JCC (±0.50 or ±0.75) can sometimes elicit better subjective responses, and these changes are more easily made with a trial frame than with a phoropter. Many phoropters have a ±0.25 JCC that cannot be changed.

- Patients with high refractive error: The back vertex power (BVP) of a combination of lenses in the trial frame or phoropter is not necessarily the algebraic sum. It depends on the power, thickness, form and position of the lenses used. After refracting a patient with high ametropia in a trial frame, you should

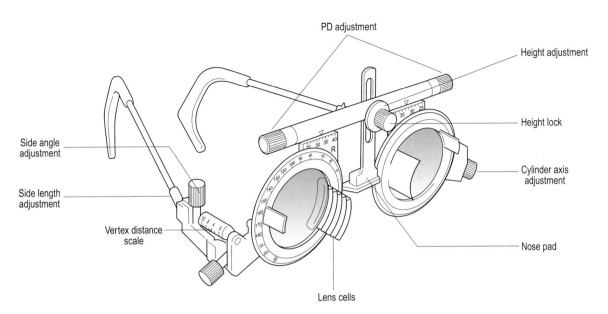

Fig. 4.7   Diagram of a trial frame.

measure the BVP using a focimeter. This is not possible with a phoropter. Indeed, for all phoropter lens powers and their combinations, you are placing your trust in the manufacturer. In addition, the pantoscopic angle and vertex distance can be controlled more easily with a trial frame. Any changes in head position could vary these parameters in a phoropter, but do not in a trial frame as it is fitted to the patient's head.

■ Patients with low vision: Large dioptric changes in sphere and a high-powered Jackson cross-cylinder (±0.75 or ±1.00 D) are required in the subjective refraction of low vision patients to enable them to appreciate a difference in vision. These can be used very easily during a trial frame refraction. In addition, the trial frame can provide larger aperture lenses and allow unusual head and eye positions that may be necessary for low vision patients using eccentric fixation.

■ Patients with binocular vision problems and children: The trial frame can stimulate less proximal accommodation than a phoropter. In addition, it is possible to perform the cover test with large aperture lenses in a trial frame, but not with a phoropter. Children can also see their parent/guardian more easily.

■ Patients with hearing problems: The phoropter obscures the patient's view of the examiner and therefore prevents communication with sign language or simple hand signals.

■ Patients with large angle strabismus: Retinoscopy can be done on the line of sight with a trial frame without occluding the fellow eye, allowing for a more accurate measure of refractive error and particularly astigmatism.

4.7 STATIC RETINOSCOPY

Retinoscopy provides an objective measurement of a patient's ametropia. Static retinoscopy provides an assessment of the distance refractive correction. Video clips showing a selection of retinoscopy reflexes and how their appearance changes during neutralisation are provided on the website 📚.

4.7.1 Objective measurement of refractive error

An objective measurement of refractive error is the only assessment available in patients who are unable to cooperate in a subjective refraction, such as young children. It is also heavily relied upon when subjective responses are limited (patients who do not speak the same language as you and those whose subjective responses are poor) or unreliable (malingerers). In more routine patients, it provides an objective first measure of refractive error that can be refined by subjective refraction.

4.7.2 Advantages and disadvantages

Retinoscopy provides a more accurate result of refractive error in a greater array of patients than autorefraction, although autorefraction (section 4.8) is a useful and reliable alternative in many 'standard' adult patients. Retinoscopy also provides a sensitive assessment of the ocular media (e.g. early detection of cataracts, keratoconus), can be used to determine refractive error at distance and near, identify accommodative dysfunction, and is portable and less expensive. Its major disadvantage is that it requires several years of training to become proficient at using it. When a subjective refraction is not possible, limited or unreliable, it is preferable to have more than one assessment of objective refractive correction.

There appears to be no research literature that compares the accuracy of streak or spot retinoscopes or refractions using negative or positive cylinders. The procedure will be described for streak retinoscopy, but spot retinoscopy appears an acceptable alternative. Streak retinoscopy is designed to be superior in detecting and correcting small amounts of astigmatism. As the name suggests, spot retinoscopy uses a spot of light rather than a streak. There is therefore no need to rotate the streak to determine the astigmatic meridians. In an astigmatic eye, the spot retinoscopic reflex is elliptical rather than circular, and the long and short axes of the ellipse determine the two astigmatic meridians. Otherwise the procedure is the same as for streak retinoscopy.

Positive cylinders have the advantage of making retinoscopy easier to learn, as 'with' movement is typically easier to see than 'against' movement. However, negative cylinders are preferred as they are standard in phoropters. In addition, there is the possibility of stimulating accommodation during subjective refraction when removing a plus cylinder from a trial frame to replace it with one of another power. For these reasons the procedure will be described using negative cylinders.

4.7.3 Procedure

A concise summary of the procedure is provided in Box 4.1.

1. Prior to the retinoscopy procedure, you should attempt to estimate the refractive correction from relevant case history (section

Box 4.1   Summary of retinoscopy procedure

1. Estimate the refractive correction from relevant case history and VA information and focimetry/lensometry.

2. Position the phoropter or trial frame appropriately and set the PD.

3. Dial in the working distance lenses if appropriate.

4. Switch on the duochrome (bichromatic), spotlight or a similar large target.

5. Explain the test to the patient.

6. Dim the room lights.

7. Set the retinoscope mirror to the plano position and align yourself with the visual axis of the patient's right eye.

8. Look across to the left eye and if 'with' movement is observed, add positive lenses until 'against' movement is obtained.

9. Determine if the refractive error of the right eye is spherical or astigmatic.

10. If the reflex is dim and the movement is relatively slow, use an appropriate lens to get nearer to neutrality, and check again for astigmatism.

11. If astigmatic, determine the principal meridians.

12. Neutralise the most plus/least minus meridian first.

13. Check the neutral point by moving forward and backward slightly from your normal working distance, and check the reflex movement.

14. Along the second meridian, add minus cylinder in a bracketing technique to achieve neutrality.

15. Repeat for the patient's left eye.

16. Remove the working distance lenses or subtract 1.50 or 2.00 D from your final result.

17. Measure the patient's visual acuities with the net retinoscopy result.

4.1) and visual acuity information (section 4.2) and focimetry/ lensometry (section 4.4). What is the expected refractive error given the patient's symptoms and visual acuity in their present spectacles? In the early years of clinical training, it may be best not to use the information from focimetry prior to retinoscopy until your retinoscopy skills have reached a competent level (during this time you should perform focimetry/ lensometry after subjective refraction to allow a comparison).

2. Set the patient's distance PD in the phoropter or trial frame. Position the phoropter or trial frame before the patient so that the lenses will be in the patient's spectacle plane (approximately 12 mm from the cornea) and make sure that it is level.

3. Either
   a) Dial in the +1.50 DS retinoscope lens into the phoropter or place working distance lenses in the back cells of the trial frame (+2.00 DS for a 50 cm working distance, +1.50 DS for 67 cm). This technique has the advantage that all 'with' movements indicate hyperopia and all 'against' movements indicate myopia. It also provides a 'fogging' lens to both eyes that will relax accommodation in a low hyperope.

   or

   b) Do not add a working distance lens. The working distance power (+1.50 D or +2.00 D usually) must later be subtracted from your final retinoscope result. This technique has the advantage that you avoid introducing two reflection surfaces from the working distance lens, which can make retinoscopy easier in some cases.

4. Switch on the duochrome (bichromatic), spotlight or a similar target that is easy to see when blurred and does not provide a stimulus to accommodation.

5. Explain the test to the patient: 'I'm going to shine a light in your eye and get an indication of the power of the glasses you may need. Please look at the red and green target, and let me know if my head blocks your view. Don't worry if the chart is blurred.' You must ensure that your head does not block the patient's view at any time, otherwise they are likely to accommodate to it.

6. Dim the room lights to provide a higher contrast, brighter view of the pupillary reflex, while providing enough light to allow easy viewing of the phoropter/ trial case. A totally dark room may induce a dark focus response (Mohindra retinoscopy, section 4.20.7).

7. Sit or stand off to the side of the patient so that manipulation of the trial frame/ phoropter is easy. Use a comfortable working distance from the patient so that you can change lenses in the spectacle plane easily (a comfortable arm's length is often 67 cm or 50 cm). You should be on the patient's right side and use your right hand and right eye to check the patient's right eye and vice versa for the left eye.

8. Set the retinoscope mirror to the plano position (maximum divergence, with the retinoscope collar at the bottom of its range) and position the retinoscope so that you are looking along the visual axis of the patient's eye (their other eye is fixating the duochrome; Fig. 4.8a). If the patient is looking slightly upwards to view the duochrome, which is common if the target is above the patient's head and viewed through a mirror, to look along their visual axis you will need to be slightly higher than the patient (Fig. 4.9).

9. Position the streak so that it is vertical. Look through the aperture of the retinoscope and direct the light at the patient's pupil and you should see the red retinoscope reflex. Sweep the retinoscope streak across the patient's pupil horizontally and compare the movement of the reflex in the pupil with the movement of the retinoscope. If the reflex moves in the same direction as the movement of the retinoscope streak, this is known as 'with' movement. If the reflex moves in the opposite direction to the

(a)

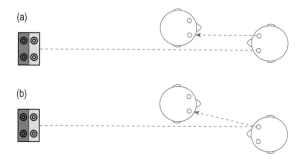

(b)

Fig. 4.8 Plan view of the position of the examiner and patient when performing retinoscopy. (a) The examiner is viewing along the visual axis of the patient's right eye, while the patient's left eye fixates the duochrome target. (b) The examiner views off-axis in the 'good' eye of a patient with strabismus. For the strabismic eye, retinoscopy could be performed along the angle of strabismus, or the good eye could be occluded and retinoscopy performed off-axis.

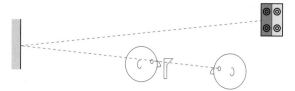

Fig. 4.9 Side view of the position of the patient and examiner when performing retinoscopy.

(a)   (b)

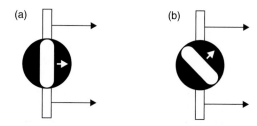

Fig. 4.10 Determining the two astigmatic meridians: (a) If you are 'retting' on axis, the reflex will move in the same direction as the retinoscopy streak. (b) If you are off-axis the reflex will move in a different direction from the direction of the retinoscopy streak. You should then rotate your streak to align with the reflex.

movement of the retinoscope streak, this is known as 'against' movement.

10. Before you begin retinoscopy on a patient younger than 60 years of age, you must try to ensure that they will not accommodate while looking at the target. If you are assessing the right eye first, look across to the left eye and if 'with' movement is observed, add positive lenses until 'against' movement is obtained. This will ensure that the left eye (which is viewing the target) is blurred by at least +1.50 D.

11. Sweep the retinoscope streak across the patient's right pupil and compare the movement of the reflex in the pupil with the movement of the retinoscope. Mentally note the direction of movement with the streak vertical and also observe the reflex's brightness, speed and width. Now rotate the

retinoscope streak so that it is horizontal and sweep across the pupil vertically and finally observe the reflex movement when the streak is oriented obliquely (45 and 135). For all four streak positions, mentally note the direction of the reflex movement and the relative brightness, speed and width of the reflex movements.

12. Determine if the refractive error is spherical (the observed reflex has the same direction, speed, brightness and thickness in all meridians) or astigmatic (the reflex differs in different meridians). If the reflex movement is relatively slow and any difference between the reflex speed and thickness is difficult to determine, place an appropriate spherical lens in the trial frame to get nearer to neutrality, and check again for astigmatism.

13. If astigmatic, determine the principal meridians by rotating the streak axis until the angle of the reflex movement coincides with the angle of the streak in two meridians; one perpendicular to the other (Fig. 4.10). If the principal meridians are hard to pinpoint, adjust the mirror position slightly to narrow the streak width.

14. Determine the spherical component by 'neutralising' (adding plus lenses to 'with' movement and minus lenses to 'against' movement until the reflex fills the entire pupil and all perceived movement stops) the most plus/least minus meridian first (the meridian with the slowest, dullest 'with' or fastest, brightest 'against' movement). The

meridian being neutralised is the meridian in which the streak is being moved. For example, to neutralise the vertical meridian, the streak is horizontal and moves vertically. If the cylinder amount is small and the most plus/least minus meridian is difficult to determine, then neutralise one meridian and then check the other. If the most plus/least minus meridian was neutralised first, then the second meridian should be showing 'against' motion for the plano mirror position. Use a bracketing technique to determine neutrality.

15. Check the neutral point by moving forward slightly and observing the movement of the reflex. A 'with' movement should be seen. If you move backward slightly from your normal working distance, an 'against' movement should be seen.

16. Set the minus cylinder axis parallel with the streak orientation of the least plus/most minus meridian. Move the retinoscope with the streak in this position and you should observe 'against' movement. Add minus cylinder in a bracketing technique to achieve neutrality. As 'with' movement can be easier to see than 'against' movement, you may wish to add minus cylinder until 'with' movement is just seen and then reduce the cylinder by 0.25 D. Alternatively, you may wish to neutralise the cylinder with the retinoscope in the concave mirror position (with the retinoscope collar moved to the top position), in which case you will add minus cylinder to neutralise 'with' movement.

17. Briefly, recheck the sphere and cylinder components for neutrality. The axis can be checked using Copeland's 'straddling' technique. This involves comparing the speed of rotation and alignment of the reflex at the cylinder axis +45° with that at the cylinder axis −45°. The cylinder axis should be changed until the reflex at these two positions is the same. In spot retinoscopy, the cylinder axis can be checked and refined by sweeping the beam along the axis of the cylindrical trial lens. If the trial cylinder is oriented at the correct axis, the reflex should be in alignment with the spot of light in the trial frame. The

axis of the trial cylinder can be adjusted until this is the case. The power of the cylindrical lens should be rechecked following an adjustment of cylinder axis.

18. Repeat steps 10 to 16 on the patient's left eye.

19. Recheck the right eye. This step may not be necessary if you have ensured that no accommodation has taken place throughout the procedure (see step 10).

20. Remove the +1.50 (or +2.00) working distance lenses (or subtract 1.50 or 2.00 D from your final result).

21. Measure the patient's visual acuities with the net retinoscopy result.

4.7.4 Adaptations to the standard technique

Monocular examiners

If you have normal visual acuity in one eye only, you may find the method of retinoscopy suggested by Barrett useful:

1. A small, bright, featureless fixation target is fixed to the retinoscope, near to the mirror. Ask the patient to observe this target.

2. Conduct retinoscopy on both eyes, using your 'good' eye to examine both eyes of the patient.

3. Once both eyes have been neutralised, recheck the endpoint of one eye using your good eye with the patient fixating a distance target. For example, if you have a 'good' right eye, then assess the patient's right eye using your good eye.

4. Any difference in spherical component in the eye that has been rechecked should be applied to the fellow eye. Note that the difference in cylindrical component should be negligible.

Dim reflex

If the reflex is very dim or hard to interpret, the patient either has media opacities, small pupils or high ametropia. If the patient is a high myope, moving increasingly closer to the patient's eye will move the retinoscope closer to the patient's far point and the reflex will become increasingly brighter and faster. Alternatively, you could just add a medium to large powered positive or negative lens and repeat retinoscopy at the normal distance.

Media opacities and/or small pupils

With patients with media opacities and/or small pupils, you will see a dim reflex as a reduced amount of light reaches the retina and even less returns to your retinoscope. In some retinoscopes you can alter the sight hole size. For small pupils and patients with media opacities you should make sure you are using the large aperture sight hole to see as much light as possible. To retain as much light as you can, use as small a number of lenses as possible as you will lose 8% of the reflex for each lens used due to reflections. Do not use a working distance lens (see step 3 in section 4.7.3) and refract each meridian using a sphere only and convert to a sphere–cylinder combination for the subjective refraction. You may also be able to obtain a brighter reflex by performing retinoscopy at a reduced working distance of, say, 25 or 33 cm (sometimes called 'radical retinoscopy'). You will have to subtract a larger value from your retinoscopy result to compensate for the reduced working distance (4.00 or 3.00 D respectively for the two distances mentioned above). Remember that there is a greater chance of error when using a close working distance. For example, if you work at 62 cm rather than a correct 67 cm when using a +1.50 DS working distance lens, the error is 0.10 D. The same 5 cm error when assuming a working distance lens of +4.00 D (25 cm) is 1.00 D.

'Scissors' reflex

This reflex moves like the action of a pair of scissors, moving simultaneously in opposite directions from the centre of the pupil, and accurate neutralisation can be very difficult. The reflex can be due to optical aberrations, particularly coma in a normal eye or due to abnormalities in the media such as keratoconus or corneal scarring. Use lens steps larger than 0.25 DS and try to bracket the neutral point. Increasing the room light level can help as it reduces the patient's pupil size and cuts down the peripheral aberrations.

Large pupils

Spherical aberration can provide a more against movement in the periphery of the lens compared to the centre. You must concentrate on the central reflex and ignore the remainder. Once again, increasing the room light level can help as it reduces the patient's pupil size and cuts down the peripheral aberrations.

Patients with strabismus

Retinoscopy is ideally performed along the patient's visual axis. In a patient with strabismus, this can be difficult, particularly when using a phoropter. Retinoscopy on the 'good' eye must be performed slightly off-axis (Fig. 4.8b). For the strabismic eye, it can be easier to change the fixation point for the 'good' eye, so that retinoscopy along the visual axis of the strabismic eye is easier. Alternatively, occlude the 'good' eye and perform retinoscopy slightly off-axis (Fig. 4.8b).

Accommodative fluctuations

During accommodative fluctuations, the pupil will be seen to vary in size and the reflex movement and brightness will rapidly change. This can be seen with young children who change fixation (typically to look at the retinoscope light or their parent/guardian) and the patient needs to be reminded to keep looking at the duochrome. If these changes do not appear related to changes in fixation, then accommodative fluctuations that could be due to latent hyperopia or pseudomyopia should be suspected and a cycloplegic refraction (section 4.20) and assessments of accommodation (sections 5.17 to 5.19) should be performed.

4.7.5 Recording

Record the spherocylindrical correction that neutralised the patient's refractive error after removing your working distance lenses. Do not use a degree sign as ° can look like a 0 and make an axis of 15° look like 150 degrees. Use 'x' rather than the word 'axis'. Record the spherical and cylindrical power to the nearest 0.25 D, and the cylinder axis to the nearest 2.5 degrees. The axis should be between 2.5 degrees and 180 degrees. Use 180 rather than 0 degrees. Also record the monocular visual acuity with the retinoscopy result. For example:

RE: $-2.00/-0.50 \times 105$ 6/4.5

LE: -2.25 DS $6/4.5^{-2}$

OD: $+2.00/-1.00 \times 105$ $20/20^{+3}$

OS: $+1.75/-0.75 \times 70$ 20/25

4.7.6 Interpretation

On average, retinoscopy provides a refractive result slightly more positive than subjective refraction in young patients. This decreases with age, so that retinoscopy and subjective results are similar in presbyopic patients. As the stimulus to accommodation is greater in subjective refraction than in retinoscopy, the retinoscopy result in young hyperopes can be much more positive than accepted in subjective refraction. Errors can occur in retinoscopy if it is performed off-axis, which will induce an astigmatic error, or if it is performed at an incorrect working distance, which will induce a spherical error. The most common working distance error is to work too close, particularly when the reflex is dim. Note that cylinder axes in the two eyes are often mirror images of each other (Solsona 1975). For example, right axis 175°, left 5°; right axis 20°, left 160°; right axis 45°, left 135°, etc.

4.7.7 Most common errors

1. Performing retinoscopy at an incorrect working distance, e.g. working at about 50 cm, while using a 1.50 D working distance lens.

2. Performing retinoscopy off-axis.

3. Blocking the patient's view of the distance chart, thereby probably stimulating accommodation.

4. Confusing the retinoscope collar positions (plano-mirror and concave-mirror positions).

5. Not concentrating on the movement in the centre of the pupil in a patient with large pupils.

4.8 AUTOREFRACTION

Autorefractors are automated optometers that provide an objective measure of a patient's distance refractive error.

4.8.1 Objective measurement of refractive error

In routine patients, autorefraction provides an objective first measure of refractive error that can be refined by subjective refraction. Autorefractors may be of the closed-view type, where an internal fixation target is viewed via a fogging lens system to relax accommodation, or of the open-view type, where the patient can view an external fixation target at any given distance. An objective measurement of refractive error is the only assessment available in patients who are unable to cooperate in a subjective refraction, such as young children. It is also heavily relied upon when subjective responses are limited (patients who do not speak the same language as you and those whose subjective responses are poor) or unreliable (malingerers). It is ideal to obtain two objective estimates of refractive error, one from autorefraction and one from retinoscopy, when a subjective refraction is not possible and when spectacles are going to be prescribed on the basis of the objective results.

4.8.2 Advantages and disadvantages

Autorefractors provide a reliable alternative to retinoscopy in many 'standard' adult patients (Elliott & Wilkes 1989, McCaghrey & Matthews 1993) and can be particularly accurate at determining astigmatism (Walline et al. 1999). When used with cycloplegia in children, it is as accurate, if not more so, than retinoscopy (Elliott & Wilkes 1989, Walline et al. 1999). Autorefraction can be performed by clinical assistants and therefore free up a little of the optometrist's time and some autorefractors can be directly linked to an automated phoropter, so that the autorefractor result is dialled into the phoropter if required. Finally, the high-tech nature of autorefractors can appeal to some patients.

However, autorefractors should not be used with young children without cycloplegia because of proximal accommodation errors producing significantly more minus results than subjective refraction (Elliott & Wilkes 1989, Zhao et al. 2004), particularly in young hyperopes. Results can also be unreliable or unobtainable in patients with poor fixation, high refractive errors, small pupils, cataracts, pseudophakia, nystagmus, and amblyopia and in some cases age-related maculopathy (Elliott & Wilkes 1989). In addition, autorefraction lacks the assessment of the ocular media (e.g. early detection of cataracts, keratoconus) provided by retinoscopy and autorefractors are typically non-portable and more expensive than retinoscopes. Finally, they are also more likely to break down than a retinoscope (Steele et al. 2006).

4.8.3 Procedure

The measurement procedure will not be described as it basically involves sitting the patient comfortably at the machine, aligning the instrument with the patient's visual axis using a monitor and pressing a button. It is usually helpful to take several readings that are then averaged. If the refractive error is hyperopic and successive readings are more plus then it can be useful to continue readings until a plateau is reached.

4.8.4 Results

Refraction results are normally displayed on a screen, and there is commonly a printout facility. Other information such as interpupillary distance is also displayed on some models.

4.8.5 Interpretation

The refraction result obtained from the autorefractor may be used as a starting point for subjective refraction, similar to the use of a retinoscopy result. Note, however, the potential to miss hyperopia in a young adult patient with active accommodation.

4.8.6 Most common errors

1. Alignment error with the visual axis, inducing oblique astigmatism, when using an open-view type autorefractor.

2. Assuming that the result from the instrument is always accurate in younger subjects.

4.9 MONOCULAR SUBJECTIVE REFRACTION

Subjective refraction is the determination of the refractive correction of the patient based on their responses to the addition of various lenses. During monocular subjective refraction, one eye is occluded while the refractive correction of the other eye is determined.

4.9.1 Subjective refraction

During subjective refraction, the examiner communicates with the patient and, using the patient's responses to the vision provided with various lenses, determines the optical correction that best suits the patient. It is therefore only possible to perform subjective refraction with patients who can communicate effectively with you. When a subjective refraction is not possible, limited or unreliable, it is preferable to have more than one assessment of objective refractive correction (e.g. retinoscopy and autorefraction). Subjective refraction should be performed under conditions that simulate the patient's normal viewing situation as closely as possible. For example, pupil size during refraction should ideally resemble the patient's pupil size when they are using their spectacles for detailed viewing tasks, when optimum visual acuity and comfort is required. Normally this would be the pupil size under room illumination with binocular viewing conditions. Given its importance to the primary care examination, it is surprising that there is relatively little research comparing the various tests used in the subjective refraction. This may be partly because there is no 'gold standard' test to compare it with, so that validity testing is difficult (section 1.1.2).

4.9.2 Advantages and disadvantages

Monocular subjective refraction is a slightly easier technique for students to learn than binocular refraction and it is not as easy to get confused. In particular, binocular refraction works most effectively if the starting point is reasonably close to the optimal refractive correction and this cannot be guaranteed with novice retinoscopists. Therefore, monocular subjective refraction is the preferred technique when you start to learn subjective refraction.

Monocular subjective refraction is limited in that the occluder can lead to less relaxation of accommodation compared to binocular refraction. This can lead to possible over-minusing or under-plussing the refractive correction in patients with hyperopia, pseudomyopia and antimetropia. Monocular refraction should also not be used in patients with latent nystagmus and any cyclodeviation. The occluder used in monocular refraction manifests latent nystagmus and makes subjective refraction difficult. The occluder can also manifest any cyclophoria that could lead to an incorrect assessment of astigmatism. Finally, monocular refraction is slightly slower than binocular refraction because a binocular balance of accommodation is required after monocular subjective refraction is completed.

4.9.3 Procedure

1. Explain the procedure to the patient: 'During this test, I will place various lenses in front of your eye to find the lenses that give you the best vision. Don't worry about giving a wrong answer as everything is double checked.'

2. Sit or stand off to the side of the patient so that manipulation of the trial frame/phoropter is easy.

3. Begin with the net retinoscopy sphere–cylinder before each eye. The patient's distance PD should already be set in the phoropter or trial frame, which should be level and positioned appropriately.

4. The subjective refraction traditionally begins on the right eye. Occlude the left eye.

5. Determine the Best Vision Sphere (section 4.10 for phoropter-based refractions and section 4.11 for trial frame-based refractions). This must be performed to ensure that the circle of least confusion is on the retina prior to the use of the Jackson cross-cylinder (JCC).

6. Check that the circle of least confusion is in an appropriate position prior to JCC using the duochrome test (section 4.12).

7. Determine the cylinder axis using the JCC, section 4.13.

8. Determine the cylinder power using the JCC, section 4.13.

9. If you have changed the cylinder power or axis significantly, repeat the Best Vision Sphere assessment (step 5).

10. Measure visual acuity (VA).

11. Repeat steps 5–10 for the other eye.

12. If your patient has some accommodation left (i.e. they are younger than about 60 years old; Charman 1989) perform a binocular balance of accommodation (sections 4.15 to 4.18).

13. Compare the monocular VAs with the present subjective refraction result with the patient's vision or habitual VAs (as appropriate). If the VA is better with the patient's spectacles, then it is likely that your subjective result is incorrect. Repeat the subjective refraction (students should perhaps call their supervisor).

14. Compare the VA with the present subjective refraction with age-matched normal data (Table 3.2). If the VA is worse than expected, or worse in one eye compared to the other, remeasure the VA with a pinhole aperture. If the VA improves with the pinhole, either the patient has media opacity, typically cataract that is being bypassed by the pinhole, or the subjective refraction is not optimal and should be repeated. Note that visual acuity will not always improve with cataract, particularly if the opacity is dense and central.

15. If the final refractive correction in either eye is above 4.00 D mean sphere equivalent (MSE, the sphere plus half the cylinder, e.g. $-3.75/-1.50 \times 180$ has a MSE of -4.50 D, $+4.50/-2.00 \times 90$ has a MSE of $+3.50$ D),

then measure the vertex distance. This is the distance from the back surface of the lens nearest the eye to the apex of the cornea. Back vertex distance can be read from the millimetre scale on the side of the trial frame, from the back vertex distance periscope on the side of the phoropter, or by using a vertex distance gauge.

4.9.4 Recording

Record the refractive correction using the same format described for retinoscopy (section 4.7.5). Do not use a degree sign as ° can look like a 0 and make an axis of 15° look like 150 degrees. Use 'x' rather than the word 'axis'. Record the spherical and cylindrical power to the nearest 0.25 D, and the cylinder axis to the nearest 2.5 degrees. The axis should be between 2.5 degrees and 180 degrees. Use 180 rather than 0 degrees. Also record the monocular VAs. If pinhole VA is measured and reveals no improvement in VA, record PHNI ('pinhole no improvement'); otherwise record the VA with the pinhole. For refractive corrections above 4.00 D (equivalent sphere) record the vertex distance.

Make sure that the prescription details that you provide to patients are clearly legible. Illegible prescription forms have been reported as a surprisingly common error in optometric practice (Steele et al. 2006).

Examples of recording:

Monocular refraction (vertex distance 11 mm)

RE: $+6.00/-1.00 \times 35$ $6/6^{+1}$

LE: $+6.25/-0.75 \times 145$ $6/6$

OD: $-2.75/-0.50 \times 180$ $20/15$

OS: -3.00 DS $20/15^{-1}$

RE: $-3.00/-0.50 \times 100$ $6/12$ PHNI

LE: $-2.50/-1.00 \times 75$ $6/4$

(Vertex distance 12 mm)

OD: $-7.50/-2.25 \times 35$ $20/70$ PH $20/30$

OS: $-8.00/-1.50 \times 150$ $20/20$

4.9.5 Interpretation

The subjective results should be compatible with the retinoscopy results in most cases, although young patients may provide a more positive (less minus) correction than retinoscopy. Inconsistent results may be due to technique error or the patient may be an unreliable observer for behavioural or visual reasons. A subjective result that is significantly less positive (more negative) than the retinoscopy result or a subjective result more minus than suggested by unaided visual acuity could indicate latent hyperopia or pseudomyopia and a cycloplegic refraction may be required (section 4.20).

The difference between the patient's own spectacles and the subjective refraction should be compatible with the difference between the habitual (with own spectacles) and optimal visual acuities in patients without eye disease. For example, if the patient has a visual acuity of 20/40 in their spectacles and 20/15 after subjective refraction, you could expect the subjective refraction to be 1.00 DS more myopic than the spectacle correction ($-0.25 \approx 1$ line of logMAR visual acuity). Thus, a refractive correction of -1.25 DS would become -2.25 DS. If the subjective refraction was 2.75 DS or even -3.00 DS this could suggest you have over-minused the subjective refraction. Changes in hyperopic correction are more difficult to explain in this way as they are dependent on the amount of accommodation the patient has (and therefore their age). Changes in astigmatism that are not due to pathology are usually small. Patients with refractive error change that is a result of cataract or other eye disease will not typically follow the same rules for improvement in visual acuity (e.g. nuclear cataract can cause a 1.00 D myopic shift with only a 1–2-line improvement in visual acuity).

4.9.6 Most common errors

1. Not monitoring the visual acuity to ensure that a change in lens power results in the expected change in visual acuity.

2. Using poor patient instructions or leading questions.

3. Losing control of accommodation.

4. Allowing the patient to direct the examination.

5. Not checking a subjective refraction that leads to sub-optimal visual acuity with a pinhole.

6. Not recording the vertex distance with a refractive correction over 4.00 DS.

7. Not rechecking the results with an alternative technique when the visual acuities, habitual correction and refraction are not consistent.

4.10 MAXIMUM PLUS TO MAXIMUM VISUAL ACUITY (MPMVA)

The maximum plus to maximum visual acuity (MPMVA) technique is used to determine the best vision sphere as part of the subjective refraction and to determine the optimal spherical correction. In the MPMVA technique the patient is initially fogged or blurred by adding plus sphere lenses to the retinoscopy result. Visual acuity is then improved to a maximum as the plus sphere lens is decreased or the minus sphere lens is increased.

4.10.1 Best vision sphere assessment

The best vision sphere assessment is used at the beginning of the subjective refraction and ensures that the circle of least confusion is on the retina prior to the use of the Jackson cross-cylinder (JCC) technique. In younger patients the circle of least confusion can be left slightly behind the retina as they can accommodate to bring it onto the retina during the JCC procedure. The best vision sphere technique can also be used after JCC to ensure that the letter chart target is precisely focused on the retina to ensure the optimal refractive correction has been found.

4.10.2 Advantages and disadvantages

There is no research literature that indicates that any best vision sphere procedure is better than another and an experienced practitioner could use a different technique for different patients or may

always use a preferred approach. However, the MPMVA technique has the advantage that accommodation is well controlled when examining young patients. This technique is particularly easy when using a phoropter as the lens changes can be made quickly and easily. A disadvantage is that care must be taken to ensure that the best vision sphere is not under-minused or over-plussed prior to the use of the Jackson cross-cylinder as inaccurate determinations of astigmatism can then occur (Bennett and Rabbetts 1998).

4.10.3 Procedure

1. Occlude the left eye.

2. Determine the visual acuity of the right eye.

3. If the VA is near normal: Add +1.00 DS to the spherical lens determined in retinoscopy and check the visual acuity. The VA should be reduced by about four lines. If the visual acuity only worsens by one or two lines (or gets better!), add additional positive power to the sphere until four lines of acuity are lost to ensure the eye is 'fogged'. Experienced practitioners will typically use a smaller fogging lens such as +0.50 DS.

4. If the VA is 6/12 or worse:
   a) In young patients, it is very unlikely that the retinoscopy result is under-plussed or over-minused, as a young patient would be able to accommodate under such conditions to obtain good distance VA. A poor VA in a young patient will likely be because the retinoscopy result is over-plussed or under-minused so that there is no need to add any more plus lenses. The eye is already fogged. Go to step 5.
   b) In patients aged 55 and over who have no accommodation, the retinoscopy result could be reducing VA because it is too minus or too plus. Use ±0.50 DS lenses to determine whether the result is over-plussed/under-minused or over-minused/under-plussed. If the eye is already fogged, go to step 5. If the eye is over-minused/under-plussed, then add plus lenses until it is fogged to about 6/12.

5. Reduce the amount of fog by 0.25 DS and check that visual acuity improves.

6. Continue to reduce the amount of fog in 0.25 DS steps and stop when there is no improvement in visual acuity.

7. Obtaining an improvement in VA beyond the 'bottom line' of your chart is, of course, impossible. This can create problems if the 'bottom line' truncates the visual acuity. For example, if your chart has a bottom line of 20/15 (6/4.5), yet the patient can read 20/10 (6/3), the patient would be over-plussed/under-minused by approximately 0.50 DS if they were only unfogged to 20/15. Remember that the *average* acuity of a 20-year-old is 20/13 (6/4; Table 3.2). Using the JCC when the circle of least confusion is in front of the retina, as it would be in this case, can lead to an incorrect determination of astigmatism (Bennett & Rabbetts 1998). If the patient can read the bottom line of your chart (and this is larger than 6/3, 20/10), you must allow extra minus/less plus that makes your bottom line of letters 'clearer'. Ensure that the bottom line of letters is 'definitely clearer and not just smaller and blacker'. This would typically be no more than -0.50 DS more than that obtained to allow 20/15 (6/4.5) to be first read.

4.10.4 Adaptations to the standard technique

Patients do not give perfect answers: The techniques listed above and described in the following sections assume that the responses provided by patients are always correct. Of course, it is seldom that they are always perfect and you need to be aware of this. This can be detected during the subjective refraction when responses to the same changes in spherical power can be different at different times and can be expected in patients whose responses to other procedures within the eye examination have been poor. Present lens changes several times until you obtain reliable responses.

Patients providing unreliable responses: Make sure your instructions are accurate and your technique is good. Particularly in the early stages of training, it is more likely to be your poor technique than unreliable patient responses. Ask a supervisor to help. If a patient is providing unreliable responses or is unable to tell any difference with ±0.25 DS, then use ±0.50 DS or even larger steps.

Patients with reduced visual acuity: If a patient with reduced monocular or binocular VA is unable to tell any difference with ±0.25 DS, then use ±0.50 DS or even larger steps. It is well understood that such procedures should be used for patients with low vision. However, the same applies for any eye with reduced vision (e.g. patients with a unilateral amblyopic eye or unilateral cataract).

4.10.5 Recording

The results of MPMVA are not recorded as the technique is just part of the subjective refraction.

4.10.6 Most common errors

1. Not monitoring the visual acuity to ensure that a change in lens power results in the expected change in visual acuity.

2. Using a truncated VA chart with a 'bottom line' of 20/20 or, to a lesser degree, 20/15 and only unfogging VA to that level. For example, if your chart has a bottom line of 20/20, yet the patient can read 20/15, the patient would be slightly over-plussed/under-minused if they were only unfogged to 20/15. Remember that the average acuity of a 20-year-old is 20/13 and some patients can see 20/10 (Table 3.2). Using the JCC when the circle of least confusion is in front of the retina, as it would be in this case, can lead to an incorrect determination of astigmatism (Bennett & Rabbetts 1998).

4.11 THE PLUS/MINUS TECHNIQUE FOR BEST VISION SPHERE DETERMINATION

The determination of the best vision sphere is part of the subjective refraction and is used to determine the optimal spherical correction. In this technique low-powered plus sphere and minus sphere lenses (typically 0.25 DS) are added in a systematic manner to the patient's retinoscopy result until the best visual acuity is obtained.

4.11.1 Best vision sphere assessment

The best vision sphere assessment is used at the beginning of the subjective refraction and ensures that the circle of least confusion is on the retina prior to the use of the Jackson cross-cylinder (JCC) technique. If it is not then an inaccurate determination of astigmatism can occur (Bennett & Rabbetts 1998). In younger patients the circle of least confusion can be left slightly behind the retina as they can use accommodation to bring it onto the retina during the JCC procedure. The best vision sphere technique can also be used after JCC to check that the letter chart target is precisely focused on the retina to ensure the optimal refractive correction has been found.

4.11.2 Advantages and disadvantages

There is no research literature that indicates that any best vision sphere procedure is better than another and an experienced practitioner could use a different technique for different patients or may always use a preferred approach. The plus/minus technique is easier than MPMVA when using a trial frame as fewer lens changes are typically required. However, it does not provide as good control of accommodation in young patients as the MPMVA technique. For this reason, one or more check tests (duochrome and/or the +1.00 blur check) are typically used with the plus/minus technique in pre-presbyopic patients.

4.11.3 Procedure

1. Occlude one eye. Direct the patient's attention to the best acuity line. Add +0.25 D and ask: 'are the letters clearer, more blurred or the same?'

2. If the acuity improves or *remains the same* with the additional plus, then exchange the

spherical lens that is in the trial frame for one that has +0.25 DS added. For example, if the patient has −3.00 DS in the trial frame and the letters look clearer with +0.25 DS, then exchange the lens for a −2.75 DS lens. When exchanging plus lenses in a young hyperope, do not remove the plus lens until the new lens has been inserted, otherwise accommodation could be stimulated. For example, if you have +2.00 DS in the trial frame and the patient indicates that additional plus power is required, insert the +2.25 DS lens first, and then remove the +2.00 DS lens.

3. Using the same approach, continue adding plus lens power in +0.25 DS steps, until the acuity first blurs. Stop at the most plus/least minus lens that does not blur the visual acuity.

4. If the visual acuity blurs with a +0.25 DS lens, then do not add it.

5. Direct the patient's attention to the best acuity line. Add −0.25 DS and ask: 'are the letters clearer, more blurred or the same?'

6. If visual acuity improves with the lens, then exchange the spherical lens that is in the trial frame for one that has −0.25 DS added. For example, if the patient has −3.00 DS in the trial frame and the letters look clearer with −0.25 DS, then exchange the lens for a −3.25 DS lens. When exchanging plus lenses in a young hyperope, do not remove the plus lens until the new lens has been inserted, otherwise accommodation could be stimulated. For example, if you have +2.00 DS in the trial frame and the patient indicates that additional minus power is required, insert the +1.75 DS lens first, then remove the +2.00 DS lens.

7. Add further minus lenses (in −0.25 D steps) *only as long as the visual acuity improves.*

8. If a young patient (with accommodation) reports that vision is improved with the lens, but there is no improvement in visual acuity, ask, 'Do the letters definitely look clearer, or just smaller and blacker?' If the letters just look smaller and blacker, do not add the

−0.25 DS. This is particularly a problem with visual acuity charts that are truncated.

9. If the patient reports no change or a worsening of vision, do not add the −0.25 DS.

10. Duochrome check: The duochrome (section 4.12) can be used as part of this technique as a check test. If the duochrome suggests that extra plus power is required, you should go back to the acuity chart and see if the patient prefers an extra +0.25 DS. If the duochrome suggests more minus is needed, go back and check with −0.25 DS. The vision obtained with the ±0.25 DS is the final arbiter of the best vision sphere and *not* the duochrome. If more than ±0.50 DS is needed to balance the clarity of the rings (or letters) on the duochrome, this usually indicates that the duochrome test is unreliable for this patient and the results should be ignored.

11. The +1.00 blur check: Place a +1.00 DS trial case lens over the final best vision sphere correction. If the original VA is about 6/4 (the average VA for a young patient; Table 3.2), then VA will blur to about 6/12$^+$ with a +1.00 DS (Elliott & Cox 2004). If VA is better than 6/12 with the +1.00 DS, then the patient may have been over-minused or under-plussed and the best vision sphere should be rechecked. Note that the four-line loss of VA with the +1.00 blur is an average and VA loss with +1.00 DS can reliably be as small as one to two lines or as large as seven lines (Elliott & Cox 2004). The vision obtained with the ±0.25 DS is the final arbiter of the best vision sphere and not the +1.00 blur test.

4.11.4 Adaptations to the standard technique

Patients do not give perfect answers: The techniques listed above and described in the following sections assume that the responses provided by patients are always correct. Of course, it is seldom that they are always perfect. This can be detected during the subjective refraction when responses to the same changes in spherical power can be different at different times, or with experience it can be expected in patients whose responses to other procedures within the eye examination have been poor. It can be useful in such patients to give some 'training' to help patients provide more accurate responses. This can be done by repeatedly presenting the same spherical lens change to the patient until they repeatedly provide the same response. Alternatively you can provide a comparison with +0.25 DS and −0.25 DS until the patient repeatedly reports the same preference. If accurate responses are never obtained, you may need to change the power of the spherical lens changes as indicated below.

Difficulty with 3 options: It can be difficult for some patients to make a decision when there are three possible options of 'clearer', 'more blurred' or 'the same'. Some clinicians just present two options to the patient and ask whether the chart is 'clearer' or 'more blurred' or 'better with the lens or . . . without it'. If the patient pauses and is clearly having difficulty deciding between the two options, the clinician can then ask whether they look about the same. The patient will sometimes report that there is no difference even without the prompt. Another option used by some clinicians when refracting young patients and close to the final correction (as indicated by a good VA) is to ask whether a +0.25 DS is 'worse' or 'the same' and whether a −0.25 DS is 'better' or 'the same' on the basis that a +0.25 DS should either blur or relax accommodation and a −0.25 DS should either improve acuity or induce accommodation. There is no research literature to indicate whether one of these options is better than any other.

Patients providing unreliable responses: Make sure your instructions are accurate and your technique is good. Particularly in the early stages of training, it is more likely to be your poor technique than unreliable patient responses. Ask a supervisor to help. If a patient is providing unreliable responses or is unable to tell any difference with ±0.25 DS, then use ±0.50 DS or even larger steps.

Patients with reduced visual acuity: Similarly, if a patient with reduced monocular or binocular VA is unable to tell any difference with ±0.25 DS, then use ±0.50 DS or even larger steps. It is well understood that such procedures should be used for patients with low vision. However, the same applies for any eye with reduced vision (e.g. patients with a unilateral amblyopic eye or unilateral cataract).

4.11.5 Recording

The results of the best vision sphere are not recorded as the technique is just part of the subjective refraction.

4.11.6 Most common errors

1. Not monitoring the visual acuity to ensure that a change in lens power results in the expected change in visual acuity.

4.12 DUOCHROME (OR BICHROME) TEST

The duochrome test is based on the principle of longitudinal chromatic aberration, where light of shorter wavelength (e.g. green light) is refracted more by the eye's optics than light of longer wavelength (e.g. red light). Duochrome tests traditionally use a red filter (peak wavelength 620 nm) and a green filter (peak wavelength 535 nm). The dioptric distance between the foci of these wavelengths is around 0.44 D (Bennett & Rabbetts 1998). An eye in a mildly myopic state (e.g. −0.25 DS) will see the target on the red filter more clearly; an eye in a mildly hypermetropic state (e.g. +0.25 DS) will see the target on the green filter more clearly.

4.12.1 Checking the spherical refractive correction

The duochrome or bichromatic test is commonly used as a check on the best vision sphere during monocular refraction. It can be used at two points during the subjective refraction. First, it can be used after the initial determination of the best vision sphere and prior to the use of the Jackson cross-cylinder (JCC). The JCC technique requires the circle of least confusion to be on the retina and the duochrome can be used to check that this is the case. The best vision sphere may also be rechecked after JCC and prior to finalising the refractive correction. The test is more rarely used as a binocular balancing technique in which the two eyes are dissociated using vertical prism (e.g., 3^{Δ} down right

eye and 3^{Δ} up left eye) or a septum (see sections 4.15 and 4.18).

4.12.2 Advantages and disadvantages

This technique is very quick and easy and works in a majority of patients. However, note that some patients give poor results with the duochrome and always prefer one colour (often red), regardless of the changes you make to the spherical refraction. Older patients, due to small pupils and the increased absorption of low wavelength light by the lens (particularly in nuclear cataract), also tend to prefer red and can give unreliable duochrome results. Colour defective patients can use the test, although the red side of the test will appear duller to protans. In addition, not all charts provide appropriate red and green wavelength light. Students can find it difficult to know when to ignore the results and should not use the test as a final arbiter of the best vision sphere.

4.12.3 Procedure

1. Occlude one eye. Turn off the room lights. This dilates the pupil and slightly increases the chromatic aberration of the eye. It also reduces the veiling glare on projected charts.

2. Ask the patient: 'Are the rings (or letters/dots) clearer and blacker on the red or on the green, or are they are about the same?' If they look the same this suggests that the best vision sphere has been obtained and the circle of least confusion is on the retina.

3. If the rings on the green look clearer, add +0.25 DS until you obtain a balance. Note the additional spherical power required to obtain a balance.

4. If the rings on the red look clearer, add −0.25 DS until you obtain a balance. Note the additional spherical power required to obtain a balance.

5. If more than ±0.50 DS is needed to balance the clarity of the rings (or letters) on the duochrome, this usually indicates that the

duochrome test is unreliable for this patient and the results should be ignored.

6. Prior to the use of the Jackson cross-cylinder: If the clarity of the rings changes from 'green' to 'red' with +0.25 DS or 'red' to 'green' with −0.25 DS, leave a young patient on the 'green' as they will be able to accommodate to bring the circle of least confusion onto the retina.

7. After the use of the Jackson cross-cylinder and prior to finalising the refractive correction: If the clarity of the rings changes from 'green' to 'red' with +0.25DS or 'red' to 'green' with −0.25DS, note the additional spherical power required to leave a young patient 'on the red'.

8. Use the additional lens power suggested by the duochrome test and double-check whether this additional power is preferred by the patient using MPMVA (section 4.10) or the plus/minus technique (section 4.11). Note that the duochrome should be used to indicate that you should double-check your result and should not be used as the arbiter of the final refractive correction.

NB: Some practitioners prefer to add +0.50 DS or +0.75 DS to the spherical correction so that the bichromatic test is initially 'on the red' and then reduce the plus power (or increase the minus power) in 0.25 DS steps until the targets on the red and green look equally black and clear.

4.12.4 Recording

The result of the duochrome test when used prior to the JCC is typically not recorded. However, some practitioners record the result of the duochrome at the end of the monocular refraction. For example:

R: −1.00/−0.50 × 170   R = G   6/4

L: −1.25/−0.25 × 10   R = G   6/4

OD: −1.25/−0.75 × 20   R > G   20/15

OS: −1.75/−1.00 × 165   R > G   20/15

4.12.5 Most common errors

1. Relying on the result obtained with the duochrome test as the final arbiter of the spherical endpoint.

2. Using this test on a patient with nuclear sclerosis.

4.13 THE JACKSON CROSS-CYLINDER

The Jackson cross-cylinder (JCC) test is based on the theory of obliquely crossed cylinders. The cross-cylinder lens has two cylindrical elements of typically 0.25 DC power and opposite signs, with axes crossed at 90 degrees. The lens can be rotated so that two different cylindrical lens powers can be presented to the patient, while the mean power of the lens remains zero. For example, the lens could be rotated from +0.25/−0.50 × 180 to +0.25/−0.50 × 90 (which is the same as −0.25/+0.50 × 180). The determination of cylinder power is easiest to explain. The crossed cylinder allows you to present two lenses to the patient: one will increase the interval of Sturm and the other will decrease it. The zero mean power of the crossed cylinder ensures that the circle of least confusion remains on the retina for both presentations. For example, assume that the patient's refractive error is −2.00/−1.50 × 30. After retinoscopy, best vision sphere and JCC assessment of cylinder axis you have found −2.25/−1.00 × 30. The mean sphere equivalent of each is −2.75 DS, so that the circle of least confusion is on the retina. The crossed cylinder will be used to present +0.25/−0.50 × 30 (lens or picture 1) and −0.25/ +0.50 × 30 (lens or picture 2). Lens 1 will reduce the interval of Sturm and lens 2 will increase it, so that the patient should prefer lens or picture 1. When used to determine the appropriate cylinder axis, the JCC combines with the correcting cylinder to produce an effective cylinder. When the JCC is rotated, the patient is presented with two effective cylinder axes, one of which will be closer to the patient's real axis than the other, which is the lens presentation that they should prefer. The effective axis shift is greater if the power of the correcting cylinder is low: a ±0.25 JCC will shift the effective axis by

Table 4.1 Estimated rotation of the cylinder axis for different cylinder powers when using the ±0.25 Jackson cross-cylinder. This is based on the effective cylinder axis shift created (Bennett & Rabbetts 1998).

Power of the correcting cylinder (DC)	Estimated initial rotation required (±0.25 JCC)
0.25	30°
0.50	20°
0.75	15°
1.00–2.00	10°
2.25+	5°

±22.5° when combined with a −0.50 DC, but will only shift the effective axis by about 7° when combined with a 2.00 DC (Bennett & Rabbetts 1998). Therefore, when making changes based on patient responses to the JCC, the amount of rotation of the correcting cylinder must consider the power of that cylinder (Table 4.1). A series of clips of the Jackson cross-cylinder technique is provided on the website.

4.13.1 Astigmatism

Most patients have a slight amount of astigmatism. This could be due to astigmatism of the anterior and posterior surfaces of the cornea and/or lens and/or due to lens tilt and/or decentration. Large amounts of astigmatism appear to be hereditary (Clementi et al. 1998). Typically, younger patients will have 'with-the-rule' astigmatism, with a steeper vertical meridian (minus cylinder axis between 160–20), probably due to pressure from the eyelids. This lid tension decreases slowly with age, so that 'with-the-rule' astigmatism slowly disappears and older patients typically have 'against-the-rule' astigmatism (minus cylinder axis between 70–110; Baldwin & Mills 1981). Note that this change with age is very slow and any significant refractive correction changes between eye examinations 1–3 years apart are likely to be largely spherical in nature. Significant changes in astigmatism over a 1–3-year period are likely to be due to refraction error at test or retest or possibly due to ocular pathology such as keratoconus, cortical cataract, chalazion, etc. causing significant astigmatic changes (Locke 1987).

4.13.2 Advantages and disadvantages

The JCC provides the practitioner with a sensitive method of determining the power and axis of a cylindrical lens for the correction of both low and high astigmatism. The key disadvantage of this method is that some patients may have difficulty with the sequential presentation of the JCC. On most JCCs (either on phoropters or hand-held), the minus axis is indicated by a red dot and the plus cylinder axis by a white dot. Unfortunately, some UK manufactured JCCs have the minus axis indicated by a white dot and the plus cylinder axis by a red dot.

4.13.3 Procedure

1. Ensure that the best vision sphere is in place so that the circle of least confusion is on the retina: Use the MPMVA (section 4.10) or plus/minus technique (section 4.11) and check the endpoint using the duochrome/bichromatic test (section 4.12). Some practitioners leave younger patients slightly over-minused/under-plussed as they are able to accommodate and bring the circle of least confusion onto the retina.

2. Isolate/indicate a circular letter or a line of letters one row above the present visual acuity. Alternatively, illuminate the Verhoeff rings (wall chart; Fig. 4.11) or the collection of dots target (projector chart). Move the JCC in front of the trial frame/phoropter aperture (Fig. 4.12).

3. Instruct the patient: 'I am going to show you two pictures of the … Both pictures may be slightly blurred, but I want you to tell me which is the clearer of the two pictures, or whether they look the same'.

4. If cylinder was found with retinoscopy, proceed with step 6.

5. If there has been no cylinder found with retinoscopy, then set the JCC so that its minus cylinder axis (red dot) and the perpendicular plus cylinder axis (white dot) assume the 90° and 180° positions. It does not matter which dot is at 90° and 180°. Refer to the current JCC orientation as 'Lens

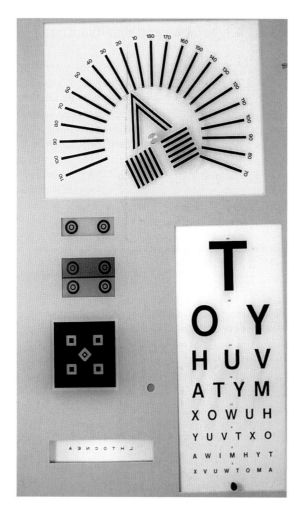

Fig. 4.11   A wall chart. The chart includes (from the top) the fan & block test, the Verhoeff circles for assessment of astigmatism with the Jackson cross-cylinder, the duochrome, a Snellen visual acuity chart, a fixation disparity measurement device, a spotlight and a drum that can be rotated to display other visual acuity lines.

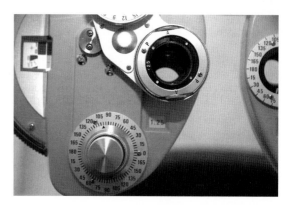

Fig. 4.12   The Jackson cross-cylinder (JCC) on a phoropter. The JCC is set up to assess the correcting cylinder axis.

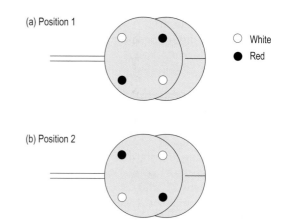

(a) Position 1

○ White
● Red

(b) Position 2

Fig. 4.13   Orientation of the cross-cylinder for axis determination in (a) 'picture (or lens) 1' and (b) 'picture (or lens) 2'.

(or picture) 1'. Flip the JCC to reverse the positions of the minus and plus axes. Refer to this latter orientation as 'Lens (or picture) 2' (Fig. 4.13). Note the orientation of the minus cylinder axis in the position which the patient reported that vision was best. Rotate the JCC so that the plus and minus cylinder axes assume the 45° and 135° positions. Repeat the above comparison and note the orientation of the minus cylinder axis of the chosen lens. If all the lenses seem equally clear, then there is no cylinder. If

certain lens positions are preferred, then set the phoropter cylinder axis at or between the indicated axes (e.g. if minus cylinder was preferred at 180° and 45°, then set the correcting cylinder axis to the approximate midpoint, i.e. 25°). Place −0.25 or −0.50 D cylinder power in the phoropter and proceed with the next step. If you add −0.50 DC in older presbyopes, you should add +0.25 DS to the spherical lens to keep the circle of least confusion on the retina (younger patients should be able to accommodate to maintain the circle of least confusion on the retina).

6. Set the JCC so that the minus cylinder axis and the plus cylinder axis straddle the correcting cylinder axis (Fig. 4.13). With modern phoropters the JCC will click into place at this correct orientation. Ask the patient to compare this initial lens position 'Lens 1', to its flipped counterpart, 'Lens 2' (Fig. 4.13).

7. Adjust the correcting cylinder axes toward the minus cylinder axis (red dot) of the preferred lens position (1 or 2). The amount of rotation typically depends on the size of the cylinder (Table 4.1). This can be tempered by the response from the patient. For example, if the JCC response with a 1.00 DC was very strongly in favour of one lens/picture (and particularly if the visual acuity was reduced so that you suspect the astigmatism after objective refraction was incorrect by a significant amount), it may be better to rotate the cylinder by 10° or 15° rather than the 5° suggested in the table. Similarly, if the JCC response was weak and hesitant, you could make less of a change than that suggested in Table 4.1 (see examples in video clips on the website).

8. Repeat the comparison (use 'Lens 3 . . . or Lens 4', etc.) and continue to adjust the axis dependent on the results. The amount of rotation of the cylinder should be reduced (approximately halved) at each change of the direction of rotation. For example, if a 0.25 DC was initially at 90°, and the JCC indicated a clockwise rotation was required, move it to 60° (Table 4.1). If the JCC then indicates that an anti-clockwise rotation was required, move the cylinder by 15° to the 75° position. Try to keep a mental note of previous decisions made with the JCC to help you 'zero-in' on the final axis. In the example above, if the JCC suggested another anti-clockwise movement was required, there would be little point in rotating the cylinder to 90° as the JCC has already been used at this position. Either 80° or 85° would be more appropriate. Continue

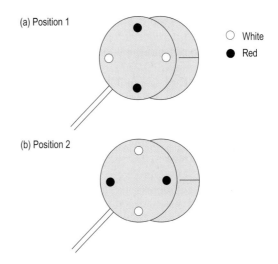

(a) Position 1

○ White
● Red

(b) Position 2

Fig. 4.14 Orientation of the cross-cylinder for power determination in (a) 'picture (or lens) 1' and (b) 'picture (or lens) 2'.

until the patient notices no difference between the two lens positions (or until you have bracketed the axis). Various examples are shown on the website.

9. If the two *initial* lens positions appear the same, confirm that the current axis is the correct one by rotating the cylinder axes off by about the amount suggested in Table 4.1 and have the patient compare Lenses 1 and 2. The patient should return you to the initial axis orientation if it was correct. If they do not, they may have a range of cylinder axes positions in which the JCC positions look the same. In this case, you need to determine the extent of this range and place the cylinder axis in the middle of it (e.g. if the patient reports that the JCC positions look the same at 20° through to 40°, place the cylinder axis at 30°). You could also use a ±0.50 JCC with such patients.

10. Check the cylinder power: Adjust the JCC so that either the minus axis (red dot) or plus axis (white dot) parallels the trial frame/phoropter cylinder axis (the JCC will click into place with modern phoropters). Have the patient compare the relative clarity of Lens 1 to Lens 2 (Fig. 4.14).

11. If the patient reports that there is no perceived difference between the images shown, do not assume you have the correct power. Remove −0.25 D from the cylinder and repeat the comparison. If the initial lens was correct the patient will call for more cylinder by choosing the lens that has the minus cylinder axis (red dot) parallel to the phoropter axis. In this case, increase the cylinder power to its original amount. However, if you remove −0.25 DC and the patient again reports that there is no difference between the two pictures, the patient may have a range of cylinder powers in which the JCC positions look the same. In this case, you need to determine the least amount of cylinder for which the patient notices a difference with the JCC. You could also use a hand-held ±0.50 JCC with such patients.

12. If there is a difference between Lens 1 and 2, then add minus cylinder (−0.25 D) if the patient prefers the minus cylinder axis (red dot) parallel to the phoropter axis. Remove −0.25 DC if the patient prefers the plus cylinder axis parallel to the phoropter axis. Continue this process until no difference between Lens 1 and 2 can be detected or until the power has been bracketed to less than a 0.25 D (choose the least minus cylinder).

13. For each 0.50 D change in cylinder power, change the sphere power by 0.25 D in the opposite direction (e.g. if you add −0.50 DC, then add +0.25 DS before comparing the lens positions). This is to ensure that the circle of least confusion remains on the retina.

4.13.4 Adaptations to the standard technique

Patients do not give perfect answers: The technique described above assumes that the responses provided by patients are always correct. Of course, it is seldom that they are always perfect. This can be detected during the subjective refraction when responses to the JCC can be different at different times, and it can be expected in patients whose responses to other procedures within the eye examination have been poor. It can be useful in such patients to give some 'training' to help patients provide more accurate responses. This can be done by repeatedly presenting the same JCC task to the patient until they start providing the same response each time. If accurate responses are never obtained, you may need to change the power of the JCC as indicated below.

Patients providing unreliable responses: Make sure your instructions are accurate and your technique is good. Particularly in the early stages of training, it is more likely to be your poor technique than unreliable patient responses. Ask a supervisor to help. If a patient is providing unreliable responses or is unable to tell any difference with the ±0.25 JCC, then use a ±0.50 JCC or even larger. A hand-held ±0.50 JCC can be used with a phoropter. If a patient still cannot provide reliable answers, then you may need to use an alternative assessment of astigmatism such as the fan and block test (section 4.14).

Difficulty with three options: It can be difficult for some patients to make a decision when there are three possible options of 'Lens 1', 'Lens 2' or 'the same'. Some clinicians just present two options to the patient and ask whether the image seen with Lens 1 or Lens 2 is better. Using such a technique, the patient often indicates at some point that the two presentations look the same. Alternatively, after the patient has confidently provided several responses of 'Lens 1' or 'Lens 2', they may hesitate and appear unsure. At this point you could ask whether the two presentations look the same.

Patients with reduced visual acuity: If a patient with reduced VA is unable to tell any difference with the ±0.25 JCC, then use a ±0.50 JCC or even a ±1.00 JCC with a trial frame. It is well understood that such procedures should be used for patients with low vision. However, the same applies for any eye with reduced vision (e.g. patients with a unilateral amblyopic eye or unilateral cataract).

Checking the need for a small cylindrical correction: Occasionally, you may be uncertain about the need for a small cylindrical correction. For example, it may be clearly present in retinoscopy but removed during JCC or vice versa. In these situations it can be helpful to simply ask the patient to compare the smallest VA line they can see with and without the cylindrical correction.

4.13.5 Recording

The results of the JCC are not recorded as the technique is just part of the subjective refraction (section 4.9).

4.13.6 Interpretation

Solsona (1975) retrospectively analysed 51 000 patients with astigmatic corrections greater than or equal to 0.75 D and found that 67% had mirror symmetry within 10°. This means that the two axes should add up to approximately 180°: both axes could be 90° or both axes 180° (i.e. 0° and 180°); one axis 175°, the other 5°; one axis 20°, the other 160°; one axis 45°, the other 135°, etc. You may wish to recheck astigmatic axes that do not follow this pattern, particularly if one axis has changed significantly from a previous examination or is significantly different from the retinoscopy result. Although astigmatism changes with age, it rarely changes significantly between eye examinations that are only a few years apart. Significant changes in astigmatism over a 1–3-year period are likely to be due to refraction error at test or retest or possibly due to ocular pathology such as keratoconus, cortical cataract, chalazion, etc. causing significant astigmatic changes (Locke 1987).

4.13.7 Most common errors

1. Using a fast presentation time in older patients whose reaction times may be slightly slower than younger patients. More reliable responses are gained if presentation times are longer and if they are repeated until a consistent response is gained. For this reason, slower presentation times in older patients actually lead to a more efficient and ultimately faster JCC process.

2. Using different presentation times for the two positions. For example, presenting the target for longer in position 2 compared to position 1. The patient should see the two presentations for the same amount of time.

3. Poor alignment of the JCC with the correcting cylindrical lens in the trial frame. This can lead to problems in determining the cylinder axis. Check that the handle of the JCC is in alignment with the axis of the correcting cylindrical lens when determining the cylinder axis.

4. Making large changes to the axis of the trial cylindrical lens in an eye with high astigmatism.

4.14 THE FAN AND BLOCK TEST

The fan and block test (Fig. 4.11) was developed to increase the sensitivity of the earlier fixed astigmatic dials, such as the 'clock' and 'sunburst' dials, and the rotary dials, such as the 'Rotary T'. All lack sensitivity, particularly in determining the cylinder axis. The relatively large 30° gaps between adjacent sets of lines on the clock dial test, for example, significantly limit its sensitivity, and any present-day use appears to be based on tradition (Borish & Benjamin 2006). The fan and block test is only available with wall charts and includes a fixed dial with a rotating arrowhead and blocks and combines the techniques used in the earlier tests.

4.14.1 Alternative procedure for the assessment of astigmatism

The Jackson cross-cylinder (JCC) should not be the only subjective test for the determination of astigmatism that a practitioner has available. Not all patients will be able to respond accurately to the demands of the JCC and the fan and block or similar technique should be used in these cases. In patients where the subjective assessment of astigmatism is poor, it is advisable to consider multiple objective measures of astigmatism from retinoscopy, autorefraction, and (to a lesser degree and if the cylinder is not lens-induced) keratometry. The astigmatism present in the patient's old spectacles should also be considered.

4.14.2 Advantages and disadvantages

An advantage of the test is that, unlike the JCC (where the circle of least confusion is on the retina and one focal line behind the retina), accommodation is well controlled as the patient is fogged prior to the use of the procedure ensuring that the circle of least confusion and both focal lines are in front of the retina. Logic would suggest that the fan and block technique is more accurate than simple cylinder axis rotation (4.14.6), but there are no research studies to confirm this. The fan and block test is believed to be less accurate at determining small cylinders than the Jackson cross-cylinder (JCC), but again there is no firm evidence to support this view.

4.14.3 Procedure

The technique described assumes that you perform the test using the information gained from an objective refraction.

1. Determine the best vision sphere as described in sections 4.10 and 4.11. This ensures the circle of least confusion is on the retina.

2. Occlude the untested eye (i.e. LE, OS).

3. Remove the cylinder determined from retinoscopy from the right eye, and add +0.50 DS to the sphere. The circle of least confusion is now in front of the retina. If the retinoscopy cylinder was correct or overestimated, then both focal lines will be in front of the retina.

4. Draw an analogy between the lines on the fan and the hours of a clock, and ask the patient if any of the lines on the fan appear clearer and darker than the other lines.

5. If the patient reports that all the lines are equally clear (or blurred) then fog by a further +0.50 D and ask the patient again if any lines are clearer and darker. If they remain equally clear or blurred, then this suggests there is no astigmatism present.

6. If some lines are reported as clearer, point the arrow that joins the blocks towards the clearest line. Adjust the arrow until its two barbs appear equally clear. One block (with its lines running parallel with those on the fan which are clearest) should be clearer than the other.

7. Ask the patient to look at the clearer block and add +0.50 DS and ask if the block blurs. If it does blur, continue to step 8. If the block does not blur, it is possible that the retinoscopy result provided a significantly under-corrected cylinder, leaving the back focal line behind the retina after step 3. In this case, additional +0.50 DS lenses should be added until the clearer block just blurs.

8. Set the cylinder axis in the trial frame/phoropter at the axis indicated by the arrow. Add negative cylinder at this axis until the blurred block *just* becomes as clear as the other. If there is a reversal, in that the more blurred block becomes clearer, take the lower cylinder power.

9. Reduce the plus fogging sphere to determine the best sphere as previously explained.

10. Repeat steps 1 to 9 for the left eye.

4.14.4 Recording

The results of the fan and block test are not recorded as the technique is just part of the monocular subjective refraction (section 4.9).

4.14.5 Most common errors

1. Failure to place both sets of focal lines in front of the retina before commencing the fan and block procedure.

4.14.6 Alternative technique: simple axis rotation

Occasionally a patient may provide very inconsistent responses with the JCC. If you are confident of the need for cylinder power (astigmatism noted in retinoscopy and/or autorefraction; reduced VA with the best sphere result), but uncertain about the cylinder axis, simple axis rotation may be useful. The technique simply involves asking the patient to view the smallest line of VA they can see and rotating the

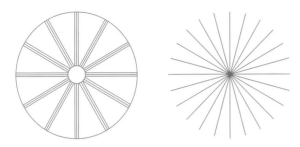

Fig. 4.15   The clock dial and sunburst targets.

correcting cylinder axis clockwise until the patient reports that the letters start to blur. This point should be noted. Then rotate the axis anti-clockwise until the patient again reports that the letters start to blur and note this point. The cylinder axis indicated by the technique is the midpoint between these two blur points. For example, if the two blur points are at 25° and 55°, the indicated cylinder axis is 40°.

4.14.7 Alternative technique: clock dial test

This technique is similar to the fan and block technique, but only consists of the 'fan' (i.e. clock dial) part of the technique (Fig. 4.15a). The technique begins in the same manner as the fan and block steps 1 to 5 (section 4.14.3). The suggested axis is determined by multiplying the smaller of the two clock dial values of the most clear lines by 30. For example, if the patient thinks that the 2 and 8 o'clock lines are the clearest, then put the cylinder axis at 60° (2 × 30). If the patient thinks that the 4 and 10 o'clock lines are clearest, place the cylinder axis at 120°. If the patient believes that two clock dials are clearest, then the axis should be placed midway between the two values indicated. For example, if the patient believes that the 1 o'clock and 2 o'clock lines are clearest, then place the cylinder axis at 45° (1.5 × 30). The cylinder power is then increased until the most blurred lines are brought to the same level of clarity as the most clear lines. The sunburst or fan dial test (Fig. 4.15b) uses a similar technique, but lines are provided at 15° intervals rather than 30°.

4.15 PRISM-DISSOCIATED BLUR BALANCE OF ACCOMMODATION

Prisms are used to provide two images of the test chart, and the test then ensures accommodation in the two eyes is balanced. A video clip of prism-dissociated blur balance is provided on the website.

4.15.1 Binocular balance of accommodation

After a monocular refraction, a binocular balance is required to ensure that accommodation is balanced in the two eyes. This test should not be performed if the patient is monocular, strabismic or has unequal visual acuity and is not necessary if they have no accommodation (patients older than approximately 60 years of age or pseudophakics). A binocular balance of accommodation is also not required after a binocular refraction.

4.15.2 Advantages and disadvantages

There has been little comparison of the various binocular balancing techniques in the research literature (West & Somers 1984). The prism dissociated binocular balance balances accommodation between the two eyes while accommodation is relaxed in both eyes and is widely used with phoropters, where it is relatively easy to use. When using a trial frame, the large number of lens changes needed makes the test awkward and other tests are preferred (section 4.16). Clinical use suggests that the alternate occlusion test for binocular balancing is relatively crude and the prism dissociated (or polaroid dissociated) duochrome test includes all the pitfalls of the duochrome test (section 4.12).

4.15.3 Procedure

1. Occlude the left eye (or ask the patient to close their eyes; the increasing diplopia produced by the prisms can be distressing) and isolate the 20/40 (6/12, 0.5) row of letters.

2. Introduce the Risley prisms before both eyes, so that there is $3^\triangle$ base down before one eye and $3^\triangle$ base up in front of the other eye. It is important that equal prism before each eye is used to equalise any image degradation by the prisms.

3. Add +1.00 DS to the right eye and check whether the 20/40 line is blurred. They should be blurred, but readable. Add further plus power in +0.25 D steps until the 20/40 is just blurred.

4. Remove the occluder (or ask the patient to open their eyes) and ask the patient if they see two 20/40 (6/12, 0.5) lines of letters, one above the other.

5. If the patient cannot see both lines, first check that both apertures are open. If they are, cover each eye in turn, so that the patient can see the position of the line seen by each eye. The patient should then be able to see both targets at the same time. If the patient still cannot see two lines, then one eye is probably suppressing and a binocular balance is not required.

6. Add plus lenses in +0.25 DS steps to the left eye until both eyes have equally blurred images.

7. If a balance cannot be achieved, use the lenses that provide the closest match.

8. Remove +0.25 DS from both eyes, and ask whether the two images remain equally blurred (you may need to isolate the 20/30, 6/9 line for this comparison). If one image is clearer, add +0.25 DS to the eye with the clearer image until both eyes have equally blurred images. If a balance cannot be achieved, use the lenses that provide the closest match.

9. Remove the Risley prisms (ask the patient to close their eyes while this is done) and display the bottom part of the visual acuity chart. Check the visual acuity to ensure that the best acuity line *has not* been achieved.

10. Remove the fog in binocular 0.25 DS steps until you obtain maximum visual acuity. If the patient can read the bottom line of your chart (and this is larger than 20/10, 6/3),

you must allow extra minus/less plus that makes your bottom line of letters 'clearer'. Ensure that the bottom line of letters is 'definitely clearer and not just smaller and blacker'. This must be no more than −0.50 DS more than the refractive correction used to see 20/15 (6/4.5).

11. Measure monocular and binocular VAs, especially if the binocular difference is more than 0.25 D from the monocular subjective. If monocular visual acuity is reduced in one eye following this procedure recheck the results.

4.15.4 Adaptations to the standard technique

The prism-dissociation test balances the images when the eyes are blurred and this may not mean that they are balanced when vision is clear. Goodwin (1966) suggested a modified technique, which uses minimal prism dissociation and balances the images with clear vision or minimal fog (one line worse than best visual acuity).

4.15.5 Recording

The monocular subjective refraction result and the correction after prism dissociated balance can both be recorded with the accompanying VA results. Alternatively, the change in spherical power made with the binocular balance can be recorded. The binocular VA is also measured after the prism balance. For example:

Monocular subjective refraction

OD: +2.75/−0.75 × 175   20/15
OS: +1.75/−0.50 × 10   20/15

Prism balance

OD: +3.00/−0.75 × 175   20/15
OS: +2.00/−0.50 × 10   20/15
OU: 20/15

Monocular subjective refraction

RE: $-1.50/-1.25 \times 160$ 6/4.5

LE: $-1.25/-1.00 \times 20$ 6/4.5

Prism balance: $+0.25$ DS RE

BE: 6/4.5

4.15.6 Interpretation

Typically, binocular balance tests either find no change in refractive correction from the monocular refraction result or find a small amount of additional positive lens power in one eye, or more rarely both. With latent hyperopia there can be a significant increase in the amount of plus accepted with this technique. This is because monocular subjective refraction can lead to possible over-minusing or under-plussing, particularly in patients with hyperopia, pseudomyopia and antimetropia, as the occluder can stimulate accommodation in the non-tested eye and thus an equivalent increase in accommodation in the eye being tested.

The maximum plus to maximum visual acuity (MPMVA) approach used in the prism-dissociation test is designed to take advantage of a patient's depth of focus to provide the maximum range of clear vision (Wang & Ciuffreda 2006). For example, after refraction, the retinal image should be conjugate with the distance VA chart at 6 m (20 ft). However, this does not take advantage of the depth of focus. For example, if the depth of focus was $+0.50$ D and the retinal image was conjugate with the distance VA chart so that 0.25 D of the depth of field was in front of the VA chart and 0.25 D behind it, the chart would be clear from 2.4 m (8 ft) to 'beyond' infinity. Using the MPMVA technique places the distal edge of the depth of focus conjugate with the VA chart (Wang & Ciuffreda 2006). Therefore, if the depth of focus is $+0.50$ D, use of the MPMVA technique ensures that the range of clear vision is from 1.5 m to 6 m (5 to 20 ft). However, using this technique does mean that patients are slightly under-minused or over-plussed by 0.16 D as the distance VA chart is at 6 m (20 ft) and not infinity. This can be offset in young patients due to a lead of accommodation ($+0.25$ DS) during distance refraction (Wang & Ciuffreda 2006), but this does not occur in older patients who have lost accommodation. This effect can be aggravated if a truncated VA chart is used and/or if the patient has a large depth of focus (such as older patients with small pupils) as there will be very slight retinal defocus over the entire range except at the precise point of conjugacy (Wang & Ciuffreda 2006). Over-plussed/under-minused refractive corrections are more commonly found in older patients than under-plussed/over-minused ones (Hrynchak 2006). An indication that this has occurred is that the measured addition is lower than expected in the presbyope.

4.15.7 Most common errors

1. Binocularly balancing pseudophakes or patients over 60 years of age who have no accommodation to balance.

2. Binocularly balancing patients who do not have binocular vision or who have unequal visual acuity.

3. Using a truncated VA chart and not allowing extra minus/less plus that makes your bottom line of letters 'clearer'. This can lead to an over-plussed/under-minused refractive correction, particularly when associated with a MPMVA technique in older patients (Hrynchak 2006).

4.16 MONOCULAR FOGGING BALANCE (MODIFIED HUMPHRISS)

Essentially, this technique uses the plus/minus technique of 'best vision sphere' determination (section 4.11) under binocular conditions after first fogging rather than occluding the non-tested eye.

4.16.1 Binocular balance of accommodation

After a monocular subjective refraction, a binocular balance is required to ensure that accommodation is balanced in the two eyes. This test should not be performed if the patient is monocular or if they have no accommodation (patients older than approximately

60 years of age or pseudophakics). A binocular balance of accommodation is also not required after a binocular refraction.

4.16.2 Advantages and disadvantages

There has been little comparison of the various binocular balancing techniques in the research literature (West & Somers 1984). The monocular fogging technique is preferred for balancing accommodation in a trial frame as the prism dissociation balance technique is awkward to use due to multiple lens changes. Fogging of one eye by a small amount (typically +0.75 DS or +1.00 DS) has several advantages in that it relaxes accommodation and suppresses central vision whilst maintaining peripheral fusion. The dissociation is therefore minimal and various factors such as pupil size and muscle balance remain in their normal binocular state, unlike during monocular refraction. The fogging binocular balance technique is not a true binocular balance technique as it does not compare images from the two eyes and accommodative balance is assumed because the best vision sphere assessment is made in a binocular situation with accommodation relaxed in both eyes due to fogging lenses.

4.16.3 Procedure

1. Fog the left eye until the visual acuity is reduced by three or four lines less than the tested eye. Typically +0.75 DS or +1.00 DS is required.

2. Repeat the best vision sphere assessment for the right eye using the plus/minus technique (section 4.11).

3. If significant positive power needs to be added, such as some patients with latent hyperopia, it is likely that this will relax accommodation in both eyes. To ensure that the amount of fogging lens is still effective add additional plus power to the left eye.

4. Remove the fog from the left eye then fog the right eye by three or four lines and repeat the plus/minus best vision sphere technique for the left eye.

4.16.4 Recording

The amount of any additional plus or minus lenses needed to balance accommodation in each eye is typically recorded after the monocular subjective refraction result. For example:

Monocular subjective refraction

RE: $+2.50/-0.75 \times 175$ 6/4.5

LE: $+1.75/-0.50 \times 10$ 6/4.5

Monocular fogging balance: +0.50 RE, +0.25 LE

BE: 6/4.5

Monocular subjective refraction

OD: $-1.50/-1.25 \times 160$ 20/15

OS: $-1.25/-1.00 \times 20$ 20/15

Monocular fogging balance +0.25 OD

OU: 20/15

4.16.5 Interpretation

Typically, monocular fogging balance either finds no change in refractive correction from the monocular refraction result or finds a small amount of additional positive lens power in one eye, or more rarely both. With latent hyperopia there can be a significant increase in the amount of plus accepted with this technique. This is because monocular subjective refraction can lead to possible over-minusing or under-plussing, particularly in patients with hyperopia, pseudomyopia and antimetropia, as the occluder can stimulate accommodation in the non-tested eye and thus an equivalent increase in accommodation in the eye being tested. It is unusual to find additional minus being required to balance accommodation and usually indicates that there was an error in the monocular refraction.

4.16.6 Most common errors

1. Using too large a fogging lens, such as +1.50 DS or +2.00 DS (as used as a working distance lens

during retinoscopy). It is possible that this degree of retinal image degradation could cause the accommodation system to adopt an open-loop response leading to stimulation of accommodation by around 1.00 D, rather than a relaxation of accommodation (Rosenfield et al. 1994).

4.17 HUMPHRISS IMMEDIATE CONTRAST (HIC)

The HIC is often used as a binocular balancing technique (section 4.16.1) to ensure that accommodation is balanced in younger subjects after monocular subjective refraction. The technique uses a fogging lens in front of the non-tested eye to relax accommodation, but also uses the effects of binocular summation and inhibition of VA to determine the appropriate lens to add to the tested eye. Binocular summation indicates the improvement in VA when viewed binocularly and is relatively small (about 0.1 logMAR or one line of acuity). It occurs when the monocular VAs are normal and equal. As the difference in monocular VA increases, the binocular summation decreases until at some point binocular VA is worse than the best monocular VA (binocular inhibition).

4.17.1 Advantages and disadvantages

As indicated by Humphriss (1988), the HIC technique is not a true binocular balance technique as it does not compare images from the two eyes and accommodative balance is assumed because the best vision sphere assessment is made in a binocular situation with accommodation relaxed in both

eyes due to fogging lenses. The advantages and disadvantages are similar to those of the monocular fogging balance test (section 4.16.2).

4.17.2 Procedure

The following procedure is based on the technique described by Humphriss (1988), although his suggestion of using a 6/12 letter H as the target is omitted. When used as a binocular balance technique a target of maximum visual acuity is preferred.

1. Fog the left eye until visual acuity is reduced by three or four lines less than the tested eye. Young patients with normal vision would usually require adding +0.75 DS or +1.00 DS to give a visual acuity of 6/9 to 6/12 (20/40).

2. Ask the patient to look at the smallest line of letters they can read.

3. Place a +0.25 DS lens in front of the right eye for about 1 second (or longer if the patient appears to need more time) and then replace this with a −0.25 DS for about 0.5 seconds (or half the time given to the +0.25 DS lens).

4. Ask the patient 'Are the letters clearer with Lens 1 . . . or Lens 2?'

5. Examples of the situation occurring in a fully corrected, slightly over-minused and slightly over-plussed eye are shown in Table 4.2. The image seen with each lens is determined by the clarity of the image in the clearer eye, modified by the effects of binocular summation.

Table 4.2 An indication of the changes made to the clearer eye and the interocular difference when either +0.25 DS or −0.25 DS is used with a +1.00 fogging lens in the Humphriss immediate contrast technique.

	With the +0.25 DS lens		With the −0.25 DS lens	
	Clearer eye	Interocular difference	Clearer eye	Interocular difference
Corrected	+0.25 DS	+0.75 DS	−0.25 DS	+1.25 DS
Overminused by −0.25 DS	Plano	+1.00 DS	−0.50 DS	+1.50 DS
Overplussed by +0.25 DS	+0.50 DS	+0.50 DS	Plano	+1.00 DS

6. If the patient immediately reports that the −0.25 DS is definitely clearer, repeat the demonstration of the lenses and ask if the −0.25 DS 'is definitely clearer or just smaller and blacker'. Only add −0.25 DS if the patient immediately reports that the lens is definitely clearer.

7. If the patient reports after some consideration, that the −0.25 DS lens is clearer, do not add −0.25 DS.

8. If the patient reports that the +0.25 DS is clearer or that there is no difference, add +0.25 DS to the refractive correction.

9. Because you have added +0.25 DS to the right eye, it is assumed that accommodation will have been relaxed in both eyes. To ensure that the amount of fogging lens is still effective add +0.25 DS to the left eye.

10. Continue to compare the −0.25 DS and +0.25 DS until the +0.25 DS is immediately rejected.

11. Repeat the procedure on the left eye with the right eye fogged.

4.17.3 Recording and interpretation

The same recording and interpretation as for monocular fogging balance is used (sections 4.16.4 and 4.16.5).

4.17.4 Most common errors

1. Presenting the +0.25 DS and −0.25 DS for an equal amount of time.

2. Failure to modify the fogging lens when a change to the sphere of the fellow eye has been made.

4.18 TURVILLE INFINITY BALANCE (TIB)

The TIB is another binocular balancing technique (section 4.16.1) to ensure that accommodation is

balanced in younger subjects after monocular subjective refraction. It allows comparison of the VA from both eyes when they are dissociated by a septum that is positioned halfway between the patient and the eye chart, typically in the middle of a mirror. In this way, the right eye can only see the right-hand side of the chart and the left eye can only see the left side. This allows simultaneous comparison of the VA chart by the right and left eyes.

4.18.1 Advantages and disadvantages

There has been little comparison of the various binocular balancing techniques in the research literature (West & Somers 1984). The Turville Infinity Balance (TIB) has the advantage that the measurement procedure inherently includes a screening test for decompensated heterophoria and suppression. However, it requires physical movement of the septum on the mirror, which makes it slightly cumbersome.

4.18.2 Procedure

1. Remove the occluder from the trial frame.

2. Ask the patient to occlude their left eye and keep their head steady.

3. Move the septum on the mirror until it covers half the visual acuity chart.

4. Ask the patient to now occlude their right eye and check that they can only see the other half of the chart.

5. With both eyes open, ask the patient to compare the relative clarity of the two sides of the VA chart.

6. If one half of the chart is missing, recheck the position of the septum. If one half is still missing, then one eye is suppressing. Any misalignment of the two halves of the chart may indicate a significant heterophoria. These misalignments should be further investigated using appropriate tests.

7. If one half of the chart is clearer than the other then perform a best vision sphere assessment

(section 4.11) of the eye with the least clear vision.

8. If the two halves of the chart are still not equally clear, perform a best vision sphere assessment of the other eye.

4.18.3 Recording and interpretation

The same recording and interpretation as for monocular fogging balance is used (sections 4.16.4 and 4.16.5). The 6/18 (20/60) letters F & L, which are often provided on the rotating drum on a wall chart, are associated with this test. However, they should not be used when using the TIB to binocular balance, but only when using it as a test to assess heterophoria. If the patient reports seeing a letter E with the TIB F and L targets, they have significant exophoria.

4.18.4 Most common errors

1. Using the F and L letters when binocular balancing using the TIB. These letters are too large to allow subtle differences in accommodation between the two eyes to be detected.

2. Poor alignment of the septum.

3. Allowing the patient to move laterally during the procedure, placing the patient's eyes in the wrong position relative to the septum and visual acuity chart.

4.19 BINOCULAR SUBJECTIVE REFRACTION

4.19.1 Subjective refraction

See section 4.9.1.

4.19.2 Advantages and disadvantages

Subjective refraction should be performed under conditions that simulate the patient's normal viewing situation as closely as possible. For example, pupil size during refraction should ideally resemble the patient's pupil size when they are using their spectacles for detailed viewing tasks, when optimum visual acuity and comfort is required. Normally this would be the pupil size under room illumination with binocular viewing conditions. Larger pupil sizes due to dim room illumination or occlusion of one eye during refraction (such as with monocular refraction) may lead to refractive changes due to spherical aberration. Another major advantage of binocular refraction over monocular refraction is better control over, and greater relaxation of, accommodation. This is particularly important when measuring the refractive error in patients with hyperopia, pseudomyopia and antimetropia. Binocular refraction is also preferred in patients with latent nystagmus and any cyclodeviation. The occluder used in monocular refraction manifests latent nystagmus and makes subjective refraction difficult. The occluder can also manifest any cyclophoria that could lead to an incorrect assessment of astigmatism. Finally, binocular refraction has the advantage of being slightly quicker than monocular refraction because no binocular balancing is required.

Unfortunately, binocular refraction is not possible with a small number of patients. For example, some patients with highly dominant eyes find it very difficult to give good subjective responses with their non-dominant eye during binocular refraction, and these patients are better refracted monocularly. In addition, some binocular refraction techniques provide difficulties for some patients. For example, patients with cataracts can find polaroid binocular refraction difficult because of the reduced illumination provided by the polarised filters. It may not be obvious to inexperienced refractionists which patients will find difficulty with binocular refraction. Finally, binocular refraction only works efficiently if the refractive corrections are reasonably close to the optimal correction at the start of the procedure. Therefore, inexperienced students, whose retinoscopy skills still need practice, should use monocular refraction until their retinoscopy skills improve. Clearly, the technique can only be used with patients who have binocular vision. Refraction can be performed binocularly using monocular fogging (modified Humphriss), Humphriss Immediate Contrast (HIC), and polaroids and using the Turville Infinity Balance (TIB).

The monocular fogging, HIC and TIB techniques for binocular balancing have already been described and their advantages discussed. Monocular fogging refraction can only be used with the plus/minus technique (section 4.11) and JCC, as MPMVA determination of the best vision sphere and fan and block determination of astigmatism require the tested eye to be blurred. Polaroid refraction, with, for example, the AO Vectographic system, uses a chart that has letters on one half polarised at, say, 90 degrees and letters on the other half polarised orthogonally (in this example at 180 degrees). The patient views the chart with Polaroid filters that transmit the letters from one half of the chart to one eye and the other half of the chart to the fellow eye. Light from the background of the chart and a central vertical bar is transmitted to both eyes. This technique provides all the advantages of binocular refraction. Disadvantages include that the light transmitted by the polarising filters is reduced by 50%. This makes the letters of slightly lower contrast than normal and this can be a problem when refracting patients with some conditions such as cataract. Another problem is that it can be difficult to produce polarised letters economically in very small sizes below 20/20 or 20/15 (Borish & Benjamin 2006).

4.19.3 Procedure

1. Explain the procedure to the patient: 'During this test, I will place various lenses in front of your eye to find the lenses that give you the best vision. Don't worry about giving a wrong answer as everything is double checked.'

2. Sit or stand off to the side of the patient so that manipulation of the trial frame/phoropter is easy.

3. Begin with the net retinoscopy sphere–cylinder before each eye. The patient's distance PD should already be set in the phoropter or trial frame, which should be level and positioned appropriately.

4. The subjective refraction traditionally begins on the right eye (or the poorer eye if you determine there may be a poor eye from the case history).

Monocular fogging procedure

1. After retinoscopy, fog the left eye until the visual acuity is reduced by three or four lines less than the tested eye. Typically +0.75 DS or +1.00 DS is required.

2. Determine the best vision sphere using the plus/minus technique (section 4.11) and cylinder power and axis using the JCC (section 4.13). Check the end result sphere using the duochrome (section 4.12) and measure VA.

3. Remove the fogging lens from the untested eye and fog the right eye. Determine the optimal subjective refractive correction in the left eye using the plus/minus technique and JCC and measure VA.

4. Remove the fogging lens.

5. Do not perform a binocular balance as accommodative balance can be assumed. Go to step 6 below

Polaroid refraction procedure

1. Place the polarised filters before both eyes and direct the patient to the chart that is seen by the right eye.

2. Determine the optimal subjective refractive correction in the right eye using your preferred techniques (sections 4.9 to 4.13) and measure VA.

3. Repeat for the left eye after directing the patient to the chart that is seen by the left eye.

4. Remove the polarised filters.

5. Do not perform a binocular balance as accommodative balance can be assumed.

6. Measure binocular VA.

7. Compare monocular VAs with the present subjective refraction result with the patient's vision or habitual VAs (if appropriate). If the VA is better with the patient's spectacles, then it is likely that your subjective result is incorrect. Repeat the subjective refraction (students should perhaps call their supervisor).

8. Compare the VA with the present subjective refraction with age-matched normal data

Table 4.3 Normal age-matched visual acuity data for various notations (from Elliott et al. 1995). The average is shown with 95% confidence limits in brackets.

Age (years)	LogMAR	VAR	Snellen (metric)*	Snellen (imperial)*	Decimal
20–49	−0.14 (−0.02 to −0.26)	107 (101 to 113)	6/4.5 (6/6 to 6/3)	20/15 (20/20 to 20/10)	1.4 (1.0 to 1.8)
50–59	−0.10 (0.00 to −0.20)	105 (100 to 110)	6/5 (6/6 to 6/4)	20/15 (20/20 to 20/12)	1.25 (1.0 to 1.6)
60–69	−0.06 (0.04 to −0.16)	103 (98 to 108)	6/5⁻ (6/6⁻ to 6/4)	20/15⁻ (20/20⁻ to 20/12)	1.15 (0.9 to 1.45)
70+	−0.02 (0.08 to −0.12)	101 (96 to 106)	6/6 (6/7.5 to 6/4.5)	20/20 (20/25 to 20/15)	1.0 (0.8 to 1.3)

* Numbers rounded for simplification.

(Table 4.3). If the VA is worse than expected, or worse in one eye compared to the other, remeasure the VA with a pinhole aperture. If the VA improves with the pinhole, either the patient has media opacity, typically cataract that is being bypassed by the pinhole, or the subjective refraction is not optimal and should be repeated. Note that visual acuity will not always improve with cataract, particularly if the opacity is dense and central.

9. If the final refractive correction in either eye is above 4.00 D mean sphere equivalent (MSE, the sphere plus half the cylinder; e.g. $-3.75/-1.50 \times 180$ has a MSE of -4.50 D, $+4.5 /-2.00 \times 90$ has a MSE of $+3.50$ D), then measure the vertex distance. This is the distance from the back surface of the lens nearest the eye to the apex of the cornea. Back vertex distance can be read from the millimetre scale on the side of the trial frame, from the back vertex distance periscope on the side of the phoropter, or by using a vertex distance gauge.

4.19.4 Adaptations to the standard technique

Patients do not give perfect answers: The techniques listed above and described in the previous sections assume that the responses provided by patients are always correct. Of course, it is seldom that they are always perfect. This can be detected during the subjective refraction when responses to the same changes in spherical power or JCC can be different at different times, or with experience it can be expected in patients whose responses to other procedures within the eye examination have been poor. It can be useful in such patients to give some 'training' to help patients provide more accurate responses. This can be done by repeatedly presenting the same task to the patient (in the best vision sphere assessment or JCC) until they start providing the same response each time. If accurate responses are never obtained, you may need to change the power of the spherical lens changes and/or JCC as indicated below.

Patients providing unreliable responses: Make sure that your instructions are accurate and technique is competent. If a patient is providing unreliable responses or is unable to tell any difference with ±0.25 DS or a ±0.25 JCC, then use ±0.50 DS or a ±0.50 JCC or even larger steps. If responses remain unreliable you may need to use other techniques. It would also be advisable to obtain additional objective information if available.

Patients with reduced visual acuity: Similarly, if a patient with reduced monocular or binocular VA is unable to tell any difference with ±0.25 D, then use ±0.50 DS or a ±0.50 JCC or even larger steps using a trial frame. It is well understood that such procedures should be used for patients with low vision. However, the same applies for any eye with reduced vision (e.g. patients with a unilateral amblyopic eye or unilateral cataract).

Hyperopes, pseudomyopes and antimetropes: In these patients perform a binocular add technique after the binocular balance: place +0.25 DS in front of *both* eyes, and ask if the letters become clearer, more blurred or are unchanged. As before, if the acuity improves or remains the same with the additional plus, then continue adding +0.25 DS binocularly until the acuity first blurs. Stop at the most plus/least minus lens that does not blur the visual acuity. If the binocular visual acuity blurs with the +0.25 DS lenses, then do not add them.

4.19.5 Recording

For example:

Binocular refraction (vertex distance 12 mm)

RE: $-8.00/-1.00 \times 45$	$6/5^{+2}$	
LE: -7.25 DS	$6/5$	BE: $6/5^{+3}$

OD: $+2.75/-0.50 \times 95$	$20/15^{-3}$	
OS: $+2.00/-1.25 \times 82.5$	$20/20^{+1}$	OU: $20/15$

(Vertex distance 12 mm)

OD: $-7.50/-2.25 \times 35$	$20/70$	PHNI
OS: $-8.00/-1.50 \times 150$	$20/20^{+2}$	

Make sure that the prescription details that you provide to patients are clearly legible. Illegible prescription forms have been reported as a surprisingly common error in optometric practice (Steele et al. 2006).

4.19.6 Interpretation

A subjective result that is significantly less positive (more negative) than the retinoscopy result or a subjective result more minus than suggested by unaided visual acuity could indicate latent hyperopia or pseudomyopia and a cycloplegic refraction may be required (section 4.20).

The difference between the patient's own spectacles and the subjective refraction should be compatible with the difference between the habitual (with own spectacles) and optimal VAs. For example, if the patient has a visual acuity of 6/12 in their spectacles and 6/4.5 after subjective refraction, you could expect the subjective refraction to be 1.00 DS more myopic than the spectacle correction ($-0.25 \approx 1$ line of logMAR visual acuity).

Thus, a 6/12 VA with a spectacle correction of $-1.00/-0.50 \times 180$ would suggest a refractive correction of $-2.00/-0.50 \times 180$. If the subjective refraction was $-2.50/-0.50 \times 180$ or even $-3.00/-0.50 \times 180$ this could suggest you have over-minused the subjective refraction. Changes in hyperopic refractive errors are more difficult to explain in this way, as they are dependent on the amount of accommodation the patient has (and therefore their age). Changes in astigmatism that are not due to pathology are usually small.

4.19.7 Most common errors

1. Not monitoring the visual acuity to ensure that a change in lens power results in the expected change in visual acuity.
2. Using poor patient instructions or leading questions.
3. Not checking a subjective refraction that leads to sub-optimal visual acuity with a pinhole.
4. Not recording the vertex distance with a refractive correction above 4.00 DS.

4.20 CYCLOPLEGIC REFRACTION

This involves a determination of the refractive error when the patient's accommodation has been totally or partially paralysed using a cycloplegic drug.

4.20.1 When is a cycloplegic refraction necessary?

A cycloplegic refraction may be necessary if there are any indications of excessive or fluctuating accommodation during the refraction. Accommodative fluctuations can lead to wholly incorrect results of objective and subjective refraction. In addition, excessive accommodation, particularly during subjective refraction, can lead to a very over-minused (or under-plussed) refractive correction. Indeed, a myopic refractive correction can be found in a hyperopic patient due to excessive accommodation during refraction and such patients are defined as pseudomyopes.

The following can indicate the need for a cycloplegic refraction:

■ Accommodative problems suggested in the case history (for example, difficulty changing focus, distance vision blur after a lot of near work).

■ Patients with esotropia or convergence excess esophoria.

■ Accommodative fluctuations indicated by a fluctuating pupil size and/or reflex during retinoscopy.

■ A retinoscopy result significantly more positive (>1.00 DS) than the subjective result.

■ A subjective result significantly more minus (>1.00 DS) than suggested by unaided visual acuity.

■ A patient with myopia and esophoria.

■ Patients with accommodative problems suggested by amplitude of accommodation, dynamic retinoscopy or accommodative facility testing.

Of course, cycloplegic refractions are only used with patients who have accommodation, and usually with those who have the most accommodation: children. The least toxic drug and the lowest dosage (concentration and number of drops) that will produce sufficient cycloplegia should be used. Other assessments of the accommodative system are required (sections 5.17 to 5.19) if the cycloplegic refraction result is unrevealing.

4.20.2 Advantages and disadvantages

Cycloplegic refraction offers the clinician a firm base for objective refraction, as the accommodative system cannot have influence on the refraction result under these conditions. In addition, the dilated pupils occurring due to the cycloplegic provides a superior view of the fundus during ophthalmoscopy. The key disadvantages of cycloplegia are the temporary symptoms of blurred vision and photophobia experienced by patients. The degradation of vision is caused by the abolition of the accommodation response and increase in ocular aberrations as a result of dilated pupils. Adverse effects and allergic reactions to cyclopentolate are rare (Jones & Hodes 1991) and the severe reactions such as psychosis, hallucinations, ataxia and incoherent speech have only been reported for the 2% concentration (or multiple drops of 1%), which should be avoided. In all cases, choose the drug with the least possible adverse effects and the lowest concentration that will allow you to efficiently attain the cycloplegia that you require. For example, research has suggested that cyclopentolate 1% is sufficient to produce good cycloplegia, with an effect similar to atropine 1%, in patients with accommodative esotropia (Celebi & Aykan 1999) and that tropicamide 1% is as effective as cyclopentolate 1% for the measurement of refractive error in most healthy, non-strabismic infants (Twelker & Mutti 2001).

4.20.3 Procedure

1. It is often useful to attempt a 'dry' (non-cycloplegic) binocular refraction first as this can provide very useful information (see interpretation, 4.20.5).

2. Obtain informed consent: Explain why you want to use a cycloplegia and explain the visual effects (near vision blur, pupil dilation and increased light sensitivity) and their duration (dependent on the drug used and the dosage). Also tell the patient that the drops will sting a little initially, but that the stinging will disappear.

3. Unless there are indications that suggest the possibility of a narrow anterior angle (such as high hyperopia or anterior segment abnormality), it may be unnecessary to conduct a full examination of the anterior angle prior to cycloplegic installation. Cycloplegia is typically performed on young children who will have wide anterior angles due to the thin nature of the lens in childhood. The 'shadow test' (section 6.12) is easier to perform with young children and will often suffice.

4. Instil an appropriate cycloplegic drug (section 6.17).

5. Ask the patient to sit in the waiting room for about 20 (tropicamide) to 30 minutes

(cyclopentolate) until the drug has obtained maximum or near maximum effect. Check that sufficient reduction in accommodation has been obtained by quickly checking the patient's amplitude of accommodation. Anisocoria could indicate unequal cycloplegia. Add another drop if sufficient accommodation reduction has not been obtained.

6. Perform retinoscopy and/or autorefraction in the usual way. If subjective refraction is not possible, it is useful to have both objective measures. When performing retinoscopy, you must concentrate on the central 3–4 mm of the pupil. The peripheral part of the pupil may show a different reflex motion due to aberrations and these should be ignored. Often, a cycloplegic refraction is performed on young children, so that the refraction ends after retinoscopy and/or autorefraction.

7. Subjective refraction should be attempted if possible.

4.20.4 Recording

Record the cycloplegic used and the time of installation. Then record the refraction results (retinoscopy and subjective if both used) in the standard manner, with the approximate time of the refraction. As an alternative to noting the times of installation and refraction, you could note the period of time the refraction was performed after installation of the cycloplegic. For example:

2.30 p.m.: 2 drops cyclopentolate 0.5%.

Retinoscopy, 3.00 p.m.:	RE: +2.00 DS	$6/6^{-2}$
	LE: +1.75/−0.50 × 180	$6/6^{-3}$

1 drop tropicamide 1%, refraction 20 minutes after installation.

Retinoscopy:	OD: +1.75/−1.00 × 170	$20/20^{-2}$
	OS: +1.25/−0.50 × 7.5	$20/20^{-1}$

Subjective:	OD: +1.50/−1.00 × 170	$20/20^{-1}$
	OS: +1.00/−0.50 × 7.5	20/20

4.20.5 Interpretation

Clearly there are limitations to many of the measurements made in 'dry' (non-cycloplegic) refractions of patients with excessive or fluctuating accommodation, but there are also limitations in 'wet' (cycloplegic) refractions and all must be considered when prescribing and deciding on the best patient management. During wet retinoscopy it is vital to concentrate on the reflex in the central 3–4 mm and ignore the reflex in the periphery that is influenced by peripheral aberrations. For this reason it can be particularly useful to obtain two objective measures of cycloplegic refractive and use both retinoscopy and autorefraction. Autorefraction provides a particularly accurate assessment of refractive correction under cycloplegia in children (Walline et al. 1999, Zhao et al. 2004). Also note that the cycloplegic VA is likely to be slightly reduced compared to the VA after a dry refraction due to the peripheral aberrations.

In some patients, the VA after dry retinoscopy can provide useful information about the VA the patient will likely obtain in new spectacles if the full cycloplegic refraction is prescribed. During retinoscopy there is little stimulus for patient accommodation, unlike during subjective refraction, so that the retinoscopy result is typically significantly more hyperopic (or less myopic) than subjective. Therefore, the VA measured after dry retinoscopy is often reduced. However, note that this is because the patient cannot appropriately relax their accommodation during the subjective refraction and the refractive correction found with retinoscopy is likely to be more accurate. It is important to record both the retinoscopy result and the subsequent VA as it can give an indication of the likely distance VA with any new spectacles. Here is an example.

The 12-year-old patient complains of distance vision blur and frontal headaches after a lot of close work.

Dry retinoscopy:	RE: +1.50/−0.50 × 165	$6/18^{-1}$
	LE: +1.75/−0.75 × 15	$6/12^{-2}$

Dry subjective:	RE: −0.25/−0.50 × 170	6/5
	LE: Plano/−0.75 × 15	$6/5^{-2}$

Autorefraction:	RE: Plano/−0.50 × 170	$6/6^{-1}$
	LE: +0.25/−0.75 × 12.5	$6/6^{-2}$

This large reduction in hyperopia from retinoscopy to dry subjective is indicative of active accommodation during the subjective refraction. In this particular case the subject has become a slight pseudomyope. The difference between a pseudomyope and latent hyperope is small; both are due to accommodative spasm, but the latent hyperope is hyperopic in the dry subjective and the pseudomyope is myopic. Due to proximal accommodation effects, these types of patients provide autorefractor results more similar to the dry subjective results than to retinoscopy. Clearly a cycloplegic refraction is required:

Grade IV (Shadow test), 2 drops cyclopentolate 0.5% (2.30 pm):

3.00 p.m. wet refraction:

Retinoscopy:	RE: +2.00/−0.50 × 180	$6/6^{-3}$
	LE: +2.00 /−0.50 × 180	$6/6^{-2}$
Subjective:	RE: +1.75 /−0.50 × 175	6/6
	LE: +1.75 /−0.50 × 5	6/6
Autorefraction:	RE: +2.00 /−0.50 × 165	$6/6^{-1}$
	LE: +1.75 /−0.75 × 10	6/6

The cycloplegic results confirm that the dry subjective and dry autorefractor results were incorrect and due to the patient's inability to relax accommodation. What should you prescribe? The dry retinoscopy results indicate that if you prescribed the full cycloplegic result, the patient would initially see about 6/18 in each eye. Without the cycloplegic, the patient would be unable to relax accommodation and would see very poorly in the distance. This would improve over time as the hyperopic spectacles helped the patient to relax accommodation, but the blur could be a disincentive to initially wearing the spectacles and this should be considered. A compromise prescription may work:

RE: +1.00/−0.50 × 165   LE: +1.00/−0.75 × 10

This is likely to initially blur distance VA to about 6/9+, which the patient should be able to cope with, yet will sufficiently relax the accommodation to improve the patient's symptoms. The patient should be seen within about a month and the prescription could be increased at that point if required. The effect on symptoms, visual acuity and binocular vision should be considered when deciding on the amount of hyperopia to correct in a young person with accommodation.

The wet subjective result could also be influenced by aberrations from the outer edges of the dilated pupil (Tuan et al. 2005) and this influence must be considered when determining what to prescribe. Even more than for routine refraction results, you should not automatically prescribe the results found in cycloplegic refraction to the patient, although this may be required for patients with accommodative esotropia. A reduced amount of plus power is usually prescribed to compensate for ciliary muscle tonus. For infants and young children, a full hyperopic correction may not be given because of the small eye error and the fact that hyperopia is normal for infants.

4.20.6 Most common errors

1. Neutralising the retinoscopy reflex seen for the whole of the pupil. The edges of the reflex should be ignored, and the practitioner should concentrate on the centre of the pupil when interpreting retinoscopy reflex movements.

4.20.7 Alternative procedure: Mohindra near retinoscopy

Mohindra near retinoscopy was developed as an alternative to cycloplegic refraction in children and infants (Mohindra 1977). It may be used when a cycloplegic refraction is contraindicated or when it is extremely difficult to instil the drops. A dim retinoscope light is used as a fixation target and seen in complete darkness it provides little stimulus to accommodation, so that patients assume their resting focus due to tonic accommodation. This is typically +0.75 DS, so that when working at 50 cm, −1.25 DS rather than the standard −2.00 DS (i.e. the working distance lens) is added to the final retinoscopy result (Mohindra 1977). You need to dim the retinoscope light as low as possible while ensuring it still provides you with an easily visible retinoscopy reflex. Turn off all room lights and perform retinoscopy using a lens rack or individual trial case lenses. An infant will only hold a steady gaze for a short period of time, so that you need to perform the test quickly. The standard technique is to occlude the non-fixating eye using your hand or the parent's hand. However, this can cause infants to become agitated and even begin to cry (Twelker & Mutti 2001), so that performing the test binocularly may be preferable in some cases. Some studies that have compared Mohindra near retinoscopy with cycloplegic retinoscopy have indicated that the test is variable and should not be used (see discussion in Twelker & Mutti 2001) and others have suggested that the test is comparable to cycloplegic retinoscopy (e.g. Saunders & Westall 1992). It would appear that to become competent with the technique, one needs to perform it regularly and this is a disadvantage for the primary care optometrist who only occasionally examines an infant (Twelker & Mutti 2001). Saunders & Westall (1992) recommend adding −0.75 DS for infants (<2 years) and −1.00 DS for children (over 2 years) rather than the original −1.25 DS.

4.21 TENTATIVE READING ADDITION USING CALCULATIONS

A determination of the reading addition begins with a tentative addition being determined prior to refinement. This is similar to using an objective measurement of refractive correction (retinoscopy, autorefraction) as a starting point for subjective refraction of the distance correction. Estimating the addition from the patient's age for near has been shown to provide a more accurate tentative addition than more time-consuming measurement techniques (Hanlon et al. 1987). Using an assessment of the patient's symptoms in combination with their habitual refractive correction is similar to the 'gold standard' technique used by Hanlon and colleagues and could be used by experienced clinicians.

4.21.1 Presbyopia and the reading addition

About the age of 40–45 years of age (earlier for some ethnic groups, people with short arms or working distances and hyperopes, later for people with long arms/working distances and myopes; Millodot & Millodot 1989, Pointer 1995) most people become presbyopic. This means that they do not have enough accommodation to be able to

read or do other near work clearly and comfortably. These patients require a positive lens addition to the distance refractive correction. This is called the reading or near addition. With increasing age and further losses in accommodation, the power of the reading addition needs to be increased. At about 55 years, accommodation is essentially zero (what can be measured clinically is probably depth of focus; Charman 1989). After this age the reading addition still needs to be increased, probably to compensate for the loss of visual acuity with age (MacMillan et al. 2001), although at a slower rate (Blystone 1999, Pointer 1995; Fig. 4.16).

4.21.2 Advantages and disadvantages

In a very useful study, Hanlon et al. (1987) determined the required reading addition of 37 dissatisfied patients who returned to a university clinic due to improper add power. From the case history information in the review (recheck) examination, it was determined whether the improper addition was too low or too high. For each patient, their reading addition was then determined using four methods (age, 1/2 amplitude of accommodation, NRA/PRA balance and binocular cross-cylinder). The percentage of additions for each test that gave the same result as

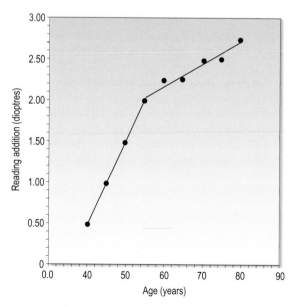

Fig. 4.16 Average near addition as a function of age from the data of Pointer (1995) and Blystone (1999).

the improper addition or worse (higher than an improper addition determined too high or lower than an improper addition determined as too low) was determined. They reported that the simplest and quickest test, asking the patient their age, accounted for the fewest errors (14%). The other techniques gave errors in 61% (binocular cross-cylinder), 46% (NRA/PRA) and 30% (1/2 amplitude) of cases. This suggests that for most patients the tentative addition should simply be based on age. Another alternative, particularly for experienced clinicians, would be to use the patient's symptoms with their old near correction, which is similar to the test used by Hanlon and colleagues to determine if additions were low or high, i.e. their gold standard test.

4.21.3 Procedure

Estimate the tentative reading addition by age and working distance.

1. For patients less than 60 years of age: Age is a good predictor of the tentative addition (Hanlon et al. 1987). Suggested values that are given in Table 4.4 were taken from the data of Pointer (1995) and Blystone (1999) and are similar to the values used by Hanlon and colleagues (1987). If the working distance is much less than 40 cm, increase the tentative addition appropriately. For example, if the working distance is about 33 cm, increase the addition by +0.50 (the difference in dioptric terms between 40 cm or 2.50 D and 33 cm or 3.00 D). If the addition is needed for computer work and therefore the working distance is about 50–60 cm, decrease the tentative addition by about +0.50 DS.

Table 4.4 Tentative near addition estimates as a function of age up to the age of 60 years. These estimates should be adjusted for working distances. Patients with longer working distances will need a slightly smaller add and vice versa.

Patient age (years)	Tentative add (D)
45	+1.00
50	+1.50
55	+2.00
60	+2.25

2. For patients over 60 years of age: After age 60, accommodation is essentially zero, and the reading addition is determined mainly by the patient's working distance, with a small reduction made to allow for depth of focus (MacMillan et al. 2001). The age norm data shown in Figure 4.16 for patients over 60 years of age essentially show the average dioptric working distance for older patients. Average near working distances get smaller with age with the reduced working distances being used as a strategy to offset the effects of age-related vision loss (McMillan et al. 2001, Millodot & Millodot 1989). Rather than use an average dioptric working distance for all patients over 60 years, it is much more efficient to estimate a tentative reading addition from an individual patient's working distance. In this way, working distances of 50, 40 or 33 cm (dioptric values +2.00, +2.50 and +3.00) indicate tentative additions of +1.75, +2.25 or +2.50 DS respectively, with higher additions allowing slightly more for depth of focus (McMillan et al. 2001). It can be useful to use a chair without arm rests or tilt the arm rests out of the way when measuring the patient's near working distance as they can influence the measurement. It can also be useful to measure the near working distance with the patient initially blurred (i.e. without a tentative reading addition) or with their eyes closed so that they hold the chart at their habitual distance and are not influenced by any tentative addition provided. You should remind the patient to hold the near VA chart at the distance they would like to read/work at rather than the distance they may have adopted to be able to see clearly.

4.21.4 Alternative procedure

This technique involves using the patient's symptoms and the power of the habitual near correction to estimate the appropriate tentative reading addition and can be used by experienced clinicians. It is best described by using some examples.

Table 4.5   Tentative addition based on patient symptoms and habitual near correction from example 1.

	Symptoms regarding near vision	Tentative addition	Tentative addition
1	Difficulty reading, blurred near vision, easier if near work held further away	One that provides NV Rx of +2.75 DS	+1.25 DS
2	No problems	One that provides NV Rx of +2.25 DS	+0.75 DS
3	Difficulty reading, has to hold too close to be able to read easily	One that provides NV Rx of +1.75 DS	+0.25 DS

Example 1

A 50-year-old patient, case history indicates they have 'difficulty reading', that it is 'easier reading further away' and that they 'need longer arms'. The patient would like to read comfortably at 40 cm.

Present spectacles:

RE: +1.00 DS   6/9

LE: +1.00 DS   6/9

Reading addition +1.25 D. N5 with difficulty R & L.

(The refractive correction for near is therefore RE: +2.25 DS, LE +2.25 DS.)

Students must remember that patients read through their near vision correction (distance refractive correction + reading addition) and *not* their reading addition. Given that the average change in distance spherical refractive correction with age in presbyopes who do not develop nuclear cataract is a hyperopic shift (Guzowski et al. 2003), a common change for the patient in the example above is for the distance correction to change to:

RE: +1.50 DS

LE: +1.50 DS.

With the new distance correction, the tentative addition would be estimated as shown in Table 4.5.
   In this case an appropriate tentative addition would be +1.25 D.
   Although the reading addition has not changed, the near vision refractive correction has increased to +2.75 DS and would likely alleviate the symptoms.

Example 2

A 60-year-old patient, case history indicates they have 'difficulty reading', that it is 'slightly easier reading further away'. The patient would like to read comfortably at 40 cm.
   Present spectacles:

OD: +1.25/−0.75 × 90   20/20

OS: +1.00/−0.50 × 90   20/20

Reading addition +1.75 D. 20/30 OD & OS @ 40 cm.

(The mean sphere equivalent of the near correction is about +2.62 OD and 2.50 OS.)

   If the distance refractive correction undergoes a very small hyperopic shift and a slight change in astigmatism, then the new distance refractive correction could become:

OD: +1.25/−0.50 × 85   20/15^{-2}

OS: +1.25/−0.50 × 95   20/20^{+3}

This changes the mean sphere equivalent of the distance refractive correction to +1.00 DS, so that appropriate tentative additions would be as shown in Table 4.6.
   In this case an appropriate tentative addition would be +2.00 D.
   Both the hyperopic distance correction and the reading addition have increased slightly and the near vision refractive correction has increased to approximately +3.25/−0.50 × 90 and would likely alleviate the symptoms. By far the most common change in refractive error with age after the age of 40 is either an increase in hyperopia (Guzowski et al. 2003) and/or presbyopia (Pointer 1995). Therefore

Table 4.6 Tentative addition based on patient symptoms and habitual near correction from example 2.

	Symptoms regarding near vision	Tentative addition	Tentative addition
1	Difficulty reading, blurred near vision, easier if near work held further away	One that provides NV Rx of ≈+3.00 DS	+2.00 DS
2	No problems	One that provides NV Rx of ≈+2.50 DS	+1.50 DS
3	Difficulty reading, has to hold too close to be able to read easily	One that provides NV Rx of ≈+2.00 DS	+1.00 DS

Table 4.7 Tentative addition based on patient symptoms and habitual near correction from example 3.

	Symptoms regarding near vision	Tentative addition	Tentative addition
1	Difficulty reading, blurred near vision, easier if near work held further away	One that provides NV Rx of +2.75 DS	+3.25 DS
2	No problems	One that provides NV Rx of ≈+2.25 DS	+2.75 DS
3	Difficulty reading, has to hold too close to be able to read easily	One that provides NV Rx of ≈+1.75DS	+2.25 DS

the most common symptoms regarding near vision are that patients have 'difficulty reading', that it is 'easier reading further away' and even that they 'need longer arms' as discussed above. This could be alleviated by an increase in hyperopia as described in Example 1 or by an increase in the reading addition if there is no change in the distance refractive correction or by a small increase in both as described in Example 2.

Example 3

Some patients develop nuclear cataract with age and this can lead to a myopic shift to the distance prescription. These patients may complain that they have to bring their near work closer than they used to, to be able to read comfortably. As the myopic shift continues they may start finding that they can read better without spectacles (the so-called 'second sight of the elderly'). For example:

72-year-old patient. Case history indicates she has 'difficulty reading', and that she 'has to bring the paper in closer to read it comfortably'. The patient would like to read comfortably at about 40 cm.

Present spectacles and habitual VA:

OD: +0.25/−0.50 × 95   20/30
OS: +0.25/−0.50 × 85   20/30

Reading addition +2.25 D. OD & OS: 20/20 @ 30 cm.

(The mean sphere equivalent of the near correction is therefore +2.25 DS.)

If the distance refractive correction undergoes a small myopic shift, then the new distance correction could become:

RE: −0.25/−0.50 × 100   20/15^{-3}
LE: −0.25/−0.50 × 90   20/15^{-2}

This changes the mean sphere equivalents of the distance refractive correction to −0.50 DS, so that appropriate tentative additions would be as shown in Table 4.7.

In this case an appropriate tentative addition would be +2.25 D.

Although the reading addition has not changed, the near vision refractive correction has decreased

Table 4.8   Tentative addition based on patient symptoms and habitual near correction for example 4.

	Symptoms regarding near vision	Tentative addition	Tentative addition
1	Difficulty reading, blurred near vision, easier if near work held further away	One that provides NV Rx of +3.50 DS	+3.50 DS
2	No problems with near vision	One that provides NV Rx of ≈+3.00 DS	+3.00 DS
3	Difficulty reading, has to hold too close to be able to read easily	One that provides NV Rx of ≈+2.50 DS	+2.50 DS

to approximately $+1.75/-0.50 \times 90$ and would likely alleviate the symptoms.

Example 4

Some patients with nuclear cataract and refractive change partly adapt to a slightly closer reading distance as the closer distance provides a little magnification to help with reduced visual acuity due to the cataract.

For example:

75-year-old patient. Case history indicates she has 'poor distance vision, but near vision is OK'.

Present spectacles and habitual VA:

OD: +0.50 DS   20/30

OS: +0.75/−0.50 × 105   20/30

Reading addition +2.50 D. OD & OS: 20/30 @ 30 cm.

The previous record may indicate that a longer near working distance was used at that time, but with the change in distance correction the effective addition in their current spectacles is +3.00 D so a nearer working distance is used.

If the distance refractive correction undergoes a small myopic shift, then the new distance correction could become:

RE: Plano   20/15^{-3}

LE: +0.25/−0.50 × 90   20/15^{-2}

This changes the mean sphere equivalent of the distance refractive correction to 0.00 DS, so that appropriate tentative additions would be as shown in Table 4.8.

In this case an appropriate tentative addition would be +3.00 D.

Although the patient has no problems with near vision, the reading addition must be increased to compensate for the cataract-induced minus shift in the distance correction to provide the same refractive correction at near in the old spectacles. Leaving the reading addition the same at +2.50 DS, under the misapprehension that this would provide the same near correction as in the old spectacles, would leave the patient under-plussed by +0.50 DS. An under-plussed near correction, particularly in patients with nuclear cataract, has been shown to be a cause of patients rejecting new spectacles (Hrynchak 2006).

4.21.5 Recording

Record the tentative addition and the method(s) of determination (when an undergraduate student). This is not usually necessary when experienced unless you are using a variety of tentative addition tests and want to keep a track of which tests were used for each individual patient. For example:

Tentative addition (age) = +2.00 DS.

4.21.6 Interpretation

Most additions are equal for the two eyes. Unequal additions require further testing: either a retest of the near addition endpoints used for each eye or a recheck of the distance binocular balance.

4.21.7 Most common errors

1. Estimating the tentative addition on the basis of the reading addition in their habitual

correction, rather than the refractive correction for near.

2. Estimating the tentative addition of a patient over 60 based on their age and not their working distance. For example, a very tall 70-year-old patient with a working distance of 50 cm (dioptric value 2.00 D) will not appreciate a reading addition of +2.50 D, as it is too strong.

3. Not considering the effect of reduced visual acuity when prescribing a sufficient near addition.

4.22 TENTATIVE READING ADDITION USING ASSESSMENTS OF ACCOMMODATION

A determination of the reading addition begins with a tentative addition being determined prior to refinement. This is similar to using an objective measurement of refractive correction (retinoscopy, autorefraction) as a starting point for subjective refraction of the distance correction. Given that a reading addition is required because of the reduction in the amplitude of accommodation with age, it seems logical that an assessment of the accommodation available would provide a useful starting point to determine the reading addition. Subjective tests to determine the tentative addition include the fused cross-cylinder, plus build-up, based on a proportion of the amplitude of accommodation and negative relative accommodation/positive relative accommodation (NRA/PRA) balance. Dynamic retinoscopy can be used when subjective responses are poor (section 5.18).

4.22.1 Presbyopia and the reading addition

See section 4.21.1.

4.22.2 Advantages and disadvantages

The subjective accommodation tests provide a tentative reading addition estimate for both eyes. Unequal estimates of the reading addition in the two eyes can indicate that the distance refractive correction has not been adequately balanced and needs to be rechecked. This 'double checking' of the distance refraction in presbyopes is not provided if the tentative addition is based on calculations (section 4.21) and can be an advantage to inexperienced refractionists. The disadvantage of the subjective accommodation tests is that they are time-consuming and do not appear to provide as accurate an estimate of the final reading addition as just asking the patient their age and using a suitable age/reading addition conversion table (Hanlon et al. 1987). Hanlon and colleagues determined the required reading addition of 37 dissatisfied patients who returned to their university clinic due to improper addition power. From the case history information in the review (recheck) examination, it was determined whether the improper addition was too low or too high. For each patient, their reading addition was then determined using four methods (1/2 amplitude of accommodation, NRA/PRA balance and binocular cross-cylinder, patient age). The percentage of additions for each test that gave the same result as the improper addition or worse (higher than an improper addition determined too high or lower than an improper addition determined as too low) was determined. They reported that the simplest and quickest test, asking the patient their age, accounted for the fewest errors (14%). The other techniques gave errors in 61% (binocular cross-cylinder), 46% (NRA/PRA) and 30% (1/2 amplitude) of cases. This suggests that for most patients the tentative addition should simply be based on age. Another alternative, particularly for experienced clinicians, would be to use the patient's symptoms with their old near correction (similar to the test used by Hanlon and colleagues to determine if additions were low or high, i.e. their gold standard test). Another study to confirm these findings, preferably with a larger sample size, would be very useful.

4.22.3 Procedure: tentative addition as a proportion of the amplitude of accommodation

This is most useful for presbyopes less than 55 years of age. In older patients, their accommodation is essentially zero and age-related pupillary miosis means that any measurement of amplitude of accommodation essentially measures their depth of focus, and the rules become less useful.

1. Measure the amplitude of accommodation using the push-up/push-down method described in section 5.17.

2. Calculate the tentative reading addition from the following calculation.

3. Tentative reading addition = working distance in dioptres $-1/2$ of the amplitude of accommodation in dioptres (some clinicians subtract 2/3 of the amplitude).

4.22.4 Procedure: binocular or fused cross-cylinder

1. Adjust the phoropter to the near PD, occlude the untested eye (typically OS) and position the cross-hatch target at the patient's working distance (or 40 cm).

2. If the patient has significant astigmatism ($>\approx1.50$ DC), check that the horizontal and vertical lines of the target appear equally clear. If they do not, the astigmatic correction should be rechecked at distance. If equal clarity can still not be achieved, the astigmatic correction should be checked at near.

3. Dial the cross cylinder ($+0.50/-1.00 \times 90$) into the phoropter.

4. If the expected addition is high ($>+2.00$ DS) add $+1.00$ DS to the distance correction. Ask the patient to close their eyes while you dial the extra power into the phoropter.

5. Ask the patient: 'Are the lines running up and down or those running from side-to-side clearer?' The presbyopic patient should report that the horizontal lines are clearer.

6. Add plus lenses in $+0.25$ DS steps until the patient reports that the vertical lines are just clearer than the horizontal.

7. Repeat steps 2 to 6 for the other eye.

8. If the tentative addition for each eye differs, recheck the results. If they remain different,

the binocular balance of the distance refractive correction should be rechecked.

9. Allow both eyes to see the target and reduce the plus power in both eyes until the horizontal and vertical targets appear equally clear.

4.22.5 Procedure: balancing negative and positive relative accommodation (NRA/PRA)

1. Adjust the phoropter to the near PD and attach the near point card. Make sure that the optimal distance refractive correction is in place and that both eyes can view the near point card.

2. Direct the patient's attention to letters one or two lines larger than their best near VA on the near point card. Ask the patient if they are clear. If they are not clear, add plus sphere power, $+0.25$ D at a time, until the patient reports that the letters are clear. This becomes the 'initial tentative near addition'.

3. Negative relative accommodation (NRA): Add plus lenses binocularly, $+0.25$ D at a time, until the patient reports the first sustained blur. 'First sustained blur' means that the patient notices that the letters are not as sharp and clear as they were initially, even if the patient can still read them. The total amount of plus added is the NRA.

4. Return the lenses in the phoropter to the 'initial tentative near addition' found in (2).

5. Positive relative accommodation (PRA): Add minus lenses binocularly, -0.25 D at a time, until the patient reports the first sustained blur. The total amount of minus added is the PRA.

6. Adjust the 'initial tentative near addition' that would provide equality for NRA and PRA. The adjusted figure is the 'final tentative addition'. For example, if the 'initial tentative near addition' was $+1.00$ and sustained blur points were found with a $+2.00$ and a $+0.50$ add, the NRA would be $+1.00$ ($2.00 - 1.00$)

and the PRA would be -0.50 ($0.50 - 1.00$). A 'final tentative near addition' of $+1.25$ DS would equalise the NRA and PRA (they would both be 0.75 DS). The change suggested by the NRA/PRA is their algebraic sum divided by two. In this example, that would be $0.50/2 = +0.25$ DS.

4.22.6 Recording

Record the tentative addition and the method(s) of determination when an undergraduate student. This is not usually necessary when experienced unless you are using a variety of tentative addition tests and want to keep a track of which tests were used for each patient. For example:

Tentative addition (X-cyl) = $+1.50$ DS

Tentative addition (NRA/PRA) = $+2.25$ DS.

4.22.7 Most common errors

1. The research literature suggests that it is more accurate to base the tentative addition on the patient's age, so that the use of these techniques does not seem to be of great value.

2. Inappropriate choice of working distance for determining the near addition.

4.23 TRIAL FRAME DETERMINATION OF A READING ADDITION AND RANGE OF CLEAR VISION

4.23.1 Presbyopia and the reading addition

About the age of 40–45 years of age (earlier for some ethnic groups, people with short arms or working distances and hyperopes, later for people with long arms/working distances and myopes; Millodot & Millodot 1989, Pointer 1995) most people become presbyopic. This means that they do not have enough accommodation to be able to read or do other near work clearly and comfortably.

These patients require a positive lens addition to the distance correction. This is called the reading or near addition. With increasing age and further losses in accommodation, the power of the reading addition needs to be increased. At about 55 years, accommodation is essentially zero (what can be measured clinically is probably depth of focus; Charman 1989). After this age the reading addition still needs to be increased (probably to compensate for the loss of visual acuity with age; MacMillan et al. 2001), although at a slower rate (Blystone 1999, Pointer 1995; Fig. 4.16).

4.23.2 Advantages and disadvantages

An incorrect reading addition is a common cause of patients' unhappiness with their new spectacles (Hanlon et al. 1987), although progressive addition lenses may have decreased the number of problems in recent years as they are more forgiving of over-plussed near corrections (Hrynchak 2006). To help to avoid such complaints, it is important to determine the range of clear near vision required by the patient and prescribe spectacles that fulfil those requirements. It is difficult to determine appropriate near working distances and ranges in a phoropter and an addition determination using a trial frame with trial case lenses is recommended. A determination of the reading addition begins with a tentative addition being determined prior to refinement.

4.23.3 Procedure

A concise summary of the complete procedure for the determination of the reading addition is provided in Box 4.2.

1. If you have determined the distance refractive correction in a phoropter, add the distance correction to the trial frame using trial case lenses.

2. Keep the room lights on, but do not use additional lighting unless this is used by the patient or is necessary. Textbooks often suggested that additional lighting should be directed toward the near card for determining the reading addition. However, it is probably

Box 4.2   Summary of the near addition procedure

1. Add the distance correction to the trial frame using trial case lenses.

2. Ask the patient if they read in normal room lighting or with an additional 'reading' light and use additional lighting if indicated.

3. Determine the near visual tasks the patient would like to perform and the relevant working distances.

4. Explain the procedure to the patient.

5. Ask the patient to hold the near VA chart at the distance they would like to read/ work at.

6. Determine a tentative addition. This is most easily obtained from the patient's age (if less than 60 years of age) or from their working distance (if over 60 years).

7. Determine the final addition by the preferred working distance or trial lens method.

8. Determine the range of clear vision with the binocular reading add.

9. If you are unable to obtain a range that encompasses all the required near working tasks, consider a progressive addition lens, compromise near addition or an intermediate addition.

10. Record the final addition(s), acuity and range of clearest vision obtained with the addition(s).

better to determine the reading addition required in lighting conditions similar to those regularly used by the patient. Ask the patient if they read in normal room lighting or with an additional 'reading' light and only use additional lighting if the patient indicates they use such lighting at home.

3. Explain the procedure to the patient: 'I am now going to determine the power you need for your reading glasses/bifocal/progressive lens.' You should know from the case history what near vision tasks the patient performs. If you do not, ask for this information now. Ask the patient to hold the reading card at their preferred near working distance(s) and measure this distance. For example, you may need to determine at what distances a patient sews, reads and uses their computer. It can be useful to measure the near working distance with the patient initially blurred (i.e. without a tentative reading addition) or with their eyes closed so that they hold the chart at their habitual distance and are not influenced by any tentative addition provided. You should remind the patient to hold the near VA chart at the distance they would like to read/work at rather than the distance they may have adopted to be able to see clearly.

4. Tentative addition determination: From one or a combination of the techniques that can be

used to estimate a tentative reading addition (sections 4.21 and 4.22), obtain an estimate of the reading addition for the indicated working distance and add these lenses to the trial frame. If the monocular tentative addition assessments (section 4.22) indicate monocular values within 0.25 DS, use the lower powered tentative addition. If the monocular values are different by more than 0.25 DS, then you may need to recheck your distance correction binocular balance.

5. Determine the final addition for the required near working distance(s). This can be performed in one of two ways:
   a) Preferred working distance method. Ask the patient to hold the near VA chart where the lenses in the trial frame provide the best vision. Ask the patient if this distance corresponds to their preferred near working distance. If it does not, then change the reading addition appropriately: increase the addition power if you wish to decrease the working distance and decrease the addition power if you wish to increase the working distance provided. Continue this process until the working distance obtained with the trial case lenses equals their preferred working distance.
   b) Trial lens method. Direct the patient's attention to the best acuity paragraph of text on the near chart. Add −0.25 DS and

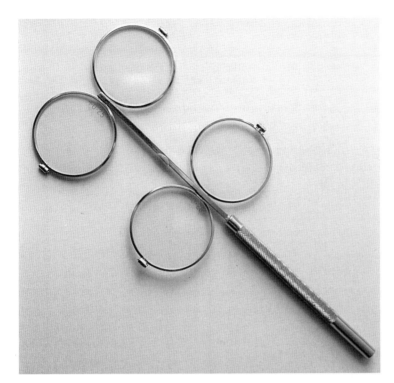

Fig. 4.17 Confirmation lenses used in subjective refraction with a trial frame.

ask if the letters become clearer, more blurred or are unchanged. Confirmation lenses (± 0.25 DS flippers) are useful for this task (Fig. 4.17). If the acuity improves with the additional minus, then continue adding −0.25 DS until the near acuity or clarity does not improve with the additional −0.25 D. If the vision is unchanged or decreased with −025 DS lenses, then do not add them. Add +0.25 DS. If the visual acuity is unchanged or decreased, then do not add the lens. If visual acuity improves with the lens, then add further plus lenses (in 0.25 D steps) only as long as the near VA or its clarity improves.

6. Determine the range of clear vision with the binocular reading add. This is important as the range decreases with higher add powers (Table 4.9). It is particularly important if you are intending that the reading addition will be used for tasks at more than one working distance.

a) To determine the near endpoint of the addition's range, ask the patient to move the reading card slowly in until they first notice blur for the best acuity paragraph. Measure this distance.

b) Determine the far endpoint of the addition range by asking the patient to move the card slowly away from them until the best acuity paragraph just blurs.

7. If you are unable to obtain a range that encompasses all the near working tasks that the patient has indicated they perform, you may consider that some form of progressive addition lens will provide the range of clear vision required. Alternatively, you could determine whether a compromise near addition would work. For example, the patient may have a preferred reading distance of 40 cm, but the addition that provides best clarity at this distance doesn't provide adequate clarity for their computer at 67 cm. A compromise addition providing best clarity at 50 cm, but adequate clarity at 40 cm and

Table 4.9 Calculations of the range of clear vision with different working distances and subjective measurements of amplitudes of accommodation.

Age	Amplitude of accommodation (D)	Near add (D)	Working distance (cm)	Range of clear vision (cm)
45	3.5	+0.75	40	133–24
		+1.25	33	80–21
50	2.5	+1.25	40	80–27
		+1.75	33	57–24
55	~1.50	+1.75	40	57–31
		+2.25	33	44–27
60+	~1.00	+2.00	40	50–33
		+2.50	33	40–29
		+3.00	29	33–25

Depth of focus effects are included in the latter measurements and are therefore included in these calculations. The near add was calculated from the equation: near add (D) = working distance (D) $-1/2$ amplitude of accommodation. The far point of clear vision (m) was calculated from the inverse of [working distance (D) $-1/2$ amplitude] and the near point of clear vision (m) was calculated from the inverse of [working distance (D) $+1/2$ amplitude]. Note the significant reductions in the range of clear vision with increased add.

67 cm may work. Alternatively, you may need to determine individual additions for their different working distances that could be provided in several pairs of single vision spectacles or trifocals.

8. Record the final addition(s), acuity and range of clearest vision obtained with the addition(s).

9. Note that if this assessment ends with the patient unable to read the smallest print on your chart (e.g., N5, 20/25, 0.4M) with their optimal near refractive correction and the patient does not have an additional 'reading' lamp at home, they should be strongly advised to obtain one.

4.23.4 Recording

Record the final addition(s), as well as the acuity attained and range of clarity for the addition. Examples:

Final add +1.50 DS @40 cm, VA: N5 R&L, range 25–67 cm.

Reading add +2.25 DS @35 cm, VA: 0.4M OD & OS, range 25–5 cm.

Intermediate add +1.25 DS @ 67 cm, VA 0.4M OD & OS, range 45–75 cm.

Make sure that the prescription details that you provide to patients are clearly legible. Illegible prescription forms have been reported as a surprisingly common error in optometric practice (Steele et al. 2006).

4.23.5 Interpretation

Most additions are equal for the two eyes. Unequal additions require further testing: either a retest of the near addition endpoints used for each eye or a recheck of the distance binocular balance. The prescribing of unequal additions between the eyes is the exception and is rarely satisfactory. Assuming no accommodative insufficiency, the power of the addition usually increases with age in patients above 40–50 years. Patients in poor general health can ask for a higher addition than is normal for their age and working distance. In some cases a reading addition that is low for a patient's age and working distance can indicate that the distance refraction has been over-plussed/under-minused (Hrynchak 2006). Practitioners rarely give additions greater than +3.00 D in patients with normal visual acuity. It is prudent to keep the addition as weak as possible to keep as large a range of clear vision as possible (Table 4.9). If possible, do not change the near refractive correction by more than +0.50 D to ease spectacle adaptation, although this may be less of an issue with progressive addition lenses.

4.23.6 Most common errors

1. Under-plussing a near correction (Hrynchak 2006). This can particularly occur with patients undergoing nuclear cataract induced refractive changes in the distance prescription that may require a significantly increased reading addition.

2. Giving extra plus when it provides no change and thus prescribing too high an addition.

3. Not determining the patient's near vision needs and subsequently prescribing an addition that gives an inadequate range of clear near vision for those needs.

4. Estimating instead of measuring the near point distances with a tape measure.

4.24 PRESCRIBING

This section provides various points regarding prescribing refractive corrections. Note that they are generalities and must not be used as hard and fast rules. In particular, they are unlikely to be valid when prescribing refractive corrections for young children or low vision patients. At the end of a primary care examination, you will commonly have to answer one of the following three questions regarding prescribing a refractive correction.

1. What prescription (Rx) should be given?

   You may consider that deciding upon the final refractive correction given to the patient is easy and that it is the result found after subjective refraction. This is not always correct.

2. Does a patient with a small refractive correction need spectacles or contact lenses?

3. Is a small change in refractive correction necessary? Does the patient need to update their lenses?

4.24.1 Demonstrate changes to the patient

The improvements in vision provided by a first refractive correction can be shown by alternately showing the patient the vision with their optimal refractive correction and without. The patient should be asked to look at a distance or near chart (whichever is appropriate) or look out of the practice window into the far distance and using trial case lenses with a trial frame. The effect of any refractive correction changes can be shown to the patient by alternately showing the patient the vision (distance and/or near) obtained with their optimal refractive correction in a trial frame compared to their current spectacles. This can be awkward and it can be easier, if there are negligible cylindrical changes (which is relatively common), to place appropriate spherical trial cases lenses over the top of their current spectacles to allow a comparison.

4.24.2 What refractive correction should you prescribe?

It would be easy to assume that the power of any new spectacles should be the subjective refraction result. This is true in a lot of cases, but is not always correct. Note that the subjective refraction result is not a perfectly repeatable measurement and both the spherical and cylindrical components can vary from test to retest by up to 0.50 D (Goss & Grosvenor 1996). Here are a few points that indicate when the Rx given should be different from the subjective refraction result. Note that these points are generalities and not strict rules. The patient's input is the best source of information when deciding what refractive correction to prescribe.

1. 'IF IT AIN'T BROKE DON'T FIX IT'. A very important rule for all age groups. If a patient is happy with their Rx, but would like a new frame, the only change you can make by changing the Rx (particular cylinder power or axis) is to make them unhappy. Remember that the subjective refraction result is not a perfectly repeatable measurement and can vary up to 0.50 D from test to retest (Goss & Grosvenor 1996).

The exception is if you can make a significant improvement in their VA, and even then it should be remembered that a patient may want slightly blurred vision (for example, the presbyopic myope may prefer to be slightly under-corrected at distance so that they can read in their distance spectacles). Ignoring this rule is one of the major causes of patients being dissatisfied with their spectacles.

2. Compare against the patient's spectacles: Changes in cylindrical correction are often minimal, so that the major change in refractive correction is spherical. It can be useful to place appropriate spherical trial case lenses over the patient's spectacles and ask the patient whether they like the change in vision (or not!)

3. Non-progressive myopes: Do not always 'push the plus' and give 'maximum plus' for non-progressive myopes. Remember that if you are refracting at 6 m or 20 ft, this is not infinity, so that patients are likely to be over-plussed by +0.17 D with a 6 m (20 ft) refractive correction. In addition, some low myopes tend to wear their Rx only for driving and especially at night. Here 'night myopia' is an additional problem. Therefore, for non-progressive myopes, it is often better to err on the side of over-minus when prescribing, rather than over-plus. In particular, be extremely careful of reducing a myopic Rx in older non-progressive myopes, especially if there are no symptoms. Over-plussing the distance correction has been reported as the most common reason for failure of spectacle lens acceptance (Hrynchak 2006).

4. Hyperopes: Only prescribe the full hyperopic Rx if the patient is presbyopic (or nearing presbyopia), esotropic or has esophoria (particularly convergence excess). Otherwise consider prescribing a partial Rx. All you need to do is prescribe a hyperopic Rx that is sufficient to remove any symptoms. The amount will depend upon the patient's symptoms, age, manifest and latent hyperopia, e.g. if fully manifest, then prescribe 1/2 to 3/4 of the Rx. The older the patient, the more likely you will prescribe ≈3/4 to full Rx. The more pronounced the symptoms, the more likely you are to prescribe more of the hyperopia. Over-plussing the distance correction has been reported as the most common reason for failure of spectacle lens acceptance (Hrynchak 2006).

5. Latent hyperopes: With a large latent component, you are likely to perform a cycloplegic refraction. Prior to cycloplegia it is important to assess the effect of extra plus over the manifest dry Rx to determine the effect of giving extra plus on distance visual acuity. This will indicate how much extra plus the patient is likely to be able to tolerate before distance blur becomes too great (section 4.20.5).

6. Heterophoria in younger patients: You must consider any significant heterophoria when prescribing in young patients (Dwyer & Wick 1995).

7. Older patients: It is easier to make big changes in Rx in younger patients. In patients over 25 years old, be wary of making changes over 0.75 D.

8. Presbyopes: Be very wary of increasing a distance or near Rx (other than the first presbyopic addition) by > 0.75 D. This is a good *general* rule for the *majority* of patients with simple increasing age-related hyperopia and/or presbyopia. Large increases in Rx in older patients tend not to be tolerated and can even lead to an increase in falls in frail elderly patients (Cumming et al. 2007).

9. Presbyopes: The near correction can often be under-plussed in a patient undergoing a minus shift in the distance refractive correction due to nuclear cataract (Hrynchak 2006). For example, consider a patient with spectacles of +1.00 DS OU with an addition of +1.50. With a minus shift making the distance correction plano in both eyes, the patient will need a +2.50 addition to retain the same near correction.

10. Presbyopes: It is vital that you know what the patient wants to see with the near vision Rx and determine their point of best focus and range of clarity. The two must overlap (section 4.23).

11. Cylinder changes:
    a) Many practitioners do not prescribe 0.25 cylinders, particularly when spheres are relatively large and/or when the astigmatism was not seen on retinoscopy. 0.25 cylinders should be prescribed when the spherical Rx is low and/or if the patient has a detail-oriented personality and responses during the subjective determination of astigmatism were precise and repeatable.
    b) When cylinder changes are moderate to large, generally make partial changes in cylinder power and axis and no more than 0.50 DC. Changes in power are more tolerable if the axes are not oblique. Changes in axis should never be large for large cylinders. Carefully look at the change in VA made by the cylinder change, and whether the astigmatic change may be the cause of any of the patient's symptoms. If there are significant VA changes and symptoms, you would be more likely to give more of the cylinder. Allow the patient to participate in the decision if possible. It can be useful to trial frame the partial Rx you are going to prescribe.
    c) Remember, if you partially prescribe a change in cylinder power, an appropriate change in sphere should be made (to give the same mean sphere). It can be useful to trial frame the partial Rx you are going to prescribe.

12. Poor adaptors: If a patient has a record of poor adaptation to new spectacles (this should always be recorded), then make small changes subsequently.

13. Anisometropia: Symptoms of aniseikonia are mainly asthenopia and headaches and very few complain of spatial distortions, etc.

    a) Generally, less than 1 D of anisometropia does not cause problems.
    b) In young patients, the first step is to prescribe the full Rx. Young patients will adapt to surprisingly large amounts of anisometropia.
    c) The best mode of refractive correction for anisometropia is often contact lenses. They remove any prismatic problems as the contact lens moves with the eye. They also may remove problems due to aniseikonia.
    d) With anisometropia ($>\approx$4D) and amblyopia of long standing (age $>$ 10, VA $<$ 6/36), then a balance lens may be appropriate for the amblyopic eye. Tell the patient that the good eye will not deteriorate because of strain.
    e) If a patient has alternating vision (e.g. RE(OD): -3.00, LE(OS): plano so that right eye is used for near work and left eye for distance) and no symptoms, then spectacles may not be necessary.
    f) Anisometropia in presbyopes: This is most commonly found with cataract-induced myopia and astigmatism and after monocular cataract surgery. Generally use a partial Rx of the more myopic eye (reduce by $\approx$ 1/3 of anisometropia). Large cylinders, especially oblique, may require partial Rx of power. Partial cylinder axis changes may also be made to reduce meridional aniseikonic effects. Make sure that using a partial correction does not reduce the visual acuity below the standard required for driving.
    g) If aniseikonia is still a problem and contact lenses cannot be fitted, then try:
        i) keeping the spectacle vertex distance as small as possible by appropriate selection of frames.
        ii) reducing the thickness of the more hyperopic Rx.
        iii) changing the blank size.
        iv) changing the base curve. You may consider prescribing equal base curves in the two lenses.
        v) using size/isogonal lenses.
        vi) using a bicentric grind to eliminate the dynamic anisophoria in the vertical meridian.

4.24.3 Should you prescribe a small Rx?

Should you prescribe a small Rx, such as 0.50 D of hyperopia or hyperopic astigmatism? This can be a very difficult question. Here are some points to consider:

1. If there are no symptoms related to the use of the eyes, then a first Rx should not be prescribed.

2. Always consider other ocular causes of the symptoms, which might not be related to the small refractive error and include inadequate convergence, accommodative facility or vergence facility and decompensated heterophoria. Also consider non-ocular causes of headaches, including tension, migraine, nasal sinusitis and hypertension. Unfortunately, tension headaches, which are a common headache, can be difficult to differentiate from ocular headaches as they are often frontal or occipital, get worse towards the end of the day and are better over the weekend.

3. If a patient has symptoms that are related to detailed vision tasks, you are more likely to prescribe a small Rx if the patient does a lot of detailed work and/or if the patient has a personality that is detail-oriented, precise or intense.

4. The relative certainty of responses should help your decision of whether to prescribe a small Rx. If glasses are to be of any value, the responses during subjective refraction should be very certain, appropriate and repeatable.

5. Usually small Rxs make little change to the VA (particularly if a truncated Snellen chart is used) and so basing decisions on VA improvements is usually not helpful.

6. The effect of the Rx on binocular vision tests can be helpful (Dwyer & Wick 1995). For example, if binocular vision tests suggest that a heterophoria is decompensated with no refractive correction and compensated with it, then the spectacles are likely to help and should be prescribed (Dwyer & Wick 1995).

7. You can view prescribing glasses as a diagnostic tool. Often the only way to be certain whether the symptoms are due to the uncorrected refractive error is to prescribe it and see if the symptoms disappear. You could offer the patient a pair of basic loan spectacles to determine whether the refractive correction will relieve the symptoms. This approach is often used in medicine. However, be aware that spectacles can provide a placebo effect and relieve the symptoms for a short period before they return.

4.24.4 Should you make small changes to the refractive correction?

1. If there are no symptoms and a small change to the refractive correction and the patient wants a new frame, it may be better to stick with their old correction unless a significant improvement in VA over their old correction can be obtained ('IF IT AIN'T BROKE DON'T FIX IT').

2. Consider the points in section 4.24.3; in particular, if a patient has symptoms which are related to detailed vision tasks, you are more likely to prescribe a small change in Rx if the patient does a lot of detailed work and/or if the patient has a personality which is detail-oriented, precise or intense. Consider the relative certainty and repeatability of responses during the subjective refraction.

3. Even if there is no change in refractive correction, a patient should always be asked if they want a new pair of glasses. They may want a change of frame or their old lenses may be scratched and need replacing.

4.24.5 Prescribing for elderly patients at risk of falling

Although falls are multifactorial, it is clear that visual impairment is linked with an increased risk of falling (Buckley & Elliott 2006). The following are points to consider when prescribing for a patient who is at high risk of falling (over 75 years of age, history of falling, using more than three medications, antidepressant use, systemic conditions that reduce mobility, cardiac problems, etc.) or who may be more dependent on their vision for balance control (patients with somatosensory system dysfunction such as diabetes and/or peripheral neuropathy; or those with vestibular system dysfunction, such as Ménière's disease):

1. Do not prescribe multifocal lenses (progressive addition lenses or varifocals, trifocals and bifocals) unless they have successfully worn them previously. Multifocal lenses double the risk of falling (Lord et al. 2002).

2. Established multifocal lens wearers should be prescribed single vision distance lenses for walking outside the home and when using stairs, etc. Multifocals should only be used for other tasks such as watching TV or driving.

3. Avoid prescribing significant changes (greater than 0.75 D) to the refractive correction as this can lead to an increase in falls in older patients (Cumming et al. 2007).

4.24.6 Most common errors

1. Changing the spectacle power, particularly the cylinder power or axis, of a patient who was happy with the vision in their old spectacles but just wanted a new frame.

2. Prescribing the refractive correction found with subjective refraction without consideration of the change in prescription or the patient's symptoms.

3. Not offering a patient who has no change in prescription the possibility of changing their frame and/or lenses.

4. Prescribing a low-powered prescription to a patient with no symptoms.

5. Not offering spectacles as a diagnostic tool to a patient whose symptoms you are not sure are caused by ametropia or a decompensated phoria.

6. Prescribing multifocal lenses or making a large change to the refractive correction of elderly patients at high risk of falling.

4.25 COUNSELLING

A small section regarding counselling is included here at the end of the refraction section, as many of the points made relate to ametropia and its correction.

4.25.1 Cause of the chief complaint

1. At the end of the examination, you must discuss your findings, particularly those that relate to the patient's chief complaint and other secondary complaints. What is the cause (if known) of the chief complaint? Give a full explanation of the diagnoses in lay terms, unless your patient works in the medical field and has some knowledge. It can be very useful to have a cross-sectional diagram of the eye to help you in this explanation.

2. Make sure you go back to the case history and try to explain each of the patient's symptoms.

3. It is generally best to discuss your findings in order of the patient's relative importance of their problems rather than your own opinion of the relative importance of the diagnoses.

4.25.2 Reassurance

1. If the cause of the chief complaint or other problem is not determined, then indicate to the patient what conditions you have not detected (Blume 1987). For example, if a patient's chief complaint was headaches and no oculovisual reason could be found on examination, present your negative findings in a positive manner: 'I do not believe that your headaches are due to a problem with your eyes or vision, Mr Smith. Your eyesight is excellent and there is no need for glasses/change in glasses; your eye muscles and focusing muscles are all working normally and are working well together and there is no sign of eye disease from any of the tests that I have performed.'

2. In all such cases, always indicate to the patient that they were correct in attending for examination (Blume 1987).

4.25.3 Treatment options

1. Discuss with the patient possible treatment options and whether referral for further assessment or treatment is necessary.

2. Be wary of overestimating the importance of price to patients and include a discussion of the highest specification (and usually most expensive) lenses. A report of a small sample of UK optometrists indicated that some omit discussion of the highest specification of lenses due to overestimating the importance to patients of price (Fylan & Grunfeld 2005).

3. Explain when the patient should wear spectacles. Do not assume that the patient will understand when to wear them. For example, if a patient's chief complaint was distance blur when driving, it may not be enough to indicate that they should wear the glasses for driving and assume they understand that they can wear them for any other distance vision task. Indicate that the glasses could be used for TV, cinema, and theatre, watching sports and when walking about outside if the patient wants to wear them for those tasks. In this regard, it is very important to inform a patient who drives without spectacles whether they are legally allowed to do so.

4. Possible problems with the treatment: For example, if making a relatively large change in refractive correction, warn the patient of possible adaptation problems. This is most important when making any cylinder changes, particularly with oblique cylinders. Take note of a patient's previous reaction to refractive correction change. It is better to overestimate the time that adaptation will take rather than underestimate the time.

5. It is useful to have information booklets available to explain the ametropias and the various treatment options available.

4.25.4 Prognosis

Explain what is the likely prognosis of the patient's condition(s). For example:

1. Explain what symptoms should disappear with the spectacles and over what time period.

2. If appropriate (e.g. early myopes and presbyopes), explain that progression is expected, and why. Advise young myopes that wearing their spectacles will not make their eyes worse, it just gives then clearer vision. Also, the patient should know that not wearing their spectacles will not make their eyes worse.

3. Explain that a gradual reduction in unaided vision is expected in hyperopia with age. It is very common for hyperopes to conclude that the glasses 'ruined their eyes' when their accommodation gradually declines and they need their spectacles more and more often.

4.25.5 Next appointment

1. Finally, indicate to the patient when you would like to see them again.

2. If this is less than a standard time (typically 2 years or 1 year for children and the elderly) explain why.

3. Always inform the patient that if they have any problems with their vision or their eyes before that time, they should make an appointment to see you.

4.25.6 Most common errors

1. Using technical language and jargon to explain diagnoses and treatment plans.

2. Not explaining to myopes, hyperopes and presbyopes the likely progression of their condition.

3. Not explaining to patients when they should wear their spectacles.

4. Not warning appropriate patients about possible adaptation problems.

4.26 BIBLIOGRAPHY AND FURTHER READING

Benjamin, W.J. (2006) *Borish's Clinical refraction*, 2nd edn. St Louis: Butterworth-Heinemann.

Carlson, N.B. and Kurtz, D. (2004) *Clinical procedures for ocular examination*, 3rd edn. New York: McGraw-Hill.

Eskridge, J.B., Amos, J.F. and Bartlett, J.D. (1991) *Clinical procedures in optometry*. Philadelphia: J.B. Lippincott.

Grosvenor, T. (2002) *Primary care optometry*, 4th edn. Boston: Butterworth-Heinemann.

4.27 REFERENCES

Baldwin, W.R. and Mills, D. (1981) A longitudinal study of corneal astigmatism and total astigmatism. *American Journal of Optometry and Physiological Optics* **58**, 206–211.

Bennett, A.G. and Rabbetts, R.B. (1998) *Clinical visual optics*, 3rd edn. Oxford: Butterworth-Heinemann.

Blume, A.J. (1987) Reassurance therapy. In: *Diagnosis and management of vision care* (ed. J.F. Amos). Boston: Butterworth-Heinemann.

Blystone, P.A. (1999) Relationship between age and presbyopic addition using a sample of 3,645 examinations from a single private practice. *Journal of the American Optometric Association* **70**, 505–508.

Borish, I.L. and Benjamin, W.J. (2006) Monocular and binocular subjective refraction. In: *Borish's Clinical refraction* (ed. W.J. Benjamin). St Louis: Butterworth-Heinemann, pp. 790–872.

Brown, W.L. (1991) Interpupillary distance. In: *Clinical procedures in optometry* (eds J.B. Eskridge, J.F. Amos and J.D. Bartlett). Philadelphia: J.B. Lippincott, pp. 39–52.

Buckley, J.G. and Elliott, D.B. (2006) Ophthalmic interventions to help prevent falls. *Geriatrics and Ageing* **9**, 276–280.

Celebi, S. and Aykan, U. (1999) The comparison of cyclopentolate and atropine in patients with refractive accommodative esotropia by means of retinoscopy, autorefractometry and biometric lens thickness. *Acta Ophthalmologica Scandinavica* **77**, 426–429.

Charman, W.N. (1989) The path to presbyopia: straight or crooked? *Ophthalmic and Physiological Optics* **9**, 424–430.

Clementi, M., Angi, M. and Forabosco, P. et al. (1998) Inheritance of astigmatism: evidence for a major autosomal dominant locus. *American Journal of Human Genetics* **63**, 825–830.

Cumming, R.G., Ivers, R., Clemson, L. et al. (2007) Improving vision to prevent falls in frail, older people: a randomized trial. *Journal of the American Geriatrics Society* **55**, 175–181.

Dwyer, P. and Wick, B. (1995) The influence of refractive correction upon disorders of vergence and accommodation. *Optometry and Vision Science* **72**, 224–232.

Elliott, D.B. and Cox, M.J. (2004) A clinical assessment of the +1.00 blur test. *Optometry in Practice* **5**, 189–193.

Elliott, D.B. and Wilkes, R.D. (1989) A clinical evaluation of the Topcon RM-6000 autorefractor. *Clinical and Experimental Optometry* **72**, 150–153.

Elliott, D.B., Yang, K.C. and Whitaker, D. (1995) Visual acuity changes throughout adulthood in normal, healthy eyes: seeing beyond 6/6. *Optometry and Vision Science* **72**, 186–191.

Elliott, M., Callender, M.G. and Elliott, D.B. (1994) Accuracy of Javal's rule in the determination of spectacle astigmatism. *Optometry and Vision Science* **71**, 23–26.

Fylan, F. and Grunfeld, E.A. (2005) Visual illusions? Beliefs and behaviours of presbyope clients in optometric practice. *Patient Education and Counseling* **56**, 291–295.

Goodwin, H.E. (1966) Optometric determinations of balanced binocular refraction corrections. *Optometry Weekly* **57**, 47–53.

Goss, D.A. and Grosvenor, T. (1996) Reliability of refraction – a literature review. *Journal of the American Optometric Association* **67**, 619–630.

Grosvenor, T. and Scott, R. (1991) Comparison of refractive components in youth-onset and early adult-onset myopia. *Optometry and Vision Science* **68**, 204–209.

Grosvenor, T., Quintero, S. and Perrigin, D.M. (1988) Predicting refractive astigmatism: a suggested simplification of Javal's rule. *American Journal of Optometry and Physiological Optics* **65**, 292–297.

Guzowski, M., Wang, J.J., Rochtchina, E. et al. (2003) Five-year refractive changes in an older population: the Blue Mountains Eye Study. *Ophthalmology* **110**, 1364–1370.

Hanlon, S.D., Nakabayashi, J. and Shigezawa, G. (1987) A critical view of presbyopic add determination. *Journal of the American Optometric Association* **58**, 468–472.

Holland, B.J. and Siderov, J. (1999) Repeatability of measurements of interpupillary distance. *Ophthalmic and Physiological Optics* **19**, 74–78.

Hrynchak, P. (2006) Prescribing spectacles: reason for failure of spectacle acceptance. *Ophthalmic and Physiological Optics* **26**, 111–115.

Humphriss, D. (1988) Binocular refraction. In: *Optometry* (eds K. Edwards and R. Llewellyn). Oxford: Butterworths.

Jones, L.W.J. and Hodes, D.T. (1991) Possible allergic reactions to cyclopentolate hydrochloride – case reports with literature review of uses and adverse reactions. *Ophthalmic and Physiological Optics* **11**, 16–21.

Locke, L.C. (1987) Induced refractive and visual changes. In: *Diagnosis and management in vision care* (ed. J.F. Amos). Boston: Butterworths.

Lord, S.R., Dayhew, J. and Howland, A. (2002) Multifocal glasses impair edge-contrast sensitivity and depth perception and increase the risk of falls in older people. *Journal of the American Geriatrics Society* **50**, 1760–1766.

McCaghrey, G.E. and Matthews, F.E. (1993) Clinical evaluation of a range of autorefractors. *Ophthalmic and Physiological Optics* **13**, 129–137.

MacMillan, E.S., Elliott, D.B., Patel, B. et al. (2001) Loss of visual acuity is the main reason why reading addition increases after the age of sixty. *Optometry and Vision Science* **78**, 381–385.

Millodot, M. and Millodot, S. (1989) Presbyopia correction and the accommodation in reserve. *Ophthalmic and Physiological Optics* **9**, 126–132.

Mohindra, I. (1977) A non-cycloplegic refraction technique for infants and young children. *Journal of the American Optometric Association* **48**, 518–523.

Mote, H.G. and Fry, G.A. (1939) The significance of Javal's rule. *American Journal of Optometry and Physiological Optics* **16**, 62–65.

Mutti, D.O., Mitchell, G.L., Moeschberger, M.L. et al. (2002) Parental myopia, near work, school achievement, and children's refractive error. *Investigative Ophthalmology and Visual Science* **43**, 3633–3640.

Osuobeni, E.P. and Al-Fahdi, M. (1994) Differences between anatomical and physiological interpupillary distance. *Journal of the American Optometric Association* **4**, 265–271.

Pesudovs, K. and Elliott, D.B. (2003) Refractive error changes in cortical, nuclear and posterior subcapsular cataract. *The British Journal of Ophthalmology* **87**, 964–967.

Pointer, J.S. (1995) The presbyopic Add I, II and III. *Ophthalmic and Physiological Optics* **15**, 235–254.

Rosenfield, M., Ciuffreda, K.J., Hung, G.K. et al. (1994) Tonic accommodation: a review II. Accommodative adaptation and clinical aspects. *Ophthalmic and Physiological Optics* **14**, 265–277.

Saunders, K.J. and Westall, C.A. (1992) Comparison between near retinoscopy and cycloplegic retinoscopy in the refraction of infants and children. *Optometry and Vision Science* **69**, 615–622.

Solsona, F. (1975) Astigmatism as a congenital bilateral and symmetrical entity. (Observations based on the study of 51,000 patients). *The British Journal of Physiological Optics* **30**, 119–127.

Steele, C.F., Rubin, G. and Fraser, S. (2006) Error classification in community optometric practice – a pilot study. *Ophthalmic and Physiological Optics* **26**, 106–110.

Tuan, K.A., Somani, S. and Chernyak, D.A. (2005) Changes in wavefront aberration with pharmaceutical dilating agents. *Journal of Refractive Surgery* **21**, S503–S504.

Twelker, J.D. and Mutti, D.O. (2001) Retinoscopy in infants using a near noncycloplegic technique, cycloplegia with tropicamide 1%, and cycloplegia with cyclopentolate 1%. *Optometry and Vision Science* **78**, 215–222.

Walline, J.J., Kinney, K.A., Zadnik, K. et al. (1999) Repeatability and validity of astigmatism measurements. *Journal of Refractive Surgery* **15**, 23–31.

Wang, B. and Ciuffreda, K.J. (2006) Depth-of-focus of the human eye: theory and clinical implications. *Survey of Ophthalmology* **51**, 75–85.

West, D. and Somers, W.W. (1984) Binocular balance validity: a comparison of five different subjective techniques. *Ophthalmic and Physiological Optics* **4**, 155–159.

Zhao, J., Mao, J., Luo, R. et al. (2004) Accuracy of noncyclopegic autorefraction in school-age children in China. *Optometry and Vision Science* **81**, 49–55.

ASSESSMENT OF BINOCULAR VISION

BRENDAN BARRETT AND DAVID B. ELLIOTT

5

Tests that assess the binocular vision system are included in this chapter. Rather than group these tests in terms of preliminary or pre-refraction tests and post-refraction or functional tests, the tests are grouped together depending on the aspect of binocular vision that they help to assess. This is because the organisation of the book is directed towards the assimilation of a problem-oriented approach (section 2.1.3) built upon a systems examination (section 2.1.2). In addition, this grouping of tests may help students to better appreciate the relationship between preliminary tests, such as the cover test (section 5.5) and post-refraction or functional binocular vision tests, such as subjective assessments of heterophoria (sections 5.7 to 5.10).

5.1 RELEVANT CASE HISTORY INFORMATION

The case history can provide significant information about binocular function and can help the practitioner decide, for example, that particular tests of binocular vision are not appropriate (e.g. near point of convergence with a near heterotropia) or, alternatively, that other tests, not routinely used, are warranted (e.g. determination of accommodative facility). The following areas are of relevance during examination of all patients but they may be of particular importance in a patient with a known binocular vision anomaly or in whom an anomaly of binocular vision is suspected.

5.1.1 Observations and symptoms

1. Observation of strabismus and head tilt: Simple observation of the patient as case history is being taken can highlight a strabismus or head tilt. Parents or carers may also inform you that they have noticed that their child occasionally has an 'eye turn' or perhaps, a head tilt. Any suggestion of a strabismus requires a careful cover test and stereopsis testing in addition to looking for amblyopia and possible causes of the strabismus such as hyperopia or anisometropia.

2. Symptoms of blurred vision, headaches or asthenopia at distance and/or near can indicate a decompensated heterophoria at the pertinent distance.

3. Complaints of 'double vision' could suggest a heterophoria breaking down into a heterotropia (typically horizontal diplopia, occurring especially when tired), a remote near point of convergence (section 5.15), the angle of strabismus changing so that the retinal image falls out of the suppression area or an incomitant deviation (section 5.24). An appropriate line of questioning during the case history will help in this differential diagnosis. Note that cortical cataract and occasionally posterior subcapsular cataract can cause monocular diplopia (or polyopia) and should be considered in elderly patients by determining if the diplopia persists if one eye is covered.

4. Fluctuations in distance vision and particularly distance blur after near work, suggest problems of accommodation and tests that assess accommodative function should be employed (sections 5.17–5.19).

5. Although the above symptoms may alert the practitioner to a possible anomaly of binocular vision, it is worth remembering that a lack of symptoms does not, in itself, mean that the binocular system is normal. For example, patients with suppression or long-standing heterotropia almost certainly will not experience binocular vision symptoms.

6. Poor reading ability and poor progress at school could also be due to a binocular vision problem.

5.1.2 Ocular history

The ocular history may indicate that the patient, or perhaps someone in the family, has a 'weak' or 'lazy' eye and/or strabismus. This should be followed up by asking if 'patching' or spectacles or any eye exercises have been prescribed or if 'eye muscle' surgery has taken place. Any positive response to these questions should lead to further questioning regarding the age when these interventions happened, when they stopped, their success and if the patient is still under any care for the amblyopia/ strabismus. If the latter is the case, you should be careful not to change an optical prescription or alter the current therapy in any way without permission/ agreement from the other practitioner treating the patient.

5.1.3 General medical history and family history

General health questions may indicate a systemic condition that can lead to binocular vision problems, such as diabetes, or systemic medications that can affect accommodation or binocular vision. When examining young children with or without a binocular vision abnormality it is useful to ask whether any member of the patient's family has a strabismus or 'lazy eye' as there appears to be a hereditary link, particularly for esotropia. In children diagnosed with strabismus and/or amblyopia, you should ask whether the child's siblings have been examined and, if not, inform the parent/carer that the other children should be examined to avoid the possibility of amblyopia developing.

5.1.4 Birth history

It is also useful to ask the child's parent/carer about the pregnancy and birth history. There is a high prevalence of ocular abnormality, in particular strabismus, in children born prematurely, those with low birth weight or disorders of the central nervous system, and in children with significant birth complications (e.g. forceps delivery). It is, therefore, recommended that the following questions be posed to the parent/carer during the case history examination:

- Was the child a full-term baby or were they born prematurely?

- What was the birth weight? (less than 2500 gr or 5.5 pounds is a significant risk factor for strabismus, in particular esotropia; Mohney et al. 1998).

- Were there significant complications at the child's birth?

- Is the child's current and past general health good?

- Since birth, has the child been investigated or received treatment for any medical condition?

5.2 RELEVANT INFORMATION FROM ASSESSMENTS OF OTHER SYSTEMS

5.2.1 Binocular visual acuity

In cases where the acuities in the right and left eyes are similar or identical, it is usual to find that binocular visual acuity (VA) is typically between half a line and a line better than monocular acuity (Pardhan & Elliott 1991). Of course, it is not possible to find this improvement if monocular VA equals the 'bottom line' of the Snellen chart you are using. When using a non-truncated chart, a binocular VA that is equal to or worse than the monocular VA can indicate a binocular vision problem. A poor patient reaction to the restoration of binocular vision after an occluder has been removed following monocular subjective refraction can also indicate a binocular vision problem.

5.2.2 Retinoscopy and subjective refraction

1. Fluctuations in retinoscopy: Fluctuations in spherical power during retinoscopy indicate changes in accommodation. These could be

due to variable fixation, but also possible latent hyperopia or pseudomyopia that should be investigated using assessments of accommodation (sections 5.17 to 5.19) and/or cycloplegic refraction (section 4.20).

2. Differences between retinoscopy and subjective refraction: A retinoscopy result that is significantly (>1.50 D) more positive than the subjective result could indicate latent hyperopia or pseudomyopia that should be investigated using assessments of accommodation (sections 5.17 to 5.19) and/or cycloplegic refraction (section 4.20).

3. Fluctuations in subjective refraction: Fluctuations in spherical power during subjective refraction could suggest poor control of accommodation. These could be due to the use of monocular refraction and/or poor technique, but may need to be investigated using assessments of accommodation (sections 5.17 to 5.19) and/or cycloplegic refraction (section 4.20).

5.2.3 Systemic and ocular health assessment

Information provided by the patient about systemic or ocular disease, previous or current, may explain signs or symptoms that are of a binocular vision nature. For example, diabetes or thyroid disease can lead to binocular vision problems. Similarly, particular signs or symptoms may prompt the practitioner to ask again about systemic health and/or to seek explanation within the eye. For example, a newly acquired divergent heterotropia (section 5.4) and ptosis may be observed in a palsy of the third cranial nerve and is suggestive of diabetes. Finally, cortical cataract and occasionally posterior subcapsular cataract can generate diplopia that is monocular in origin (i.e. it persists even when one eye is covered).

5.3 CLASSIFICATION OF HETEROPHORIA

Binocular vision requires that the eyes move together so that the visual axes intersect at the object of regard.

The eyes are held in alignment by a combination of the sensory and motor fusion mechanisms. If sensory fusion is prevented (for example, by occluding one eye as during the cover test), only the motor fusion mechanism is operational and a misalignment of the visual axes will occur in many patients. This misalignment is sometimes referred to as a latent deviation but is more commonly known as a *heterophoria*. Video clips of the cover test being used to assess a variety of heterophorias are provided on the website 🖱.

5.3.1 Direction

ORTHOPHORIA is present if the visual axes remain correctly aligned when sensory fusion is prevented. Heterophorias can be defined in terms of the direction of the misalignment when sensory fusion is prevented:

- ESOPHORIA: Convergence of the visual axes
- EXOPHORIA: Divergence of the visual axes
- HYPERPHORIA: One visual axis higher than the other
- HYPOPHORIA: One visual axis lower than the other.

Classification of vertical heterophorias is rather artificial in the sense that if the right visual axis is higher than the left this may be classified as a right hyperphoria or, alternatively, as a left hypophoria. In practice, it is usual to classify vertical heterophorias in terms of which eye is the hyperphoric eye; thus vertical heterophorias are normally described as either right hyperphoria or left hyperphoria in order to indicate the higher visual axis.

A relative rotation of the vertical poles of the cornea is called a cyclophoria, which can be further categorised into:

- EXCYCLOPHORIA: Outward rotation of the upper poles
- INCYCLOPHORIA: Inward rotation of the upper poles.

Cyclophorias are seldom investigated in primary eye care examinations. If a cyclophoria is present it is likely that it will be accompanied by other types of heterophoria (e.g. vertical heterophoria) and in most cases it will be possible to explain its presence by considering the actions of the elevating and depressing extraocular muscles of the eye (von Noorden 2002; e.g. the intorting actions of the superior oblique muscles and extorting actions of the inferior oblique muscles). Given the rarity with which cyclophorias alone are diagnosed in primary eye care and the fact that no treatment exists, cyclophorias will not be discussed further.

5.3.2 Magnitude and stability

Most patients have a small amount of heterophoria, especially at near. The magnitude of heterophoria is estimated or measured in prism dioptres ($^\Delta$). At distance, between 2^Δ of esophoria and 4^Δ of exophoria is considered normal. At near, between 3^Δ and 6^Δ of exophoria is considered normal. The tendency for the eyes to exhibit a small amount of exophoria at near is referred to as *physiological exophoria*. The tolerance to vertical misalignments is less than horizontal with greater than 0.5^Δ vertical heterophoria considered abnormal. While heterophoria over the course of a lifetime remains fairly constant (although physiological exophoria shows a small increase with age; Freier & Pickwell 1983), the ability of the patient to cope with their heterophoria can be influenced by stress on the visual system (e.g. excessive workload), by fatigue or by the patient's general health.

5.3.3 Comparing heterophoria at distance and at near

Heterophoria is usually evaluated with distance (6 m or 20 ft) and near (40 cm or 16″) viewing because the amount of heterophoria exhibited at the two distances is often quite different. This is because of the accommodation/convergence relationship. When a near target is viewed the eyes converge as well as accommodate. Depending upon the amount of convergence that accompanies each dioptre of accommodation (the magnitude of the AC/A ratio, section 5.11), the heterophoria at near may be very different from that which exists at distance. The following names are used to describe the possible conditions that may be present when a large difference exists between the distance and near heterophoria and where the patient is experiencing symptoms that are consistent with the presence of a binocular vision problem:

■ CONVERGENCE INSUFFICIENCY: Exophoria much larger at near than at distance. The definition indicates that exophoria must be *much* larger because of physiological exophoria at near (section 5.3.2).

■ CONVERGENCE EXCESS: Esophoria larger at near than at distance.

■ DIVERGENCE INSUFFICIENCY: Esophoria larger at distance than at near.

■ DIVERGENCE EXCESS: Exophoria larger at distance than at near.

Patients with convergence insufficiency or convergence excess will obviously experience their symptoms during near viewing whereas patients with divergence insufficiency or divergence excess will report symptoms during distance viewing.

5.3.4 Compensated versus decompensated heterophorias

The majority of patients will exhibit a heterophoria under some conditions and most heterophorias will not cause symptoms.

■ COMPENSATED HETEROPHORIA: A heterophoria that does not cause symptoms (or suppression).

■ DECOMPENSATED HETEROPHORIA: A heterophoria thought to be responsible for the patient's symptoms or for generating suppression.

It is important to stress that it is not simply the case that large heterophorias will be decompensated whereas small heterophorias will be compensated. The best example of this is the case of vertical heterophorias where even small tendencies towards vertical misalignment (e.g. 0.5^Δ) can give rise to symptoms whereas much larger horizontal heterophorias frequently exist without leading to symptoms or suppression. In order to deduce whether a particular heterophoria is compensated or decompensated it is necessary to consider factors in addition to the magnitude of the heterophoria. For example, the quality of the recovery movement on cover test (section 5.5) or the amount of fusional reserves that oppose the heterophoria (section 5.12) will also help to evaluate if the patient's symptoms or suppression stem from the presence of the heterophoria.

5.4 CLASSIFICATION OF COMITANT HETEROTROPIA (SQUINT OR STRABISMUS)

Binocular vision requires that the eyes move together so that the visual axes intersect at the object of regard and the eyes are held in alignment by a combination of the sensory and motor fusion mechanisms. If the fusion reflex fails to develop or is unable to function normally, a manifest misalignment of the eyes or heterotropia (tropia, strabismus, squint) will result. In a comitant heterotropia the angle of deviation is constant in all directions of gaze although it may differ depending upon whether the patient is viewing a near or distant target. There are considerable variations in the type of comitant heterotropia observed in clinical practice (Stidwell 1997) and consequently comitant heterotropia requires a more detailed classification than heterophoria. In addition to the direction and magnitude (in $^\Delta$) of the deviation, information is also required regarding its frequency, laterality, age of onset, influence of accommodation and cosmesis (Table 5.1). A comitant heterotropia is detected using the cover test (section 5.5). It should be differentiated from an incomitant heterotropia (section 5.24) in which the angle of deviation varies with direction of gaze and is usually caused by the malfunctioning of one of the six extraocular muscles. An incomitant heterotropia is detected using the motility test (section 5.25). Video clips of the cover test being used to assess a variety of heterotropias are provided on the website 🖱.

5.4.1 Age of onset

Congenital strabismus is used to describe deviations that are present at birth or develop during the first 6 months (von Noorden 2002). The term 'acquired strabismus' may be applied to deviations that arise after this age.

Table 5.1   Information required to classify comitant heterotropia.

Frequency	Location
Constant	Distance (6 m)
Intermittent	Near (~40 cm)
Cyclic	Age of onset
Laterality	Congenital
Right	Acquired
Left	Influence of accommodation
Alternating	Fully accommodative
Direction	(Donder's)
Esotropia	Partly accommodative
Exotropia	Non-accommodative
Hypertropia	
Hypotropia	Cosmesis
Cyclotropia	Rate as good, fair, poor
Magnitude	
Estimated or measured	
in prism dioptres at	
distance and near	

5.4.2 Frequency: constant or intermittent

The heterotropia may be constant or intermittent as patients with limited fusional ability may exhibit a manifest deviation at some times during the day but a latent deviation (i.e. a heterophoria) at other times. Under conditions of visual stress or fatigue the fusional system may break down allowing the deviation to become manifest (i.e. a heterophoria becomes a heterotropia). One relatively common example of this phenomenon is the case of the patient with significant exophoria at near. Following prolonged reading, the patient may temporarily exhibit exotropia.

5.4.3 Laterality: unilateral or alternating

Unilateral heterotropia is one in which the patient always fixates with the same eye. The visual acuity is often reduced in the deviated eye due to amblyopia. Alternating heterotropia refers to the case where the patient can use either eye to fixate. These patients usually have approximately equal visual acuity in each eye. It is much more common for patients with exotropia to be able to alternate the

deviating eye than is the case for patients with esotropia whose deviations are more frequently unilateral (von Noorden 2002).

5.4.4 Presence of amblyopia

Constant, unilateral strabismus is a known risk factor for the development of amblyopia, a condition in which there is reduced visual acuity despite optimum refractive correction and the absence of any disease of the eye or visual system. Although the precise mechanism by which amblyopia develops from the presence of strabismus is not well established, the process is thought to involve chronic, unilateral suppression of the deviating eye. Since esotropia tends to be constant and unilateral whereas exotropia is more often intermittent and alternating (von Noorden 2002), it is not surprising that amblyopia is much more prevalent in esotropes than exotropes. For example, in recent studies around 51% of children with esotropia were found to have amblyopia compared to only around 14% of exotropes (Mohney 2001, Mohney & Huffaker 2003). Because of the link between strabismus and amblyopia development, it is important that strabismus is diagnosed as early as possible in order to reduce the risk of amblyopia (von Noorden 2002).

5.4.5 Direction of heterotropia

If the visual axes manifestly deviate from alignment the following conditions result:

- ESOTROPIA: Convergence of the visual axes

- EXOTROPIA: Divergence of the visual axes

- HYPERTROPIA: If one visual axis points upwards

- HYPOTROPIA: If one visual axis points downwards.

Unlike with vertical heterophorias, which are normally classified according to which eye is the hyperphoric eye, vertical heterotropias must be labelled as either hypertropia or hypotropia, and the deviating eye must be recorded (for example: 'right hypotropia').

A rotation of the vertical poles of the cornea is called a cyclotropia, which can be further categorised into:

- EXCYCLOTROPIA: Outward rotation of the upper pole
- INCYCLOTROPIA: Inward rotation of the upper pole.

Cyclotropias seldom exist as an independent restriction of ocular motility. Instead they are most commonly caused by abnormal functioning of one or more extraocular muscles responsible for elevating or depressing the eye. They can also occur in association with A and V patterns. They can be viewed as an imbalance between the extraocular muscles that are responsible for intorsion and extorsion (von Noorden 2002).

5.4.6 Differences between near and distance viewing

Patients may present with a heterophoria at one fixation distance and a heterotropia at a different fixation distance. For example a patient with high, uncorrected hyperopia may exhibit esophoria when viewing in the distance but become esotropic when viewing at near. The underlying problem here is the fact that the hyperopia is uncorrected. It is possible for the same result to be observed (esophoria at distance, esotropia at near) in an emmetropic patient whose AC/A ratio (section 5.11) is abnormally high. It is important to remember that comitant deviations can (and frequently do) differ in type and magnitude between distance and near viewing. This does not make them an incomitant deviation, but is caused by an anomaly of the vergence system (Schor & Horner 1989). The link between accommodation, uncorrected hyperopia and the presence of heterotropia is discussed further in the next section.

5.4.7 Influence of accommodation and uncorrected hyperopia

A young, uncorrected hyperope will be able to accommodate to overcome the hyperopic defocus but the accommodation exerted will bring with it convergence which may be excessive and which might precipitate an esotropia. The chances of an esotropia being present will be increased as the viewing distance is reduced. Around 50% of esotropias have an accommodative element (Mohney 2001), whereas there is no link between accommodation/hyperopia and the presence of exotropia. Deviations that are classified as accommodative can be further sub-divided into fully-accommodative and partially-accommodative deviations. A fully-accommodative heterotropia refers to a heterotropia that is present without refractive correction but which is eliminated when the full hyperopic correction is worn. In a patient with a partially-accommodative strabismus, the angle of deviation is reduced but not eliminated when the full hyperopic correction is worn. Deviations are described as non-accommodative if they are independent of the amount of accommodation being exerted and do not change in type and magnitude between distance and near viewing.

5.5 THE COVER TEST

The cover test is one of the most important tests that you will carry out and it should be performed as part of every eye examination. The aim of the test is simply to allow you to observe what happens when binocular vision is suspended by covering one eye whilst the patient has been instructed to view a target. The cover test should be carried out when the patient fixates a distant and a near target. It is often important to determine the effect of any refractive error on the deviation, so an assessment of binocular status is often required in the unaided state and/or in the patient's own spectacles and with the optimal refractive error. There are two varieties of cover test, the cover/uncover test and the alternating cover test. In the case of the cover/uncover test, the cover is first introduced in front of one eye to prevent binocular vision, and then it is removed to allow viewing under habitual conditions. In the alternating cover test, when the cover is removed from one eye it is immediately transferred to the fellow eye thus preventing binocular viewing of the target for the full duration of the test. The cover/uncover test gives a measure of the habitual angle of deviation. In cases of heterophoria, the deviation observed during the alternating cover test is typically larger than that observed during the cover/uncover test, and is referred to as the total angle of deviation. The cover/uncover version of the test must always be performed since this is the only test that allows a heterophoria to be distinguished from a heterotropia. However, many practitioners will use both versions of the test; if the cover/uncover test has revealed that no heterotropia exists, any movements observed on the alternating cover test indicate that a heterophoria is present. Video clips of the cover test being used to assess a variety of heterotropias and heterophorias are provided on the website 📓.

5.5.1 Binocular status in the primary position

An assessment of binocular status in the primary position is required at both distance and near to determine whether a heterotropia or heterophoria is present. If present, the direction and size of the deviation should be determined and recorded. Clinical judgements about constancy or laterality (heterotropia) or control (heterophoria) may also be possible.

5.5.2 Advantages and disadvantages

The cover/uncover test is the only method by which an ocular deviation can be distinguished as either a heterotropia (tropia, strabismus or squint) or a heterophoria. The test has the advantage of being an objective test (i.e. one that requires cooperation but no response from the patient) although the subjective response of the patient while performing the test can provide valuable additional information. The cover test provides considerable information about a deviation including its direction and size. In addition, the pattern of movements observed may enable the practitioner to form an opinion about the stability, constancy, laterality or control of a deviation. The test is quick and simple to perform. One disadvantage of the test is that even experienced practitioners cannot detect very small deviations (up to 2–3$^\Delta$; Fogt et al. 2000). Since even small vertical heterophorias can be clinically significant, it is likely that you would miss these if just using the objective cover test. However, small deviations of any variety may be identified using the subjective

cover test. The only disadvantage of the cover test is that it requires considerable practice before accurate observations can be made.

An advantage of the alternating cover test in the assessment of heterophoria is that the deviation observed will normally be considerably larger (and therefore more obvious) that that which is apparent during the cover/uncover test. This is because binocular vision is suspended altogether during the alternating cover test whereas binocular vision is interrupted and then restored during the cover/uncover test. The deviation found on the alternating cover test represents the total angle of deviation as compared to the habitual angle measured during the cover/uncover test. It should also be noted that the alternating cover test can be used as a means of placing stress on the oculomotor system, and it can be useful to consider the total deviation as an indicator of the heterophoria when the patient is tired or at the end of the day. The alternating cover test can also be used to identify those heterophorias that can intermittently break down into a heterotropia. The alternating cover test cannot be used alone to evaluate whether a patient has a heterotropia as the pattern of eye movements observed during the alternating cover test in a patient with an exotropia will be indistinguishable from those observed in a patient with exophoria, etc. To detect a heterotropia, the cover/uncover test must be performed. However, the alternating cover test can be used to estimate the magnitude of any heterotropia found during the cover/uncover test.

5.5.3 Procedure

1. Keep the room lights on and, if necessary, use localised lighting so that the patient's eyes can be easily seen without shadows.

2. Explain the purpose of the test to the patient: 'I am now going to find out how well your eye muscles work together'.

3. The following targets should be used:
   a) For the distance cover test, isolate a single letter of a size one line larger than the patient's VA of the poorer eye. For example, if VAs are 6/4.5 (20/15) and 6/9 (20/30), use a 6/12 letter (20/40) as a target for the distance cover test. The

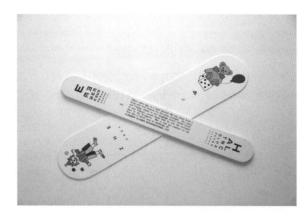

Fig. 5.1 Fixation sticks used for the near cover test and other tests requiring near fixation.

patient must be able to easily see the letter with both eyes, but it should be a target that requires accurate fixation and accommodation. If you are using a projector chart, isolate a single letter on the appropriate line. If you are using a printed chart, then ask the patient to look at a letter at the end (or beginning) of a line, as it will be easiest to locate after the eye has been uncovered. If the monocular VA in either eye is 6/18 (20/60) or worse, a spotlight may be used for fixation.

b) For the near cover test, a fixation stick should be used that contains letters or pictures of various sizes (Fig. 5.1). A single letter of a size one line larger than the patient's near VA of the poorer eye should be chosen. As most near VA charts are truncated to N5 or 0.4M (20/20), this will tend to be N6 or 0.5M (20/25). Pictures can be used for young children, but they should be of an appropriate size. Pictures (or letters) that are too large do not provide an accurate stimulus for fixation or accommodation and this is essential for an accurate cover test. The fixation stick should be held at the patient's near working distance (this may be at an intermediate distance if you wish to assess their binocular status at a distance at which they view a computer screen).

4. Irrespective of whether you are carrying out a cover test during distance or near viewing, you should sit directly in front of the patient, at a distance of 25–40 cm away. This will place you close enough to be able to critically note eye movements. When performing the cover test for distance viewing, you should be very careful not to block the patient's view of the fixation target.

a) For the distance cover test, the patient should have their head erect and eyes in the primary position of gaze.

b) For the near cover test, the eyes should be in a slight downward gaze (similar to the position for reading). It can be particularly difficult to see the patient's eyes when wearing multifocal spectacles and it can help to ask the patient to tilt their head back slightly, and then look in a slight downward gaze. The drooping upper lids of some older patients may need to be gently held up if you still cannot see the eyes easily. In this case, you should ask the patient to hold the fixation stick. Finally, if it is otherwise not possible to see the patient's eyes sufficiently well, ask the patient to hold their multifocal spectacles up slightly and to view the fixation stick with their head erect and eyes in the primary position of gaze. In this case, you should note that the near cover test has been performed in primary gaze rather than the preferred slight downward gaze.

5. Instruct the patient: 'I would like you to look at the letter … at the other end of the room (or the letter … on this stick). Please keep watching the letter as closely as you can

---

Step 1: Check for Tropia

Step1: Tropia Present (Y/N)?
Procedure: Cover one eye whilst observing fellow eye

RE moves when LE covered Dx. RE tropia	LE moves when RE covered Dx. LE tropia	RE moves when LE covered & LE moves when RE covered Dx. Alternating tropia	Neither eye moves when fellow eye covered Dx. No tropia is present, now check for phoria

Step 2: If no Tropia present, check for Phoria

Procedure: Alternating Cover Test
Observe each eye as it is being uncovered

Eyes move IN when cover switched to fellow eye Dx. EXOphoria	Eyes move OUT when cover switched to Fellow eye Dx. ESOphoria	No movement seen when cover switched but Px. reports shift in apparent target position. Dx. Phoria present (WITH in EXOphoria, AGAINST in ESOphoria)	No movement seen when cover switched & Px. reports no shift in apparent target position. Dx. ORTHOphoria

Box 5.1

while I place this cover in front of your eye. If the letter appears to move please follow it with your eyes.' In order to check compliance with your instructions, especially in the case of children, it is useful to occasionally move the stick a short distance to one side. If the eyes are seen to follow the target then you can be confident that your instructions are being followed.

6. When carrying out a cover test it is vital to be systematic in your approach. FIRST: Search for the presence of a heterotropia. If one exists, then by definition, a heterophoria cannot be present simultaneously and once you have recorded the direction and magnitude of the heterotropia you should move onto the next test in your examination procedure (e.g. cover test at a different distance).
SECOND: If there is no heterotropia, search for a heterophoria using the cover/uncover test and/or the alternating cover test. If no

heterophoria is evident you should perform a subjective cover test by asking the patient for their impression of movement as the cover is switched from eye to eye during the alternating cover test. These two sequential steps differ subtly from one another in terms of the procedures to be carried out and in their interpretation. They cannot be performed simultaneously. These steps are diagrammatically summarised in the flow chart (Box 5.1) and detailed instructions as to how to perform and interpret both of them is provided in the text that follows.

7. **Perform the cover/uncover (unilateral cover) test to look for a heterotropia** (Fig. 5.2):
   a) Place the cover before the left eye. As you do so, observe the response of the right eye that has not been covered. Repeat this procedure two or three times before you arrive at any decision. If the right eye moves when the left is covered, then a tropia is present in the right eye. The

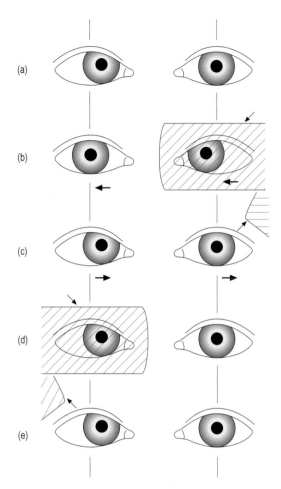

Fig. 5.2 Cover test in a patient with a right esotropia. (a) The right eye is turned inwards slightly but this may not be obvious, depending on its size and your experience. (b) As the left eye is covered, the right eye is seen to move out to take up fixation. Behind the cover, the left eye moves to the right, obeying Hering's law. (c) As the left eye is uncovered, it moves out to take up fixation as it is the non-strabismic eye. (d) When the right eye is covered, the left eye does not move. (e) When the right eye is uncovered, neither eye moves. (Reproduced with permission from Pickwell, 1989.)

movement observed occurs to take up fixation. You should allow the eye time to take up fixation, which may be 2–3 seconds. If the eye moves out to take up fixation, then in the binocular situation it must have been directed inwards and so an ESOtropia is present. If the eye moves in to take up fixation an EXOtropia is present. If the eye moves up to take up

fixation, then in the binocular situation it must have been directed downwards and so a HYPOtropia is present. If the eye moves down to take up fixation, a HYPERtropia is present.

b) Repeat the cover/uncover test by placing the cover over the right eye and look for a heterotropia in the left eye. Once again, repeat the procedure two or three times. If neither eye moves when the other is covered there is no heterotropia and you should go to step 8 below.

c) In a unilateral strabismus, when the deviating eye is covered and then uncovered, the non-tropic 'normal' eye will continue to fixate and will not move. If there is a unilateral heterotropia present, there is frequently amblyopia so that the visual acuity is reduced in that eye.

d) Eyes with strabismus and amblyopia may not take up fixation immediately when the fellow eye is covered. Give them time to fixate and actively encourage the patient to do so. Note and record any fixation instability or tremor (nystagmus) when the patient attempts to fixate with the eye that normally deviates.

e) If the visual acuity is approximately the same in the two eyes, and you believe that a heterotropia is present then the possibility of an alternating heterotropia should be investigated. Note that patients with a marked difference in VA between the eyes will not alternate. With an alternating heterotropia, the right eye will exhibit the tropia if the left eye is asked to fixate during the cover test and the left eye will exhibit the tropia if the right eye is asked to fixate during the cover test. The difficulty with diagnosing an alternating tropia is that the tropia movement only occurs during the first cover/uncover assessment. When the cover/uncover assessment is repeated a second and third time (step 7a), the eye being observed does not now move as it has now become the fixating eye. The other eye has now become the deviating eye and the tropia will appear in the first cover/uncover assessment of the other eye. When asked to view binocularly after completion of the cover/uncover test, some patients with an alternating heterotropia will continue to fixate with the eye that was last asked to fixate the target during the cover test procedure. In such cases, there is no preferred fixating eye. In other cases, there is a definite preference for fixation with one eye over the other and although the non-preferred eye might continue to fixate for a short period (e.g. a few seconds) after the cover had been removed, fixation would then switch to the preferred eye. Some patients with alternating tropia can switch eyes at will if you ask them to and some may even anticipate which eye is to be covered and switch eyes prior to you using the occluder. These tropias can be very confusing at first, so if you suspect an alternating heterotropia, ask a supervisor for help.

f) Note that some heterotropias may be intermittent. Typically these are large heterophorias that sometimes break down into a heterotropia. If you suspect an intermittent tropia, use the alternating cover test to break the tropia down.

g) Repeat the test from the beginning to confirm your diagnosis.

h) If a heterotropia is present there is no need to search for a heterophoria. You should record your result and move on to the next test (e.g. cover test in different refractive correction, or at a different viewing distance).

8. If no heterotropia was found you should now begin the search for a heterophoria. There are two possible alternatives here and both have their advocates. Some practitioners will continue to use the cover/uncover test that was used for heterotropia investigation in the search for a heterophoria. If this is your preferred approach then go to step 9 below. An alternative approach is to switch now to the alternating cover test. If this is your preferred approach then go to step 10. Some practitioners use both techniques to evaluate heterophoria. There is no research to support one approach over the other.

9. **If no heterotropia is present, perform the cover/uncover test to look for a heterophoria** (Fig. 5.3):

a) In heterophoria, the eye being covered will move out of alignment with the other eye because sensory fusion is being prevented. It will then retake fixation when the cover is removed. Some practitioners attempt to observe both the movement of the eye that is under cover and the recovery movement of that eye when the cover is removed. This requires some dexterity on the part of the practitioner and care must be taken to ensure that the 'cover' is really covering the patient's view of the target. Other practitioners only attempt to observe the eye's recovery movement when the cover is removed. If you choose to do the latter, then go directly to step (c).

b) Place the cover before the left eye in a manner that prevents the patient from viewing the target but allows you to continue viewing the covered eye. Observe the response of the left eye behind the occluder when it is first covered. If a heterophoria is present then the covered eye will drift outwards in EXOphoria, inwards in ESOphoria, upwards in HYPERphoria and downwards in HYPOphoria.

c) Observe the response of the covered eye as the cover is removed. Remove the cover in a manner that allows you to view the eye continuously as it is being uncovered. In other words don't move the occluder away from the patient's eye in a fashion that causes you to temporarily lose sight of it. For example, you can remove the cover from in front of the patient's right eye by moving the cover diagonally downwards and leftwards. Note the recovery movement of the eye will be opposite to that which took place behind the cover. For example, in EXOphoria the eye moves back in when the cover is removed as it drifted out (away from the nose) behind the cover.

d) When establishing if a heterophoria is present it is the eye being covered and uncovered that is the subject of the practitioner's attention. However, it is useful to consider what happens to the fixing (uncovered) eye as the test is carried out. If a heterophoria is present, two patterns of movement may be seen:

i) When the covered eye is uncovered, the fellow, fixating eye shows no sign of movement. Note that this pattern is not in accordance with Hering's law of equal eye movements (section 5.5.5).

ii) When the cover is removed, the eye that was covered will make a fusional recovery movement (outwards in ESOphoria and inwards in EXOphoria, etc.). In addition, the eye, which had been fixating the target, will also move. It moves in the same direction as the uncovered eye (equal version movement) and then reverses in direction to retake fixation (Fig. 5.3), This pattern of movements is more obviously in keeping with Hering's law of equal innervation (section 5.5.5) and is more frequently observed in patients with large phorias or when a highly dominant eye is uncovered. The appearance is of the fixating eye undergoing a flick or wobble as the cover is removed from the other eye.

iii) Since it is not possible to observe the two eyes at once when the cover is removed, you should repeat this cycle several times, watching first one eye and then the other and comparing the movement of the two.

e) Repeat the observations when covering and uncovering the right eye. If an esophoria was present in the left eye, it should be present and similarly sized in the right. It does not make sense to state that a patient has, for example, 'esophoria of the right eye' since esophoria of the same or very similar magnitude will almost always be present when the left eye is covered. There are some rare exceptions to this rule, such as in patients with uncorrected or residual anisometropia, where greater accommodative convergence in one eye influences the movements. Because the presence of a vertical heterophoria signals a tendency for the eyes to drift out of vertical alignment, a

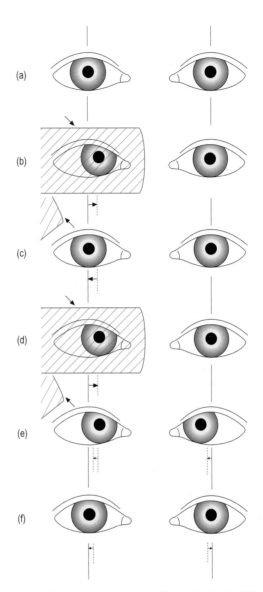

Fig. 5.3 Cover test in a patient with esophoria. (a–c) The simple pattern of movements that is usually seen. (d–f) The rarer versional pattern of movements that can occur when one eye is dominant. (a) Both eyes look straight ahead. (b) The right eye is covered and the left eye does not move, indicating that there is no strabismus in the left eye. Behind the cover the right eye moves inwards. (c) The right eye is uncovered and the right eye moves out to resume fixation with the other eye. Note that, during the movements of the right eye, the left eye has not moved and disobeys Hering's law to maintain fixation. (d) The right eye is covered as before and it moves inwards behind the cover. (e) The right eye is uncovered and both eyes move right by the same amount, obeying Hering's law. (f) Both eyes diverge by the same amount, again obeying Hering's law, and take up fixation. (Reproduced with permission from Pickwell, 1989.)

hypophoria evident in one eye will be evident as a hyperphoria in the fellow eye. Once again, however, the deviations will usually be of a similar size in the two eyes.

f) Observe the latency and the speed of the fusional recovery movement on uncovering, since this may give clues as to the strength of the fusion reflex. The movement should be smooth and fast. Poor fusion reflexes are slow and hesitant, with jerky movements.

g) Estimate or measure the magnitude of the deviation. Deviations can be measured by placing prisms of increasing power in front of one eye until no movement is observed during the cover/uncover test. The prism is normally placed in front of one eye only. Base-in prism power is used to measure EXOphorias/EXOtropias, and base-out to measure ESOphorias/ESOtropias. A prism bar is most conveniently used for this purpose, although estimates made by experienced practitioners can be in good agreement with measurements made using prism bars (Rainey et al. 1998a).

10. **If no heterotropia is present, perform the alternating cover test.**

a) Place the occluder before one eye for 2–3 seconds and then transfer it quickly to the other eye, without pausing. Keep the occluder in front of the eye for 2–3 seconds, and allow the other eye to take up fixation, and then repeat the cycle. The patient must not view the target binocularly at any time and thus rapid movement of the cover between the eyes is required. For this reason, the occluder should be moved along a horizontal line between the eyes rather than in an arc-shaped pattern. In order to facilitate swift transfer of the cover between the eyes it is best if the practitioner's hand that holds the cover is held close to the patient's forehead or close to the tip of the patient's nose.

b) If there is a deviation of the eyes, it will be seen as a re-fixation eye movement when the cover is transferred from one eye to the other. The eyes will move outwards in ESOphoria/ESOtropia, and inwards in EXOphoria/EXOtropia, etc.

c) Observe the latency and the speed of the fusional recovery movement on uncovering, since this may give clues as to the strength of the fusion reflex. The movement should be smooth and fast. Poor fusion reflexes are slow and hesitant, with jerky movements.

d) Estimate or measure the magnitude of the deviation.

11. **If no heterophoric movements are seen during the alternating cover test perform the subjective cover test**

If you cannot see any movement of the eyes during step 10 and the patient can provide good subjective responses, continue to perform the alternating cover test and ask the patient if the target moves when the occluder is switched from one eye to the other. Subjectively reported movements of the target are called 'phi' (pronounced as 'fy' as in 'why') movements. Small amounts of phoria (1–3 $^\triangle$) may be detected in this way. Any reported vertical phi movement should be further investigated using other tests, such as the modified Thorington technique (section 5.7). The type of deviation present can be inferred according to whether the target appears to move in the same or opposite direction as the cover. For example, esophoria will cause the target to move 'against' the movement of the occluder and an exophoria will cause the target to move 'with' it.

12. Estimate or measure the magnitude of the deviation. Deviations can be measured by placing prisms of increasing power in front of one eye until no movement is observed during the alternating cover test. The prism is normally placed in front of one eye only. Base-in prism power is used to measure EXOphorias/EXOtropias, and base-out to measure ESOphorias/ESOtropias. A prism bar is most conveniently used for this purpose, although estimates made by experienced practitioners can be in good agreement with measurements made using prism bars (Rainey et al. 1998a).

5.5.4 Recording

1. Record NMD (No Movement Detected) if this was the case and if no assessment of 'phi' movement was conducted. NMD is preferred to 'ortho' (i.e. orthophoria) or similar, as even experienced practitioners cannot detect very small eye movements (up to 2–3$^\triangle$; Fogt et al. 2000). Hyperphorias of this size can be significant and cause the patient problems, so you must not assume that the patient does not have a significant phoria based on detecting 'no movement' using the cover test.

2. Record 'ortho' (orthophoria) or similar (ϕ for horizontal orthophoria, $\ominus$ for vertical orthophoria and $\oplus$ for both vertical and horizontal orthophoria) only if no movement was detected using the cover test *and* no phi movement was reported.

3. If heterotropia is detected, then record:
   - The constancy (if intermittent is not recorded, the tropia is assumed to be constant. If the deviation is intermittent, note the percentage of time that the eye deviates).
   - Which eye is deviated (right, left or alternating; abbreviated to R, L or Alt).
   - The direction (exo, eso, R hyper or hypo, L hyper or hypo, excyclo, incyclo). Exo and Eso are abbreviated to XO and SO respectively.
   - Add the suffix tropia (abbreviate to T, e.g. SOT, XOT).
   - An indication of the size of the tropia, either measured with a prism bar or estimated (if estimated, precede your result with the symbol '≈'), e.g. ≈20 $^\triangle$L XOT
   - The quality of the fixation reflex in the deviating eye may be recorded if it appears to be unsteady, e.g. 10 $^\triangle$R SOT, unsteady fix.
   - Tropias can also be defined as following an A- or V-pattern or other varieties of alphabet pattern (e.g. Y or inverted Y). By definition such deviations are of the incomitant variety and their presence will emerge during the motility test (section 5.25).

Examples are given in Table 5.2.

If heterophoria is detected, then record:

- The direction (exo, eso, R/L or L/R). Exo and Eso are abbreviated to XO and SO respectively. R/L indicates a right hyperphoria, which is the same as a left hypophoria. L/R indicates a left hyperphoria/right hypophoria.

- Add the suffix phoria (abbreviate to P, e.g. SOP, XOP).

- An indication of the size of the phoria, either measured with a prism bar or estimated (if

Table 5.2   Examples of recordings from the cover test.

Abbreviation	Description
NMD	No movement detected (deviation <2–3$^\triangle$)
<3 SOP (Phi)	A small esophoria (<3$^\triangle$) not seen, but reported subjectively
~4 XOP	A small exophoria with good recovery, estimated to be 4$^\triangle$
8 SOP, slow rec.	An esophoria with slow recovery, measured to be 8$^\triangle$
~4 R/L	Right hyperphoria, estimated to be 4$^\triangle$
Int (50%) ~10 RSOT	Intermittent right esotropia (tropia present about 50% of the time), estimated to be 10$^\triangle$
8 R hyper T	Constant right hypertropia, measured with a prism bar to be 8$^\triangle$
25 Alt XOT c̄ 4 R/L	Constant alternating exotropia of 25$^\triangle$ with a vertical component. There is also an alternating right hypertropia of 4$^\triangle$ (measurements with a prism bar)

estimated, precede your result with the symbol '≈')

- Any recovery movements that were slow, hesitant and/or jerky. Normal, smooth and fast recovery movements are generally not recorded.

- Heterophorias that were found using the subjective cover test, but not seen by the practitioner should be recorded in the usual manner (size, direction) and followed by the term ('phi').

5.5.5 Interpretation

Hering's Law states that the innervation to synergist muscles of the two eyes is equal. This would imply that the eyes would always move by equal amounts (in the same direction in version movements and in the opposite direction in vergence movements). The normal cover test response, in which the fixating eye remains still and the uncovered eye makes a fusional movement, contravenes Hering's Law. Hering's Law would predict that when one eye is uncovered, both eyes would make a version movement equal to half the deviation, and then both eyes would make an equal fusional (vergence) movement, to restore bifoveal fixation. This response does occur in some patients and should not be confused with heterotropic movements (Fig. 5.3). Note that heterotropic cover test movements are in one direction and take place when the cover is *introduced* to the other eye whereas, when they occur, Hering's law movements have the appearance of a 'wobble' and take place when the cover is *removed* from the other eye.

Most children show no movement on the cover test at distance and either no movement or a just visible exophoria at near (Walline et al. 1998). There appears to be little information regarding cover test results for normal adults in the research literature. Textbooks suggest that the majority of adults will also show either no movement or a just visible exophoria or esophoria (up to about 4^Δ) on the distance cover test (Evans 2002). At near, a small amount (3^Δ to 6^Δ) of exophoria is considered normal (physiological exophoria) and this is likely to increase with age (exophoria measured with the Maddox Wing increased from a mean of zero at age

20 to 5^Δ at 65; Freier & Pickwell 1983). As even experienced practitioners *cannot* detect very small eye movements (up to $2–3^\Delta$; Fogt et al. 2000), small hyperphorias will be missed with the objective cover test, and any hyperphoria that is detected will be abnormal.

The movements made by each eye are usually similar in heterophoria. In cases where the heterophoria movement is greater in one eye than the other, this may be due to uncorrected or residual anisometropia or incomitancy (section 5.24).

5.5.6 Most common errors

1. Not positioning yourself appropriately to allow a clear and unimpeded view of the patient's eyes. You need to get close to the patient and you may need to use additional lighting. In older patients, you may need to hold up the upper eyelids when performing the near cover test.

2. Blocking the patient's view of the target that you have instructed them to fixate upon. This is only a problem during the distance cover test.

3. Covering and uncovering the eyes so rapidly that the eyes do not have time to make the movements consistent with the deviation that is present. You should leave the cover in place for at least 2–3 seconds before removing it or transferring it to the other eye.

4. Arriving at your diagnosis too quickly. Repeat the test two or three times in quick succession to confirm your diagnosis. Fixational instability can cause a misleading result on a single test.

5. Missing an esophoria in a pre-presbyopic patient by not using a small enough target to stimulate accommodation and accurate fixation.

6. Missing a heterotropia in an eye with deep amblyopia by not choosing an appropriate fixation target for the test and not actively encouraging steady fixation of the non-fixing eye.

7. Using large, sweeping lateral movement of the occluder when covering/uncovering.

This is distracting and encourages eye movements. Small vertical or lateral movements with the occluder are all that is required.

8. Diagnosing as a heterotropia the immediate loss and recovery of fixation of an eye when the other eye is covered. Because of a heterophoria movement of the covered eye behind the cover, the fixing eye may move from its original accurate foveal position due to Hering's law of equal innervation and then refixate due to the fixation reflex (Fig. 5.3).

9. Not watching for an alternating tropia when switching from covering/uncovering left eye to covering/uncovering right eye.

10. Allowing binocular fixation during the alternating cover test due to poor technique.

5.6 HIRSCHBERG, KRIMSKY AND BRUCKNER TESTS

The Hirschberg test compares the position of the corneal reflexes (the first Purkinje images) of the two eyes that are formed by a pentorch. Using prisms from the trial case, the Hirschberg test can be extended to provide more accurate measures of the angle of heterotropic deviation. When carried out in this fashion, the test is known as the Krimsky test. It is important to realise that, in most patients, the corneal reflections will be displaced slightly nasally relative to the pupil centres. This displacement arises because a separation exists between the pupillary and visual axes. The angle between these axes is referred to as the angle kappa, which is given a positive value if the reflexes are nasally displaced. Video clips of these tests being used are available on the website 🖱.

5.6.1 Objective assessment of heterotropia

In very young children, who may be unable to maintain fixation for long enough to allow the cover test to be performed, an objective assessment of oculomotor status in the primary position can provide useful information to indicate the presence or absence of heterotropia.

5.6.2 Advantages and disadvantages

The Hirschberg test is quick and easy to perform, and requires little cooperation on the part of the patient. However, it can really only be performed at near, the penlight target provides a poor stimulus to accommodation and it is relatively inaccurate. Choi & Kushner (1998) found that even experienced practitioners can obtain results that differ by up to 10 prism dioptres.

5.6.3 Procedure

1. Keep the room fully illuminated. Additional use of localised lighting is recommended so that the patient's eyes can be easily seen without shadows.

2. Remove any spectacles that the patient may be wearing. However, if it is felt that the refractive correction will alter the result (e.g. in cases of significant hyperopia), the test should also be performed through the correction.

3. Hold a penlight horizontally 40 to 50 cm from the patient with the light aimed at the bridge of the patient's nose. The back of the penlight should be very close to the tip of your nose.

4. Ask the patient to look at the light with both eyes open. Young children will automatically tend to look toward the bright light but may need a little encouragement.

5. Note the location of the corneal reflex in each eye individually. In order to do this you should briefly cover each eye in turn; you can do this with the palm of your hand. Remember that the reflex is frequently decentred about 0.5 mm nasally with respect to the centre of the pupil because angle kappa is normally positive.

6. Now compare the location of the corneal reflexes as the patient views habitually (i.e. without any occlusion). The eye that has the same angle kappa as in the monocular test is the fixing eye. The location of that reflex should be considered the reference position.

7. If there is a heterotropia present, the corneal reflex of the other eye will have shifted in a direction opposite to that of the ocular deviation. For example, in the case of an ESOtropia, the corneal reflex will be displaced temporally on the patient's cornea relative to the position of the reflex in the fellow eye.

8. The magnitude of the deviation can be estimated from the displacement of the reflex in millimetres (mm) relative to the reference position using the approximation of $1\,\text{mm} \approx 22^{\Delta}$.

9. Instead of estimating the angle of deviation as in step 8, a more reliable estimate of the magnitude of deviation can be achieved using measuring prisms. This is known as the Krimsky test and it is a simple extension of the Hirschberg test. In the Krimsky test the practitioner varies prism power in front of the fixating eye in order to place the corneal reflex in the deviated eye in the same relative position as the corneal reflex in the fixating eye. As with the Hirschberg test, the penlight is held stationary in front of the patient's eyes. The practitioner needs to be seated directly in front of the deviating eye in order to avoid problems of parallax. Measures of the angle of heterotropia obtained using the Krimsky test do rely upon the assumption that the deviating eye fixates centrally rather than eccentrically. While this assumption may not be valid in many instances, the error it introduces is likely to be small in relation to the overall size of the deviation. Furthermore, the same criticism can be applied to heterotropia measures obtained using the cover test in combination with a prism bar.

5.6.4 Recording

Record the eye that deviates, along with the direction of the deviation (see section 5.5.4 for more details). In your recording, make it clear that the observation was made using the Hirschberg or Krimsky technique. Equal nasal displacement of the corneal reflexes in each eye indicates a non-strabismic patient. For example:

Hirschberg: No Strab; Hirschberg: $\approx 11^{\Delta}$ RSOT; Krimsky: 15^{Δ} L XOT.

5.6.5 Interpretation

A reflex located nasally to the reference point suggests an exotropia; a reflex located temporally to the reference point suggests an esotropia. Superior displacement of the reflex suggests a hypotropia, and inferior displacement suggests a hypertropia. It is important to remember that a large angle kappa may result in the misdiagnosis of heterotropia or failure to detect a heterotropia. For example, a large positive angle kappa will simulate the presence of an exotropia. Similarly, an existing exotropia will appear larger than it actually is and small esotropias may escape detection.

5.6.6 Most common errors

1. Basing your decision upon the absolute position of a single reflex relative to the pupil centre rather than on a comparison of the relative locations of the corneal reflexes in the two pupils.

2. Not viewing directly behind the penlight for the Hirschberg test or from directly in front of the deviating eye in the case of the Krimsky test.

3. Placing too much emphasis on the accuracy of the estimates provided by the Hirschberg and Krimsky tests. These tests are less accurate than the cover test in combination with prism bar for estimating the magnitude of heterotropic deviations (Choi & Kushner 1998).

5.6.7 Alternative test: Bruckner test

The Bruckner test is an alternative method for detecting the presence of strabismus in infants. In a dimly lit room, direct the light from a direct ophthalmoscope from about 1 m away onto the child's face and compare the colour and brightness of the fundus reflexes. In the presence of a strabismus the reflex will be brighter and whiter in the deviating eye as compared to the reflex from the fixing eye. It is suggested that this is because the fundal reflections from a deviating eye are thought to be greater than from the darkly pigmented macular area of a normally fixating eye. Some controversy exists regarding the usefulness of this test but it appears that it can help in the diagnosis of small angle strabismus (Miller et al. 1995). When interpreting the results of the Bruckner test, it is important to remember that differences in brightness can be caused by factors other than strabismus including anisometropia and media opacities.

5.7 MODIFIED THORINGTON TEST

The modified Thorington test is used to measure the amount of heterophoria at distance and/or near. As the name suggests, the technique is a modification of the Thorington method, which used a vertical prism to produce dissociation. In the modified technique, the Maddox rod (section 5.8) is used to produce dissociation.

5.7.1 Subjective assessment of heterophoria

The cover test is objective in that it requires no direct response from the patient (although subjective responses regarding phi movement should be obtained when possible), but all other tests for heterophoria are subjective. Because the cover test can

be difficult to perform when using a phoropter or reduced aperture trial case lenses, subjective procedures may need to be used to assess any heterophoria with the optimal refractive correction. Also remember that the objective cover test is insensitive to small eye movements below about $2–3^\Delta$ (Fogt et al. 2000) and a subjective cover test or other subjective test should be used to check for small vertical heterophorias that may be clinically significant. To investigate any heterophoria, fusion must be suspended. This can be achieved by occluding one eye (cover test), distorting the image seen by one eye (Maddox rod) or by vertical separation of the images seen by the two eyes (von Graefe).

5.7.2 Advantages and disadvantages

The modified Thorington technique is a very simple and quick technique that can be used in a phoropter, trial frame or free space. It produces the most repeatable results of the most commonly used techniques (Casillas & Rosenfield 2006, Rainey et al. 1998b). The principal problem of the Maddox rod technique is the lack of control of accommodation (section 5.8.2). The modified Thorington overcomes this problem by using a target of small letters or numbers (Fig. 5.4). It is principally used at near, but Thorington cards are available for both distance and near. In view of its many advantages

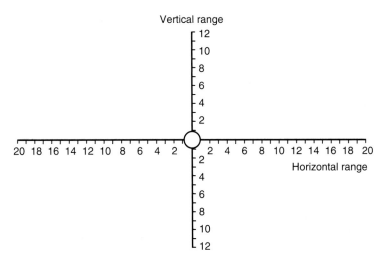

Fig. 5.4 A representation of a typical Thorington card. There is a central aperture in the middle of the card, through which you shine a pen light towards the patient's eyes.

it is somewhat surprising that it is not widely used at present. Like other subjective heterophoria tests, the modified Thorington is more repeatable with a trial frame than with a phoropter (Casillas & Rosenfield 2006).

5.7.3 Procedure

The test is typically used after subjective refraction to determine the heterophoria with the optimal correction. In pre-presbyopic patients, near phorias should be measured immediately after the distance heterophoria measurements. In presbyopes, they should be measured after inclusion of the required reading addition.

1. Inform the patient about the test: 'This test is to check how your eye muscles work together with the new spectacle prescription'.

Horizontal near heterophoria

2. Ensure the patient is wearing their optimal near refractive correction and adjust the phoropter/trial frame to the near centration distance.

3. Place the Maddox rod in front of one eye making sure that the 'grooves' are absolutely horizontal. Note that it is conventional to place the Maddox rod before the right eye. Dim the room lights.

4. Shine the light from a penlight through the central aperture of the Thorington near card.

5. Direct the patient to look at the letters and keep them clear. Ask them to then look at the spotlight, and tell you whether the vertical red line is seen to the right, left or straight through the spotlight.

6. Some patients have difficulty seeing the red line initially. If they cannot see the red line, cover each eye in turn to demonstrate that one eye sees the spotlight and the other sees the red line. Once they are aware of the test format they are often able to see the red line and spotlight simultaneously. Placing a green filter before the eye viewing the spotlight can also help the patient to perform the test. If difficulty is still experienced place the Maddox rod in front of the left eye and try again. If the

spotlight and red line cannot be seen together then suppression may be present and follow-up tests should be performed.

7. With the Maddox rod in front of the right eye the following responses may be given:
   a) If the line is seen to pass through the spotlight the patient has no horizontal phoria.
   b) If the line is to the left of the spotlight (crossed images) the patient has an exophoria. If the line is to the right of the spotlight (uncrossed images) the patient has an esophoria. Determine the size of the deviation by asking the patient which number on the horizontal series of letters on the Thorington card the line passes through. There is no need to insert prism to produce an overlap of the line and spot because the scale on the card is a tangent scale; i.e. the number read off the scale corresponds to the number of prism dioptres of horizontal heterophoria.

8. Compare the horizontal heterophoria found with the cover test result performed with the patient's spectacles. If there is no significant change in refractive error, the heterophoria should be similar to that found with the cover test. Any change in the heterophoria should be consistent with the change in refractive correction (see section 5.7.5).

Vertical near heterophoria

1. Rotate the Maddox rod so that the 'grooves' are oriented vertically.

2. Ask the patient if the red line is seen above, below or straight through the spot.

3. With the Maddox rod in front of the right eye the following responses may occur:
   a) If the line is seen to pass through the spotlight the patient has no vertical phoria.
   b) If the line is above the spotlight the patient has a right hypophoria. It is possible to specify vertical heterophorias with respect to the right or left eye. Thus, a right hypophoria can also be called a left hyperphoria. As above, the size of the deviation is determined by asking the

patient which number on the vertical series (number or letters) of letters on the Thorington card the line passes through.

Distance horizontal and vertical phorias

These can be similarly measured using a distance Thorington card and a penlight.

5.7.4 Recording

1. Record 'ortho' (i.e. orthophoria) or similar (Φ for horizontal orthophoria, ⊖ for vertical orthophoria and ⊕ for both vertical and horizontal orthophoria) if the line seen through the Maddox rod overlaps the spotlight.

2. Record the amount of deviation in prism dioptres (Δ) and the direction of the phoria, e.g. 3^Δ SOP, 5^Δ XOP, $1^{\Delta R}/_L$, $1/_2{}^{\Delta L}/_R$.

3. Note if any suppression took place during the test.

5.7.5 Interpretation

Most people with normal binocular vision have some slight degree of heterophoria. Mean distance heterophoria in children and young adults is 1^Δexophoria $\pm 1^\Delta$ and mean near heterophoria is 3^Δ exophoria $\pm 3^\Delta$ (Lyon et al. 2005, Scheiman & Wick 2002). In older adults, there is a tendency towards greater amounts of exophoria (physiological exophoria) and up to 6^Δ of exophoria is not uncommon (Evans 2002). In adults and children, only about 0.5^Δ of vertical phoria may be considered normal, and in some patients even this amount can give rise to symptoms.

The heterophoria determined using the Thorington test, measured with the optimal refractive correction, should be compared with the corresponding cover test result measured using the patient's spectacles. If there is no significant change in refractive error and the patient's spectacle correction is similar to that found during subjective refraction, the heterophoria found with the Thorington method should be similar to that found with the cover test.

If a change in refractive correction has occurred this should lead to a predictable change in the heterophoria determined using the cover test and subjective assessments. For example, if the optimal correction shows an increase in plus/ decrease in minus power from the patient's spectacles, then an increase in exophoria or a decrease in esophoria should be expected. Similarly, an increase in minus/ decrease in plus power should lead to a decrease in exophoria or increase in esophoria. The amount of change will depend upon the accommodative convergence/accommodation ratio (AC/A ratio, section 5.11).

5.7.6 Most common errors

1. Not attempting the various procedures that may be necessary to enable the patient to simultaneously perceive the red line and spot.

2. Attempting to determine the presence of heterophoria in a patient with strabismus.

3. Failing to distinguish between lens-induced deviations and true heterophorias, particularly in the case of vertical heterophorias caused by the trial frame or phoropter not being level.

5.8 MADDOX ROD

The Maddox rod is used to assess the type and size of heterophoria at distance and (much more rarely) at near. The Maddox rod is a red or clear lens composed of a series of parallel, plano-convex cylinders. When a spotlight is viewed through the Maddox rod, a line is seen with an orientation that is perpendicular to the axis of the cylinders, i.e. if the cylinders are horizontal, a vertical line will be seen. It is usually placed in front of the right eye, so that the right eye sees a line image and the left eye sees the spotlight. This prevents sensory fusion so that the eyes adopt their heterophoric position.

5.8.1 Subjective assessment of heterophoria

The cover test is objective in that it requires no response from the patient (although subjective responses regarding phi movement should be obtained when possible), but all other tests for heterophoria are subjective. Because the cover test can be difficult/impossible to perform when using a phoropter or reduced-aperture trial case lenses, subjective procedures may need to be used to assess any heterophoria after subjective refractive and binocular balancing have taken place (i.e. with the optimal refractive correction in place). Also remember that the objective cover test is insensitive to small eye movements below about 2–3$^\Delta$ (Fogt et al. 2000) and a subjective cover test or other subjective test for vertical heterophoria should be used to check for vertical deviations. In order to assess heterophoria, fusion must be suspended. This can be achieved by occluding one eye (cover test), distorting one image (Maddox rod) or displacing an image (von Graefe's method).

5.8.2 Advantages and disadvantages

The Maddox rod test can be easily performed with a phoropter, trial frame or the patient's own spectacles and with any test chart that contains a spotlight. It is widely used, easy for patients to understand, and can be performed relatively quickly. One drawback is that a spotlight represents a poor stimulus for accommodation and some clinicians consider that this limits the usefulness of the Maddox rod to the measurement of vertical heterophorias, which are assumed to be unaffected by accommodative changes. However, the Maddox rod should produce reliable assessments of horizontal heterophoria when used in patients with no accommodation, such as patients over the age of 60 or pseudophakes. The results may be influenced by a head tilt or a non-level trial frame/phoropter that may lead to an induced vertical deviation. The test should be carried out with the head held in the habitual fashion. Since use of a phoropter will limit the patient's ability to adopt an habitually abnormal head position, the measurement of vertical phorias using the Maddox rod is best performed using a trial frame or a hand-held rod in free space. Like other subjective heterophoria tests, Maddox rod results are more repeatable with a trial frame than with a phoropter (Casillas & Rosenfield 2006).

5.8.3 Procedure

■ Ensure the patient is wearing his/her optimal distance refractive correction.

■ Inform the patient about the test: 'This test is to check how your eye muscles work together with the new spectacle prescription.'

Horizontal distance heterophoria

1. Place the Maddox rod in front of the right eye making sure that the 'grooves' are absolutely horizontal.

2. Provide a spotlight target at distance using the wall/projector chart and then dim the room lights.

3. Ask the patient to look at the spotlight, and to indicate if the vertical (red) line is seen to the right, left or straight through the spotlight.

4. Some patients have difficulty seeing the red line initially. If this occurs, try the following:
   a) Make sure that there are not other sources of light that will each produce a line image.
   b) Cover each eye in turn to demonstrate to the patient that one eye sees the spotlight while the other sees the line. Once they are aware of the test format they are often able to see the line and spotlight simultaneously.
   c) Placing a green filter before the eye viewing the spotlight may also help the patient perform the test, presumably because the brightness difference between the spot and streak is reduced relative to the normal white/red condition.
   d) If the patient continues to see only the line or spot, transfer the Maddox rod to the left eye and try again.
   e) If the spotlight and red line cannot be seen together then suppression may be present and follow-up tests should be performed.

5. With the Maddox rod in front of the right eye the following responses can occur:
   a) If the line is seen to pass through the spotlight the patient has no horizontal

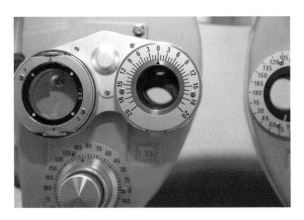

Fig. 5.5 A Risley prism in position to provide prism base-in or base-out.

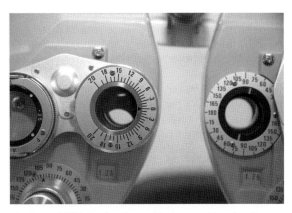

Fig. 5.6 A Risley prism in position to provide prism base-up or base-down.

heterophoria (they may have a vertical phoria).

b) If the line is seen to the left of the spotlight (crossed images) the patient has an exophoria. If the line is to the right of the spotlight (uncrossed images) the patient has an esophoria.

6. To measure the size of the phoria, place prism in front of either eye. The following approach can be adopted:

a) When using a phoropter, use the Risley prism (Fig. 5.5) and increase the power of the appropriate prism (base-in for exophoria, base-out for esophoria). Ask the patient to say when the line is seen to overlap the spot and record the prism power at this instant.

b) When using a trial frame, use loose prisms or a prism bar and increase the power of the appropriately oriented prism (base in for exophoria, base out for esophoria) until the patient indicates that the line runs through the spot or until the line is reported to have crossed to the other side of the spot. In the latter case use an interpolated score. For example, if the patient has exophoria and with 2^Δ IN the line is still to the left of the spot, but with 3^Δ IN it switches across to the right, record 2.5^Δ.

c) Some practitioners adopt a screening approach when using the test with a trial frame and place a 2^Δ prism with appropriately oriented base in front of one

eye. If the line moves to the opposite side, the heterophoria can be recorded as $<2^\Delta$. Compare the horizontal heterophoria found with the cover test result. If there is no significant change in refractive error, the heterophoria should be similar to that found with the cover test. If a change in refractive correction has occurred, any change in heterophoria should be consistent with this in terms of both the magnitude and direction of the alteration in heterophoria (see section 5.7.5).

Vertical distance heterophoria

1. Rotate the Maddox rod so that the 'grooves' are oriented vertically.

2. Ask the patient if the red line is seen above, below or straight through the spot.

3. With the Maddox rod in front of the right eye the following responses can occur.

a) If the line is seen to pass through the spotlight the patient has no vertical heterophoria.

b) If the line is above the spotlight the patient has a right hypophoria. It is possible to specify vertical heterophorias with respect to the right or left eye. Thus, a right hypophoria can also be called a left hyperphoria. The size of the deviation is determined using base-down prisms before the left eye (or base-up prism power before the right eye) using a Risley prism (Fig. 5.6) until the red line and spotlight are overlapping.

c) If the line is below the spotlight the patient has a right hyperphoria (or left hypophoria). The size of the deviation is determined using base-up prisms before the left eye (or base-down prism power before the right eye) until the red line and spotlight are coincident.

4. As a screening technique when used with a trial frame, place a $^1/_2{}^\Delta$ prism with appropriate base in front of one eye. If the line moves to the opposite side of the spot, the phoria can be recorded as $<^1/_2{}^\Delta$.

Horizontal and vertical phorias at near measured using Maddox rod

These can be similarly measured, although the near *horizontal* phorias measurements are considered unreliable in young patients due to the lack of a good accommodative stimulus. In pre-presbyopic patients, near phorias should be measured immediately after the distance phoria measurements. In presby-opes, they should be measured after inclusion of the required reading add, and the phoropter should be adjusted to the near centration distance. A penlight held at 40 cm or the patient's near working distance can be used as the spotlight. The measurement technique is otherwise exactly the same as for distance phoria measurement.

5.8.4 Recording

1. Record 'ortho' (i.e. orthophoria) or similar ($\emptyset$ for horizontal orthophoria, $\ominus$ for vertical orthophoria and $\oplus$ for both vertical and horizontal orthophoria) if the line seen through the Maddox rod runs through the spotlight.

2. Record the amount of deviation in prism dioptres ($^\Delta$) and the direction of the phoria, e.g. 3^Δ SOP, 5^Δ XOP.

3. Vertical phorias can be recorded in a variety of ways, such as:

$2^{\Delta R}/_L$ (or 2^Δ R hyper or 2^Δ L hypo), $1^{\Delta L}/_R$ (or 1^Δ L hyper or 1^Δ R hypo).

4. If the screening approach was used, record $<2^\Delta$ XOP or $<^1/_2{}^{\Delta R}/_L$.

5. Note if any suppression took place during the test.

5.8.5 Interpretation

See section 5.7.5.

5.8.6 Most common errors

1. Not attempting the various procedures that may be necessary to enable the patient to simultaneously perceive the red line and spot (see 5.8.3, step 4).

2. Attempting to determine the presence of heterophoria in a patient with strabismus. Note that the Maddox rod test can be used in strabismic patients to assess retinal correspondence and to assess overactions and underactions of elevating or depressing extraocular muscles (section 5.26.7).

3. Failing to distinguish between lens-induced deviations and true heterophorias. This is particularly important in the case of vertical heterophorias caused by the trial frame or phoropter not being level.

5.9 MADDOX WING

This hand-held device is used to measure the heterophoria at near (Fig. 5.7). The Maddox wing is a common accompaniment to the Maddox rod test for distance heterophoria. Unlike the Maddox rod, the eyes are dissociated using a septum that provides distinct, separate images for the eyes; one eye sees a tangent scale while the other sees an arrow.

5.9.1 Subjective assessment of near heterophoria

The cover test is objective in that it requires no direct response from the patient (although subjective responses regarding phi movement should be obtained when possible), but all other tests for

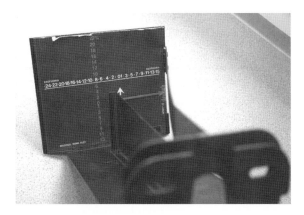

Fig. 5.7   A Maddox wing.

heterophoria are subjective. Because the cover test can be difficult to perform when using a phoropter or reduced aperture trial case lenses, subjective procedures may need to be used to assess any hetero-phoria with the optimal refractive correction. Also remember that the objective cover test is insensitive to small eye movements below about 2–3$^\Delta$ (Fogt et al. 2000) and a subjective cover test or other subjective test should be used to check for small vertical heterophorias that may be clinically significant.

5.9.2 Advantages and disadvantages

The Maddox wing provides a simple and relatively fast technique for the measurement of heterophoria at near. However, the figures used on the scale are relatively large with the result that the patient does not require accurate accommodation. This may lead to an overestimate of an exo deviation or under-estimate of an eso deviation. In addition, the eyes may not be fully dissociated because the septum may allow peripheral fusion to occur. Finally, the instrument uses a standard, fixed centration distance between the lenses and a fixed testing distance of 25 cm. The instrument cannot be used with a phoropter.

5.9.3 Procedure

1. Ensure the patient is wearing their optimal near refractive correction. If the patient is presbyopic, set the trial frame to the near centration distance.

2. The test is carried out with the room lights on. Ensure there is sufficient lighting to allow the scale on the Maddox wing to be seen with ease.

3. Direct the patient to look through the horizontal slits to view the chart, which comprises horizontal and vertical scales, and horizontal and vertical arrows. The right eye sees only the arrows whilst the left eye sees only the scales. The arrows are positioned at zero on the scales but, through the dissociation, any departure from orthophoria will be indicated by an apparent movement of the arrow along the scale.

4. Some patients have difficulty seeing the arrows and the scales simultaneously and require help to position the instrument correctly. If necessary demonstrate to the patient, by covering the aperture in front of each eye in turn, that one eye views the arrows and the other eye views the scales. If the arrows and scales cannot be seen together then suppression may be present and follow-up tests should be performed.

5. Firstly, ask the patient to say whether the arrow is to the right or left of the zero on the scale. This will inform you as to whether there is exophoria or esophoria present. Allow the patient plenty of time before asking 'which white number does the white arrow point to?' The number on the scale indicates the magnitude of the deviation in prism dioptres and the direction (even numbers correspond to exophoria, odd numbers to esophoria). If, over time, the arrow moves to higher and higher numbers on the scale, wait until the arrow has stopped moving before taking the reading. If the arrow is varying between a maximum and a minimum value, record the value of the midpoint between the extremes.

6. To measure a vertical heterophoria ask the patient 'which red number does the red arrow point to?' The number on the scale indicates the magnitude of the deviation and the direction.

7. Compare the horizontal heterophoria found with the cover test result. If there is no significant change in refractive error, the

heterophoria should be similar to that found with the cover test. Any change in refractive correction should produce a predictable change in heterophoria (see section 5.7.5).

5.9.4 Recording

See the modified Thorington (section 5.15.4) or Maddox rod (section 5.16.4) techniques.

5.9.5 Interpretation

As for the modified Thorington test (section 5.7.5).

5.9.6 Most common errors

1. Not allowing the patient sufficient time for the arrow to stop moving. This is only an issue in the case of horizontal phorias. Many patients will report that the arrow continually moves and that movement is especially pronounced immediately after a blink. If the arrow does not stabilise but varies in apparent position between two points on the scale the average value should be recorded.

2. Mistaking the direction of horizontal heterophoria present because the patient has interpolated between the numbers on the scale. For example, if the arrow is seen to be between the 11 and 13 scale positions (esophoria), the patient may state that 'the arrow is pointing to 12'. The practitioner may mistakenly record this result as 12^Δ of exophoria because even numbers are employed on the test for exo deviations. The way to avoid this problem is to initially ask whether the line is seen to the left or right of the zero position.

5.10 VON GRAEFE PHORIA TECHNIQUE

This technique may be used to measure dis tance and near heterophorias using a phoropter.

Dissociation is achieved by separating the retinal images using a prism.

5.10.1 Subjective assessment of heterophoria

The cover test is objective in that it requires no direct response from the patient (although subjective responses regarding phi movement should be obtained when possible), but all other tests for heterophoria are subjective. Because the cover test can be difficult to perform when using a phoropter or reduced aperture trial case lenses, subjective procedures may need to be used to assess any heterophoria with the optimal refractive correction. Also remember that the objective cover test is insensitive to small eye movements below about 2^Δ (Fogt et al. 2000) and a subjective cover test or other subjective test should be used to check for small vertical heterophorias which may be clinically significant. To investigate any heterophoria, fusion must be suspended. This can be achieved by occluding one eye (cover test), distorting the image seen by one eye (Maddox rod) or by vertical separation of the images seen by the two eyes (von Graefe's method).

5.10.2 Advantages and disadvantages

The technique is widely used and familiar and can be easily performed in a phoropter with a projector chart and no additional equipment. Unfortunately, it is the least reliable technique of those commonly available (Casillas & Rosenfield 2006, Rainey et al. 1998b) and its results correlate poorly with the cover test (Calvin et al. 1996), especially in the case of horizontal phoria measures. This may result from variable amounts of prism adaptation, phoropter-induced proximal accommodation, a head tilt behind the phoropter leading to an induced vertical deviation or a reduction in peripheral fusion (Casillas & Rosenfield 2006). In addition, it is a relatively lengthy procedure, can be difficult for patients to understand and cannot easily be used with a trial frame. The technique does not appear to warrant its widespread use and other more reliable techniques such as the modified Thorington (section 5.7) should ideally replace it.

5.10.3 Procedure

Inform the patient about the test: 'This test checks how your eye muscles work together in the new spectacle prescription.'

Distance lateral phoria

1. The test is performed after a phoropter-based distance refraction has been completed. For this reason, the phoropter should be set at the correct centration distance and should be properly positioned for the patient. As a projector chart is being used, either switch off the lights above the projected chart or dim the room lights to keep the contrast of the letters high.

2. Using the projector chart, isolate a letter or a vertical column of letters one line larger than the visual acuity of the poorer eye. This ensures that both eyes can easily see the letter(s). As the patient is asked to keep the letter(s) clear, this also helps to control accommodation. Direct the patient's attention to the letter(s).

3. Inform the patient: 'Please close your eyes while I make the letters go double.' Patients are asked to briefly close their eyes because some patients do not react well when the letters are seen to move as the prism is being introduced. Using the Risley prisms, place $6^\triangle$ base-up (BU) in front of the left eye. This is the dissociating prism. Place $10^\triangle$ base-in (BI) in front of the right eye. This is the measuring prism.

4. Ask the patient whether they see double. If they do not, there are a number of changes you can make to ensure diplopia is appreciated:
   a) Check the phoropter as one eye may be occluded.
   b) Ask the patient to look around. The patient may simply not have noticed the second image.
   c) Alternately occlude the eyes so that each eye's target is shown. This can help the patient find the targets and can help to eliminate slight suppression.
   d) Increase the base-up prism to $8-10^\triangle$ BU. They may have a very large vertical vergence range or large prism adaptation.
   e) Change the prism to $6^\triangle$ base-down (BD). The patient may have a vertical deviation that the original $6^\triangle$ BU is correcting/partly correcting.

5. Explain to the patient that you want them to look at the bottom letter and that you are going to line up the two letters/columns of letters 'like buttons on a shirt'. To minimise accommodative (and accompanying vergence) changes, ask the patient to keep the bottom letter clear. This is the letter viewed through the dissociating prism.

6. To ensure that prism adaptation has minimal effect, the letters should only be made visible to the patient for brief periods of about 1 second ('flashing'). Briefly occlude the right eye with a hand-held occluder, then remove the occluder and ask the patient if the top letter is seen initially to the right or left of the bottom one.

7. Given the prism used in step 3, the bottom letter is seen by the left eye and the top letter by the right eye. If the top letter is initially seen to the right of the bottom, this is uncrossed diplopia, and the deviation is less than the $10^\triangle$ measuring prism, so this should be reduced. If the top letter initially appears to be to the left of the bottom, this is crossed diplopia, and the deviation is greater than the $10^\triangle$ measuring prism, so this should be increased.

8. Repeat the occlusion and change the base-in measuring prism accordingly. Initially use about $4^\triangle$ steps and progressively reduce the step size to $2^\triangle$ as the alignment position is first passed and then use a step size of $1^\triangle$ as you approach alignment.

9. Use a bracketing technique to determine the amount of measuring prism required to make the letters line up 'like buttons on a shirt'.

10. Some clinicians get close to the end-result by asking the patient when the letters are lined up as they move the prism in the appropriate direction. They then 'fine-tune'

the result using a flashing technique. There is a greater risk of prism adaptation with this technique, and it is less repeatable than the 'flashing' procedure (Rainey et al. 1998b).

Distance vertical phorias

This is usually measured after the distance lateral phoria measurement.

1. Occlude one eye and change the prism before the right eye to 15^{Δ} BI. Leave the prism before the left eye (6^{Δ} BU). In this case, the base-in prism is the dissociating prism and the base-up prism is the measuring prism.

2. Adjust the base-up prism in front of the left eye until the patient reports that the two letters line up like 'the headlights on a car'. Use a similar technique as for the lateral phoria measurement: 'flash' the letters for 1 second only, change the prism power when the left eye is occluded, ask the patient to keep the letter to the right clear (this is the letter viewed through the dissociating prism) and use a bracketing technique to determine the required prism. Use an initial step size of 2^{Δ}, then subsequent step sizes of 1^{Δ} and finally 0.5^{Δ} as you approach alignment. Accuracy is especially important for the vertical phoria measurement as small phorias frequently give rise to symptoms.

Near lateral and vertical phorias

These can be similarly measured. In pre-presbyopic patients, near heterophorias are measured immediately after the distance phoria measurements. In presbyopes, they are measured after inclusion of the required reading addition. The phoropter should be adjusted to the near centration distance. The near-point card should be attached to the near-point rod in good illumination. The near card is traditionally set at 40 cm, but could be set at the patient's typical near working distance if this differs considerably from 40 cm. The target should be a column/row or small block of letters that are approximately one line larger than the near acuity in the poorer eye. In patients with normal visual acuity, this is usually about 0.5M or 20/30 equivalent Snellen. The measurement technique is otherwise exactly the same as for distance heterophoria measurement with the von Graefe technique.

5.10.4 Recording

As for the modified Thorington test (section 5.7.4).

5.10.5 Interpretation

As for the modified Thorington test (section 5.7.5).

5.10.6 Most common errors

1. Allowing continual viewing of both letters, which may induce prism (vergence) adaptation.
2. Not reminding the patient to keep one of the letters clear.
3. Providing an inadequate stimulus to accommodation by using a target that is too large.
4. Allowing tilting of the patient's head or not ensuring that the phoropter is level.

5.11 MODIFIED GRADIENT AC/A RATIO TEST

The modified gradient test measures the accommodative convergence/accommodation (AC/A) ratio by calculating the change in heterophoria with specific spherical lenses.

5.11.1 Accommodative convergence/ accommodation (AC/A) ratio

The coupling of accommodation and vergence allows clear stable single binocular vision across a range of viewing distances. A change in accommodation (A) is usually accompanied by a change in vergence known as accommodative convergence (AC). When accommodation is exerted the eyes are induced to converge. When accommodation is relaxed the eyes are induced to diverge. The amount of accommodative convergence in prism dioptres (Δ) evoked by 1D of accommodation is known as the AC/A ratio. As the actual accommodation response is difficult to measure in clinical practice, it is usual to

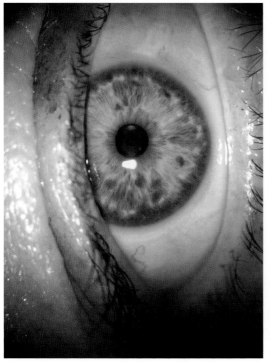

Fig. 6.2   Iris naevi.

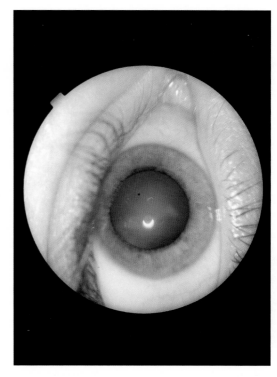

Fig. 6.4   A Mittendorf dot.

Fig. 6.1   A wedge-shaped section of hyperpigmentation (heterochromia).

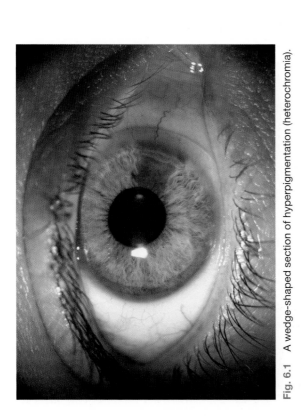

Fig. 6.3   Persistent pupillary membrane.

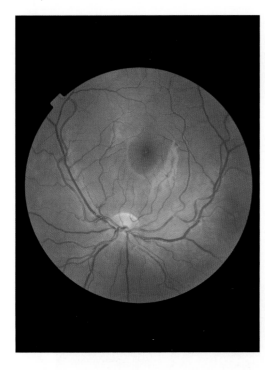

Fig. 6.6 Small optic disc with minimal cupping and a visible nerve fibre layer of a young emmetropic Caucasian patient. Some reflections can be seen in a broken ring outside the macular region.

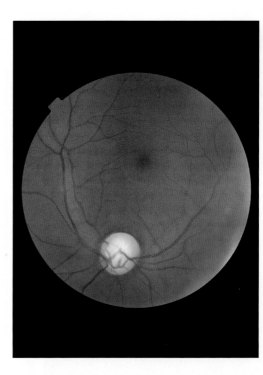

Fig. 6.8 Large optic disc and large cupping (CD ratio ≈ 0.60) and a visible nerve fibre layer of a young emmetropic Afro-Caribbean patient. The inferior edge of the photograph shows some light scatter from the edge of the undilated pupil.

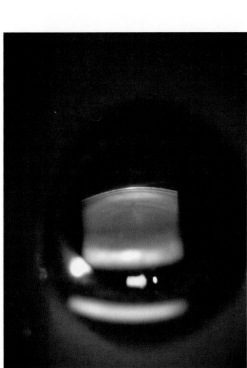

Fig. 6.5 Zones of discontinuity and a Y-suture in a posterior lens section.

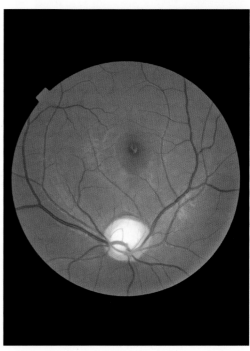

Fig. 6.7 Large optic disc and large cupping (CD ratio ≈ 0.60), a visible nerve fibre layer and macular pigmentation of a young, slightly myopic Asian patient. Some reflections can be seen in a broken ring outside the macular region and beside some of the main blood vessels.

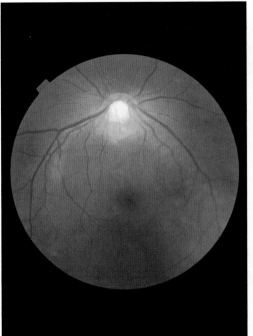

Fig. 6.9 Magnified view of a deep cup with visible lamina cribrosa (CD ratio ≈ 0.25), a choroidal crescent, visible nerve fibre layer and cilio-retinal artery of a young myopic Caucasian patient.

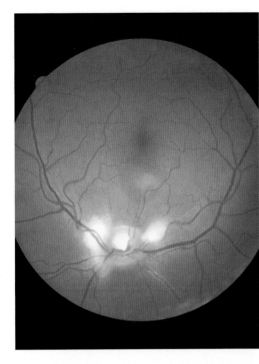

Fig. 6.10 Tilted disc with the nasal side raised and blood vessels nasally displaced. There is a temporal choroidal crescent, slightly tessellated fundus and visible nerve fibre layer. The fundus of the other eye was a mirror image of this one.

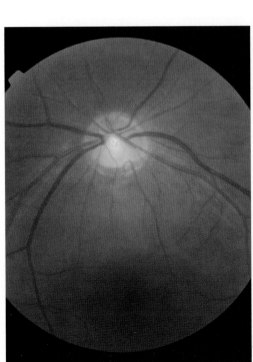

Fig. 6.11 Tilted disc syndrome and highly visible choroidal blood vessels in a young, highly myopic and astigmatic Caucasian patient. The disc is tilted inferior nasally with situs inversus.

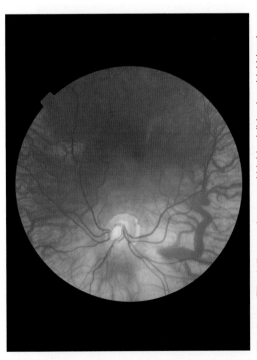

Fig. 6.12 Myelinated nerve fibres. There is a purplish reflection between the macula and disc and the inferior edge of the photograph shows some light scatter from the edge of the undilated pupil.

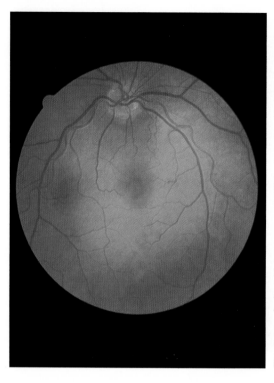

Fig. 6.14 A choroidal naevus, ≈ 1 DD in size, about 3 DD from the disc between 10 and 11 o'clock. The disc is small and flat.

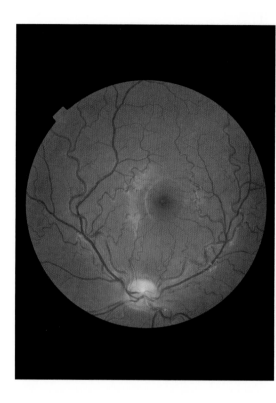

Fig. 6.16 Very tortuous retinal arteries and visible macular pigment in a young Caucasian patient. Some reflections can be seen in a broken ring outside the macular region, just above the ring and beside some of the blood vessels.

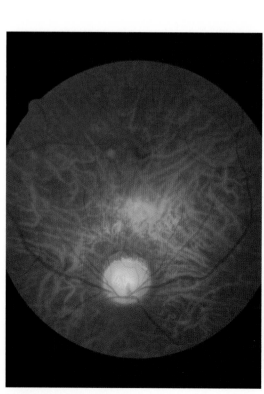

Fig. 6.13 A tigroid fundus with a large optic disc and cup (CD ≈ 0.55), visible lamina cribrosa and choroidal crescent in a young myopic patient.

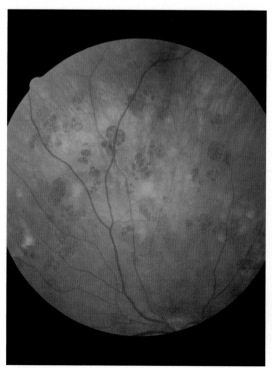

Fig. 6.15 Bear tracks in the peripheral retina.

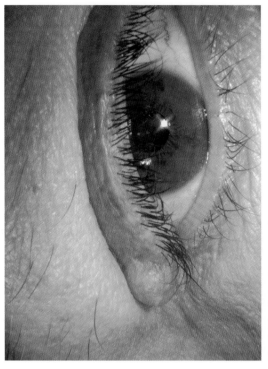

Fig. 6.17   Early dermatochalasis.

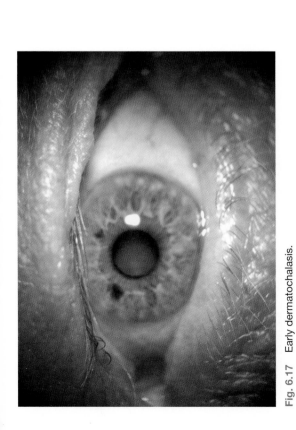

Fig. 6.18   Subcutaneous sebaceous cyst.

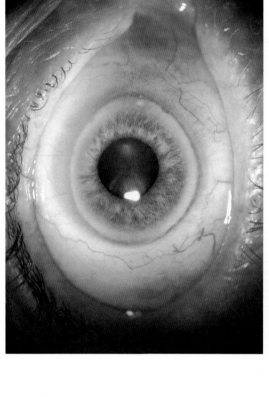

Fig. 6.19   Xanthelasma.

Fig. 6.20   Complete corneal arcus and cortical cataract viewed in direct diffuse illumination. The patient was able to maintain an unusually large palpebral aperture for the photograph.

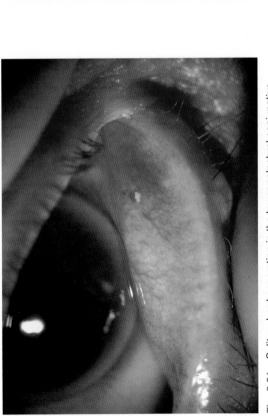

Fig. 6.21   Solitary hard concretion in the lower palpebral conjunctiva.

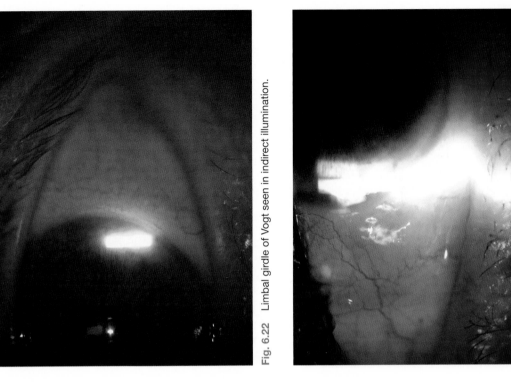

Fig. 6.22   Limbal girdle of Vogt seen in indirect illumination.

Fig. 6.23   A Hudson–Stähli line.

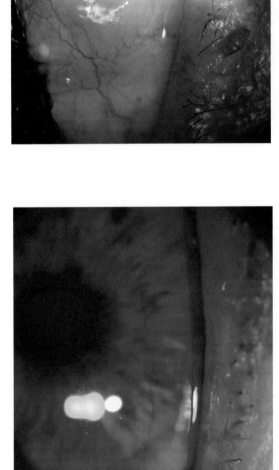

Fig. 6.24   A pinguecula seen to the left of the slit-beam in indirect illumination. A small papilloma is also visible on the lower lid.

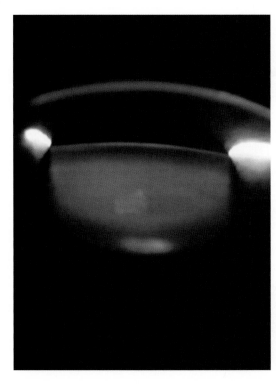

Fig. 6.25 A small posterior subcapsular cataract and several vacuoles seen in fundal retro-illumination.

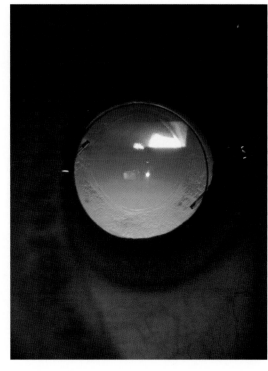

Fig. 6.26 Nuclear cataract seen by optical section. The blurred blue arc to the right is the out-of-focus cornea.

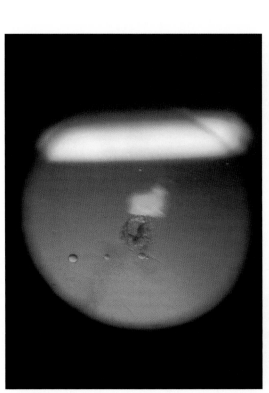

Fig. 6.27 Cortical cataract seen in fundal retro-illumination.

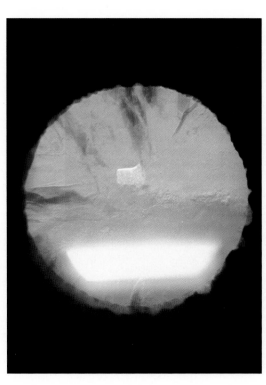

Fig. 6.28 An intraocular implant with peripheral posterior capsular remnants in a dilated pupil seen in fundal retro-illumination.

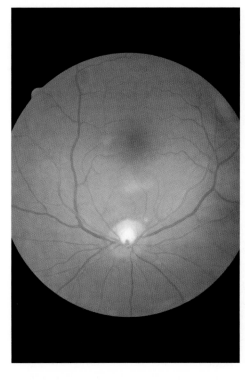

Fig. 6.30   Zone beta PPA, several 90 degree crossings and drusen in the macular area. Some choroidal vessels are visible.

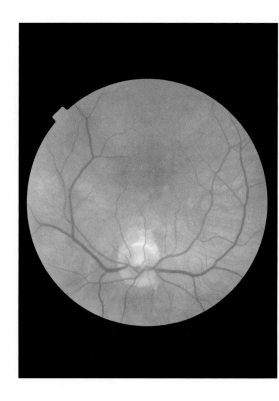

Fig. 6.32   Venous nipping of both temporal veins, several 90 degree crossings and drusen at the macula. There are two reflections, one between the macula and disc and one above the disc, and the edge of the photograph shows some light scatter from the edge of the undilated pupil.

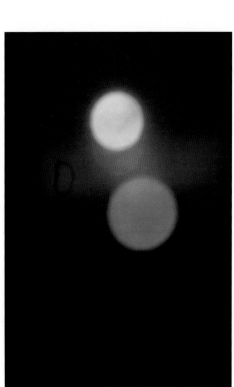

Fig. 6.29   A Weiss ring photographed using fundus biomicroscopy.

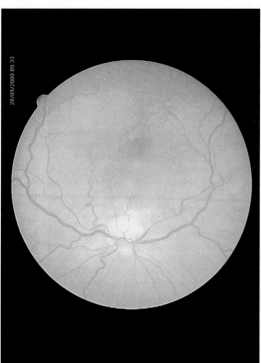

28/09/2000 09:33

Fig. 6.31   Venous nipping of the inferior temporal vein, several 90 degree crossings, drusen temporal to the disc and some pigmentary changes at the macula. The contrast of the fundus view is slightly reduced, probably due to light scatter from early cataract.

measure the change in vergence obtained with a fixed change in the stimulus to accommodation. This is formally known as the stimulus AC/A ratio but clinically it is usually just called the AC/A ratio. The AC/A ratio is a useful measure in the diagnosis and management of binocular vision anomalies. AC/A ratios that are abnormally high or low can give rise to binocular vision problems (Schor & Horner 1989). The AC/A ratio remains fairly constant throughout life until the onset of presbyopia. Measurements of AC/A after the age of 45 years are of little value (Ciuffreda et al. 1997).

5.11.2 Advantages and disadvantages

The modified gradient test allows a quick and reliable measure of the AC/A ratio using standard clinical equipment. This procedure allows proximal components of the response to be controlled as the test is performed at a fixed distance (Hung et al. 1996). The modified gradient AC/A depends on heterophoria measures at only two points, which can lead to errors (Rosenfield et al. 2000). The full gradient test overcomes this problem by measuring heterophorias with additional powers from +3D to −3D in 1.00 D steps and plotting a graph of lens power against induced phoria. The gradient of this line gives the AC/A ratio in $^\Delta$/D.

5.11.3 Procedure

1. Ensure the patient is wearing an appropriate refractive correction, either their own spectacles or, preferably, the optimal correction determined during the eye examination.

2. Measure the horizontal near heterophoria using either the modified Thorington method (section 5.7), Maddox rod (section 5.8) or Maddox wing (section 5.9).

3. Add − 2.00 DS to the refractive correction in both eyes and measure the new horizontal phoria (any pair of minus lenses can be used but − 2.00 DS provides a reasonable accommodative stimulus for most patients).

4. The above procedure is normally carried out at near. However, it is just as valid to

determine the AC/A ratio by comparing the horizontal heterophoria at 6 m when viewing with optimal refractive correction to the heterophoria that exists when the patient looks through a pair of − 2 D lenses.

5.11.4 Recording

Use the following formula to calculate the AC/A ratio. Use positive numbers for esophoria and negative numbers for exophoria.

$$AC/A = \frac{\text{Phoria with additional minus lenses} - \text{baseline phoria}}{\text{Absolute power of additional minus lenses}}$$

The calculation required to determine the AC/A ratio is the same irrespective of whether the heterophoria measurements were taken during near or distance viewing. For example, if a patient exhibits 6^Δ esophoria during distance viewing when −2.00 D lenses are added to his/her normal refractive correction but 2^Δ exophoria with the normal refractive correction in place, the AC/A ratio is calculated as:

$$AC/A = 6 − (−2)/2 = 8/2 = 4^\Delta:1 \text{ D}.$$

5.11.5 Interpretation

Normally the AC/A is $3−5^\Delta$/D. A low AC/A ratio may, depending upon the distance heterophoria, result in convergence insufficiency exophoria. Similarly, a high AC/A ratio may lead to a problem of convergence excess esophoria. Knowledge of the AC/A ratio can be useful when determining plus lens power for the correction of decompensated esophoria. As the amount of convergence induced by 1.00 D stimulus to accommodation is known, it is possible to calculate the extra plus lens power required to reduce the esophoria to an acceptable level.

5.11.6 Most common errors

1. Using the von Graefe assessment of heterophoria (section 5.10) to determine the AC/A ratio, which is less reliable than other

simpler measurements of subjective heterophoria such as the modified Thorington technique (section 5.7).

2. Attempting to measure AC/A ratio in a presbyope.

5.11.7 Alternative technique: calculated AC/A

The AC/A ratio can also be calculated from the information that is already available during a routine eye examination, specifically by comparing the distance heterophoria and near heterophoria. Unlike the methods described above which are carried out at the same test distance, this method has the disadvantage that proximal accommodation is present in one heterophoria measure (near) but not the other (distance). Also, the result is subject to error because only two measures of heterophoria are used in the calculation.

The calculated $AC/A = PD_{cm} + (n - d)/D$, where PD = interpupillary distance measured in cm; n = near phoria; d = distance phoria; D = accommodation. Exophorias are negative and esophorias are positive, e.g. PD = 6 and D = 2.5 (accommodation required at 40 cm), distance phoria is ortho and near phoria is 5 exo, $AC/A = 6 + (-5/2.5) = 4^\Delta{:}1$ D.

Without using the above formula, it is of course possible to get an impression of whether the AC/A ratio is normal or not by comparing the near and distance heterophorias. For example, an exophoria that is much greater at near than at distance will be found in a patient with a low AC/A ratio. Similarly, esophoria that is greater at near than at distance strongly suggests a high AC/A ratio. In cases where the near and distance phorias are the same, the formula above indicates that the AC/A ratio is given by the patient's PD (in cm).

5.12 FUSIONAL RESERVES (FUSIONAL VERGENCES)

There are several names attached to tests that involve determining the prism power that leads to a breakdown in fusion and the perception of diplopia. The names in common use include Fusional Reserves, Fusional Amplitudes, Fusional Vergences and Prism Vergences. The term 'fusional reserves' will be used

as it provides a clear indication of the clinical information provided by the measurement. A video clip of the technique used in free space is available on the website 🖱️.

5.12.1 Fusional reserves

The measurement of fusional reserves is an important clinical test in the assessment of binocular vision status. Heterophorias are latent deviations that are corrected by the sensory fusion reflex. It is useful to know what proportion of the fusional reserves are required to correct the heterophoria (Sheedy & Saladin 1977). For reflex muscular activity, between 1/3 and 2/3 of the fusional reserves may be used without placing the system under undue stress.

Positive and negative fusional reserves can be measured at distance and near by placing appropriate prisms before the eyes. Prism is introduced before the eyes until fusion breaks down and diplopia results (Penisten et al. 2001). Placing base-out prism before the eyes stimulates convergence and the amount required to produce diplopia is called the positive fusional reserve (PFR). Because the eyes are forced to converge, accommodation is stimulated (convergence accommodation, CA, Schor & Narayan 1982) but cannot be maintained at the correct level for the task and therefore the target usually blurs before diplopia occurs.

Placing base-in prism before the eyes stimulates divergence and the amount required to produce diplopia is called the negative fusional reserve (NFR). When measuring NFR at near, a blur point is usually reported prior to diplopia as accommodation relaxes when the eyes are forced to diverge. However, it is unusual to obtain a blur point when measuring NFR at distance as accommodation is already at a minimum and cannot relax beyond this point.

5.12.2 Advantages and disadvantages

Risley or rotary prisms are an ideal method of changing the amount of prism before the eyes in a smooth manner and they provide repeatable results in young adults (Penisten et al. 2001) although the results are somewhat less repeatable in children (Rouse et al. 2002). Although phoropters typically feature rotary prisms they have the disadvantage of enclosed conditions that do not allow a view of the patient's eyes. Fusional reserve tests in free space, typically using prism bars, more closely mimic natural viewing conditions and are particularly useful with young children as the eyes can be seen and an objective assessment of the fusional reserves can be obtained.

5.12.3 Procedure

NOTE: This description is for the measurement at 6 m. The technique can be applied for near by adjusting the trial frame/phoropter to the near centration distance and locating a fixation target at the appropriate distance.

1. Explain the test to the patient: 'This test measures the range over which your eye muscles can keep objects clear and single.' The patient should wear their distance refractive correction. Keep the room lights on.

2. Position yourself in front of the patient so that you can view the patient's eyes easily without obstructing the patient's view of the target.

3. To ensure accurate fixation and accommodation, isolate a single letter of a size equal to or slightly larger than the patient's visual acuity of the poorer eye (alternatively, a small block or a vertical line of letters can be used). For young children, a small picture may be better to hold their attention.

4. Instruct the patient: 'I would like you to look at the letter … at the other end of the room (or the letter … on this stick for near reserves).

Horizontal fusional reserves

5. Measure horizontal fusional reserves first. You should first measure the fusional reserve that opposes the heterophoria: e.g. if the patient has exophoria, measure the positive fusional reserve first. This is to ensure that an accurate measurement is obtained, as fusional reserves that are measured subsequently may be modified by vergence adaptation (Rosenfield et al. 1995).

6. If you are using a phoropter, ask the patient to close their eyes and introduce the Risley prisms (set at zero) in front of both eyes. If you are using a prism bar, position it so that horizontal prism will be introduced from a zero starting point over one eye.

7. Let us take the example of measuring PFR (measured with base-out prism): Slowly increase the amount of base-out prism placed before the eye(s). If you are using a phoropter, increase the prism in both eyes at an equal rate (about 2–3 $^\triangle$/second in total). In this case, the amount of prism being added is the sum of the two powers.

8. Instruct the patient to report the first perceptible blur. As soon as the blur is reported, stop increasing the base-out prism and instruct the patient to attempt to clear the letters. If the letters can be cleared continue to slowly increase the base-out prism power until the patient reports a blur that cannot be cleared. This is the sustained **blur point** and it indicates that the prism power has caused the patient's accommodation response to be over-exerted (base-out prism) or under-exerted (base-in prism) for the viewing distance in question. In other words, the error in accommodation response just exceeds the depth-of-focus at the blur point. Make a mental note of the prism amount before the patient's eye(s) at this point. If the patient does not report a blur but instead reports diplopia first, then there is no blur point.

9. Ask the patient to report when the letter now doubles. Increase the amount of prism until the patient reports sustained double vision. This is the **break point** and it corresponds to the situation where the eyes can no longer make the motor response to overcome the prism power and the visual axes are no longer in alignment. Make a mental note of the prism before the eye(s) at this point.

10. Increase slightly the amount of prism to ensure complete separation of the doubled image.

11. If the amount of prism that has been added seems unusually large, ask the patient if the

letter has remained centred or if it has drifted off to the side. If it has drifted this indicates that one eye has been suppressed. The direction of movement will indicate which eye has been suppressed. A versional (as opposed to vergence) eye movement will be seen objectively.

12. Slowly reduce the amount of prism until the patient reports that the two images have moved together again to form a single image. This is the **recovery point.** Make a mental note of the amount of prism in front of the patient's eye(s) and remove the prism bar.

13. If you are using a phoropter, ask the patient to close their eyes and return the Risley prism power to zero.

14. Repeat the measurement for the other horizontal fusional reserve (steps 6–13). In the example above, base-out prisms were used to measure the PFR, so base-in prisms should now be used to measure the NFR. Remember that with NFR measurement at distance there is usually no blur point.

Vertical fusional reserves

15. If you are using a phoropter, ask the patient to close their eyes and introduce a Risley prism in front of one eye only (e.g. base-up BU RE). If you are using a prism bar, position it so that vertical prism will be introduced from a zero starting point over one eye.

16. To measure vertical fusional reserves, slowly increase the amount of prism placed before the eye(s). Note that the magnitude of vertical fusional reserves is considerably less than the horizontal and the increase of the prism power should be slower than used for measuring horizontal vergences (at about 0.5–1^{Δ}/second).

17. Measure the break and recovery points for right supravergence (base-up before right eye) and infravergence (base-down before right eye). Vertical fusional reserves do not have a blur point.

5.12.4 Recording

1. If there is no blur point, record 'X'.

2. Examples of test results include: e.g. NFR @ 6 m: X/14/10; PFR @ 6 m: 12/18/10; R(OD) infra @ 40 cm: 3/1; R(OD) supra @ 40 cm: 3/1.

3. A recovery point that requires prism of the opposite base to that used to initially produce the diplopia (such as a base-in prism being needed for recovery from diplopia when using base-out prisms to produce diplopia and measure PFR) is recorded as a minus value. For example, PFR @ 6 m: 3/5/ − 1 indicates that 1^{Δ} base-in was required to achieve recovery from the diplopia that resulted when 5^{Δ} base-out had produced diplopia.

4. If the limit of the prism power is exceeded, record as >40 (or the maximum prism value).

5.12.5 Interpretation

Fusional reserves can be compared to normal data (Table 5.3). However, a wide variety of 'normal' data has been published over the years and it is preferable for each clinician to obtain their own using their own equipment and their own technique. More profitably perhaps, the fusional reserves can be compared to the heterophoria measurements. A patient with an exophoria will use part of their PFR to correct the deviation. The measured PFR therefore represents the amount of fusional vergence in reserve to maintain single binocular

Table 5.3   Approximate range of normal fusional reserves.

	Distance (range, $^{\Delta}$)	Near (range, $^{\Delta}$)
Positive fusional reserves		
Blur	12–16	20–28
Break	18–22	26–34
Recover	14–18	22–30
Negative fusional reserves		
Blur	Not applicable	6–10
Break	6–12	12–18
Recovery	4–8	8–14

vision. Similarly, a patient with esophoria will use part of the NFR to correct the deviation. Knowledge of the heterophoria size and of the magnitude of the opposing fusional reserves can be useful in the assessment of a patient's binocular status, specifically in relation to whether the heterophoria is likely to be giving rise to the patient's symptoms. The proportion of the total fusional vergence used to correct the phoria can be determined. For example:

Distance phoria	9^Δ exophoria
Measured positive fusional reserves	18^Δ
Total positive fusional reserves	$18^\Delta + 9^\Delta = 27^\Delta$.

Therefore, 1/3 (9^Δ) of the total positive fusional reserves (27^Δ) are used to correct the phoria, which is within normal limits. This approach has been formalised in Sheard's and Percival's rules, which are used to compare the fusional reserves with the heterophoria and to indicate whether the phoria is likely to be decompensated or to decompensate in the future under conditions of stress (e.g. around examination time in the case of students).

Sheard's rule proposes that the fusional reserve blur point should be at least twice the size of the phoria. Sheard's criterion works best for exophoric cases so that the PFR to blur should be at least twice the size of the exophoria in order for it to be compensated (Sheedy & Saladin 1978). Sheard's criterion further suggests that the prism required to correct a decompensated exophoria is:

Prism required = {2/3} exophoria − {1/3} PFR.

Percival's rule suggests that a patient should operate in the middle third of their binocular vergence range. Percival's rule should only be used for near phorias as normal distance PFR and NFR are typically very unbalanced and Percival's rule tends to work best for near esophoric cases (Sheedy & Saladin 1978). Percival's rule suggests that the PFR and NFR should be balanced and that one should not be more than double the other. Percival's criterion suggests:

Prism required for esophoria = {1/3} total range − NFR.

For example, if the PFR is 11^Δ and the NFR is 4^Δ, the prism required is 15/3 − 4 = 1 $^\Delta$ BO.

5.12.6 Most common errors

1. Expecting a blur point when measuring the NFR at distance or vertical fusional reserves.

2. Carrying out the test in those patients who do not have binocular vision at the test distance.

3. Assuming that the test can be done when suppression is present such as with a strabismic patient.

4. Providing an inappropriate stimulus to accommodation through poor choice of target.

5. Attempting to assess fusional reserves in young children when other, quicker tests are available to assess motor fusion (see section 5.12.7).

5.12.7 Acceptable alternative technique: 20 base-out test

This technique is suitable for use in those patients who may not be able to cooperate with fusional reserve measurement (e.g. young children) as outlined in the sections above. Rather than introduce variable prism power and obtain responses from the patient regarding the blurring or doubling of images, the test relies upon qualitative judgements made by the practitioner in response to the introduction of a high-powered prism. Typically, a 20^Δ base-out is used (though in theory any prism power or direction can be employed) and the practitioner examines whether the eye behind the prism makes a swift and smooth inwards movement in order to restore the image of the object of regard on the fovea. The test is repeated with the prism in front of the other eye. In principle the test is similar to the 4-prism base-out test (section 5.21) but it is qualitatively much easier for the practitioner to establish whether the appropriate motor fusion response has taken place following the introduction of this high-powered prism. A normal response on this test can allow the practitioner to generalise about the effectiveness of the motor fusion system and thus the ability of the visual system to maintain fusion throughout the day. A normal response on this test may be recorded in the following fashion: '20^Δ base-out overcome with either eye, and good recovery'. A positive response on this test (i.e. an appropriate motor fusion response) is a very strong indicator that peripheral fusion exists and thus the 20^Δ base test can prove useful in children who are too young to undergo formal sensory testing (Kaban et al. 1995). Unfortunately, the same is not true in reverse, because a negative result on the 20^Δ base does not guarantee that peripheral fusion is poor or absent.

5.13 THE MALLETT FIXATION DISPARITY UNIT

The Mallett unit is typically used to measure the fixation disparity at distance and near. The distance Mallett unit uses red monocular strips and a central fixation lock (OXO), but does not have a peripheral fusion lock (Fig. 5.8). The near Mallett unit uses green monocular strips, as green is usually more

sharply focused at near due to a slight lag of accommodation, a central fixation lock (OXO) and a surrounding paragraph of print providing a peripheral fusion lock. The near Mallett unit (Fig. 5.9) also contains paragraphs of text of various sizes (typically N5 to N10), a retractable ruler, a near duochrome and targets that allow investigation of stereopsis and suppression.

5.13.1 Aligning prism or associated heterophoria

When viewing an object binocularly the visual axes are directed at the object of regard so that an image falls on each fovea. However, it is possible to fixate an object without the visual axes intersecting precisely on the object and still have binocular single vision, providing the misalignment is within Panum's areas. Panum's areas are small and horizontally oval. A fixation disparity is present when one or both of the visual axes are not directed precisely on the fixation object. The advocates of fixation disparity maintain that this is likely to occur when the visual system is under stress; indeed the presence of fixation disparity is considered by some to be that part of the heterophoria that is decompensated. The amount of prism required to eliminate a fixation disparity has been called the associated heterophoria. As heterophoria can only be measured with dissociation, the term 'associated heterophoria' is somewhat contradictory, and for this reason, the term 'aligning prism' has been suggested (Evans 2002). Fixation disparity is usually assessed when the best refractive correction is in place.

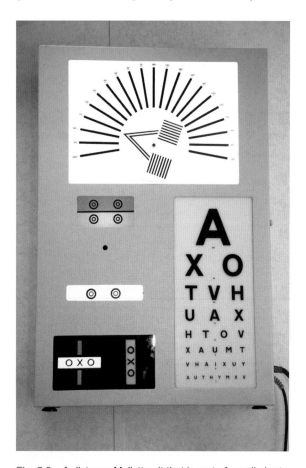

Fig. 5.8   A distance Mallett unit that is part of a wall chart.

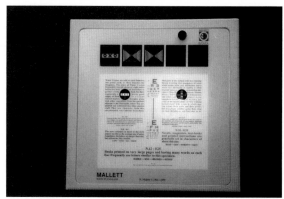

Fig. 5.9   A near Mallett unit.

5.13.2 Advantages and disadvantages

The assessment of fixation disparity with the Mallett unit is quick and simple and gives the prism or spherical lens power that can be used as the starting point for correction of binocular problems. Jenkins et al. (1989) found that 1^{Δ} and 2^{Δ} of fixation disparity was associated with symptoms in pre-presbyopes and presbyopes respectively, and it may be the best indicator that a heterophoria is decompensated (Yekta et al. 1989). Mallett (1988) reported that the aligning prism corresponded to the decompensated portion of the heterophoria, and fixation disparity has also been shown to increase under binocular stress, such as working under inadequate illumination or too close a working distance, and at the end of a working day (Yekta et al. 1989). The disadvantages of testing with the Mallett unit are that some remain unconvinced about the clinical relevance of fixation disparity and view it instead as a physiological phenomenon (von Noorden 2002). For example, if fixation disparity does reflect the decompensated portion of the heterophoria, the type of fixation disparity present should always match the direction of heterophoric deviation (e.g. an exo fixation disparity should only be present in a patient with exophoria). However, this is not always the case (Jampolsky et al. 1957). Nevertheless, others place much greater emphasis on its clinical significance and claim that fixation disparities above a particular level have diagnostic significance, particularly in relation to the negative influence it can exert upon the level of stereopsis that can be achieved by the patient (Saladin 2005).

5.13.3 Procedure for the distance Mallett unit

1. Explain the test to the patient: 'This is a test that will help to determine whether your symptoms could be due to a problem of your eye muscles not working together properly.'

2. Orient the OXO in a horizontal position with the red strips vertical. Keep the room lights on to illuminate the unit surroundings; this provides paramacular and peripheral fusion stimuli.

3. Prior to placing the polaroid visa in front of the patient's eyes, ask the patient to 'Look at the X in the middle of the OXO; do you see two red strips, one above and one below the OXO? Are the two strips exactly in line with each other and in line with the middle of the X?' This ensures that the patient is aware of what alignment looks like (Fig. 5.10a), so that any subsequent misalignment is more easily noticed.

4. Place the polaroid visor in front of the patient's eyes and check that the top red strip is seen by the left eye, and the lower strip by the right eye.

5. Ask the patient 'Can you still see the two red strips?' If only one strip is seen, show the patient the two individual strips by covering each eye in turn. If only one strip is still seen, deep central suppression may be present, and no further measurement is possible. Most patients, however, should see both strips without difficulty.

6. Ask the patient 'Are the strips in line with the middle of the X?'

7. If both of the strips are seen to be aligned with X, no fixation disparity is present (Fig. 5.10a).

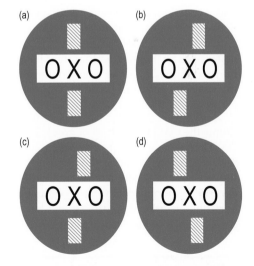

Fig. 5.10 The positions of the red strips of the Mallet unit as seen by patients with various types of fixation disparity. The right eye sees the lower strip and the left eye sees the top strip. (a) No fixation disparity. (b) Lower strip (right eye) is seen to the left of the upper strip, indicating crossed, and therefore Exo disparity. (c) Exo disparity in the left eye only. (d) Eso disparity.

8. Several results could be reported:
    a) If the lower red strip (RE) is to the left of the X and the upper strip (LE) is to the right, an EXO fixation disparity is present in both eyes (Fig. 5.10b).
    b) If the lower strip (RE) remains below the X but the upper strip (LE) moves to the right, an EXO fixation disparity is present in the left eye only (Fig. 5.10c). When the disparity is unilateral, it is usually the non-dominant eye that demonstrates the deviation. Unilateral fixation disparity is most common in vertical imbalance, whereas horizontal fixation disparities are usually bilateral.
    c) If an ESO fixation disparity is present, the lower strip (RE) will be to the right of the upper strip (LE) (Fig. 5.10d).

9. The fixation disparity should be neutralised using the lowest prism power (or in some cases of esophoria, the weakest positive spherical lens) that eliminates the fixation disparity. With a unilateral fixation disparity, it is suggested that prism should be added to the eye demonstrating the slip. Note, however, that in the case of a bilateral slip it is not necessary to introduce prism before both eyes when neutralising the disparity. Between changes of prism, instruct the patient to read a few Snellen letters from the distance chart. Remember that the Mallett unit is designed to allow you to determine the *minimum* power of prism necessary to eliminate the fixation disparity.

10. Rotate the OXO through 90 degrees. The OXO letters now appear in a vertical line with the red strips horizontal. Repeat the assessment. If both a horizontal and vertical fixation disparity exist together, the horizontal fixation disparity should be corrected before the vertical is measured.

5.13.4 Procedure for the near Mallett unit

The measures obtained using the near Mallett unit are likely to be changed by previous heterophoria measurement, particularly if von Graefe's technique (section 5.10) was employed. It is recommended, therefore, that the near Mallett unit should be used before the dissociated heterophoria is measured in patients regarded as having unstable binocular vision, past or present (Brautaset & Jennings 1999). The measurement procedure is similar, except that:

1. The patient's normal reading spectacles or optimal near correction should be worn in the trial frame.

2. The centration distance should be adjusted for near.

3. A paragraph of small text must be read prior to any fixation disparity assessment to ensure accurate accommodation on the target.

5.13.5 Recording

1. If the two strips were not visible to the patient, record the eye that was being suppressed and whether the suppression was intermittent or constant.

2. If there was no fixation disparity, record 'Mallett: No FD D & N' or similar.

3. If a fixation disparity was present, record the lowest amount of prism or spherical lens required to align the strips. If the fixation disparity was found in one eye only, this should be recorded. For example, 'Mallett, Dist: $2^\triangle$ BI; Near: $1^\triangle$ BI LE'.

5.13.6 Interpretation

Most patients will be able to simultaneously perceive both strips, and usually they are aligned without the need for any prisms. It is important to remember that the prism power required to align the markers is not predictable from the magnitude of the fixation disparity (e.g. small fixation disparities are not always eliminated by low prism powers) and two patients experiencing the same amount of fixation disparity may require very different powers to perceive the lines as aligned. Owing to prism adaptation it is advisable to leave the lowest prism power that neutralises the fixation disparity in place for a period of time (several minutes). If a slip re-appears after a period of time when the same prism power had initially neutralised the fixation disparity, it is less clear that prescribing this prism will prove beneficial. On the other hand, it is claimed that most patients with abnormal binocular vision which gives rise to symptoms do not adapt, or only partially adapt, to prisms (North & Henson 1981).

5.13.7 Most common errors

1. Decentration errors due to poorly fitting trial frame/phoropter or badly centred lenses.

2. Not starting with the lowest possible prism.

3. Making a decision to prescribe prism before checking whether the patient's visual system will adapt to the prism and thus rendering the prism less useful, or perhaps, of no use at all.

4. Not allowing a patient with a vertical deviation to adopt their customary head posture.

5.14 3^Δ BASE-IN/12^Δ BASE-OUT PRISM FLIPPERS

Prism flippers, which consist of a pair of 12^Δ base-out prisms that can be flipped to a pair of 3^Δ base-in prisms, are used to assess a patient's ability to rapidly change vergence without changing accommodation.

5.14.1 Fusional vergence facility

Measures of vergence facility may be useful in diagnosing binocular vision problems in symptomatic patients whose fusional reserves (section 5.12) are normal in the same way that measures of accommodative facility can provide additional information beyond that provided by measures of accommodative amplitude (Gall & Wick 2003). The base-out prism forces the eyes to converge and thus the patient is forced to employ their positive fusional reserves to restore bifoveal fixation following the introduction of the base-out prism pair. No change

in accommodation is needed, and any accommodation that accompanies the positive fusional effort may blur the target. Similarly, the patient needs to employ their negative fusional reserves without relaxing the accommodation to overcome the presence of the base-in prism.

5.14.2 Advantages and disadvantages

This test requires little additional equipment and is straightforward to perform. The results of the test may explain symptoms not readily explained by other tests (Gall & Wick 2003). Gall and colleagues (1998) reported that the combination of 3^Δ base-in and 12^Δ base-out prism flippers provided the best repeatability and discrimination between symptomatic and non-symptomatic patients.

5.14.3 Procedure

The test is normally carried out at near. The patient should view a vertical line of letters, which are one line bigger than the smallest letters that can be read at the test distance. The patient should wear the habitual near correction for the test.

1. Instruct the patient as follows: 'I am now going to test how well your eyes can maintain clear and single vision when I introduce some lenses.'

2. Demonstrate the task required of the patient by introducing the prisms and asking the patient to appreciate that it takes some time for the letters to become clear and single after the introduction of the prism flippers. Remind the patient that they will be required to let you know as soon as the letters are clear and single and that they should attempt to make them clear and single as quickly as possible.

3. Once the patient has understood the test, start your watch and introduce 12^Δ base-out prism before each eye. When the patient reports 'clear', flip the handle to introduce the 3^Δ base-in prism power. When the patient again reports 'clear' this represents one cycle.

4. Count the number of cycles achieved by the patient in a 60 second period.

5.14.4 Results

Record the number of cycles achieved in the following format: Fusional facility at 40 cm: 10 cycles/minute.

5.14.5 Interpretation

Normal values for this test are in the region of 15 cycles/minute.

5.14.6 Most common errors

1. Using an inappropriately sized target for the test (e.g. letters that are too large).

2. Counting the recovery from each prism introduction as a cycle and thus greatly overestimating the test performance

5.15 NEAR POINT OF CONVERGENCE

The near point of convergence (NPC) is the point along the midline where the visual axes intersect under the maximum convergence effort and while binocular single vision is retained.

5.15.1 Convergence ability

In a patient with normal binocular function, the ability of the eyes to converge when performing a near visual task is paramount to the patient's visual comfort. When we wish to view a near target, three processes take place and collectively this is referred to as the near triad of responses. The eyes converge, they accommodate and there is pupillary constriction. Convergence insufficiency is typically described as a syndrome of exophoria that is greater at near than at distance, a remote near point of convergence and poor positive fusional reserves (Rouse et al. 1999). Convergence insufficiency is an important binocular vision problem due to its high prevalence (up to 13% amongst children aged 9 to 13; Rouse et al. 1999) and because it can usually be simply and successfully treated. It is not appropriate to assess convergence ability in a patient with heterotropia at near as they will almost certainly not experience diplopia because of suppression of the strabismic eye.

5.15.2 Advantages and disadvantages

The near point of convergence is a quick and easy test to perform. It requires no special equipment and it provides a very repeatable result (Rouse et al. 2002). It is the standard test for convergence ability and has the advantage over jump convergence (section 5.16) of providing a quantitative assessment. The results of this test, together with the results of cover test at distance and near, can help to rule out the presence of convergence insufficiency. In patients who 'fail' these screening tests or in symptomatic patients, additional testing of jump convergence (section 5.16), fusional reserves (section 5.12) and fixation disparity (section 5.13) is recommended.

5.15.3 Procedure

1. Seat the patient comfortably with their head erect and eyes in slightly downward gaze. Make sure the patient is wearing their near correction. Sit directly in front of the patient so that you have a clear view of the two eyes.

2. Keep the room lights on. If necessary, position additional lighting to illuminate the patient's eyes and/or the target, thus avoiding shadows.

3. Explain the measurement to the patient: 'This test determines how well your eyes can turn in to follow a close object.'

4. Position the target (a pen tip or finger is fine; Siderov et al. 2001) at a distance of 50 cm directly in front of the patient slightly below the midline. A target with fine detail should be avoided as otherwise patients often confuse blur with diplopia. A medium-sized, coloured picture on a fixation stick can be used with children.

5. Instruct the patient: 'Please watch the ... Do you just see one? OK, now I'm going to move it towards you. Please tell me if it becomes

doubled; not blurred but doubled.' Older patients in particular should be warned that the target will blur (once the near point of accommodation has been reached) before it doubles.

6. Make sure that the patient is looking at the target with both eyes.

7. Slowly but steadily move the target toward the bridge of the patient's nose. The speed should be such that it takes approximately 10 seconds to move the target from 50 cm to the bridge of the patient's nose. To keep the patient's attention, it can be useful to move the target from side to side slightly, particularly at the beginning of the measurement, and check that the patient maintains fixation.

8. Observe the patient's eyes for loss of convergence. Measure the distance the target is from the eyes when one of the eyes loses fixation by flicking outwards (objective NPC) and/or the patient reports diplopia (subjective NPC).

9. If the target becomes doubled (subjective NPC) before it is more than 10 cm from the bridge of the nose, encourage the patient to make an extra effort to make the target single again. Moving it away slightly will help this. If single binocular vision can be re-established, advance the target again towards the patient.

10. If a patient (particularly a presbyopic patient) reports a remote NPC and both eyes

appear to be converging to the target, they may be confusing diplopia with blur. Check this by covering one eye and asking the patient if the target is still double. Continue to move the target in until the objective NPC is found.

11. Once the NPC has been reached, slowly move the target away from the patient's eyes and ask them when the target becomes single again. Measure this point and record it as the recovery NPC point. Repeat the test. If the patient can keep the target single to their nose, this is recorded as 'to nose' and a recovery point is not measured.

12. If the history indicates that the patient requires prolonged and/or excessive convergence in a specific position of gaze then repeat the procedure in that specific gaze position.

5.15.4 Recording

The break and recovery NPC points should be recorded in centimetres from the bridge of the nose. Record the break point first, followed by the recovery point. Examples are given in Table 5.4. If the subjective NPC is much larger than the objective NPC, it is likely that the patient has confused blurring with diplopia and the objective NPC should be recorded. If the patient reports that the target is still seen singly when the eyes are seen to be misaligned, suppression should be suspected and investigated further.

Table 5.4   Examples of recordings of the near point of covergence.

Abbreviation	Description
NPC: 6 cm/9 cm	A break point of 6 cm and recovery point of 9 cm (normal convergence)
(Obj.) NPC: 5 cm/8 cm	Objective NPC recording of a 5 cm break point and 8 cm recovery point
NPC: to nose	Normal convergence to the nose, no recovery point measurable
NPC: 12 cm/16 cm, RE out	Abnormal convergence, with 12 cm break and 16 cm recovery points. The right eye moves out at the break point
NPC: 14 cm/18 cm, LE out, suppression?	Abnormal convergence with likely suppression. The break point is 14 cm and the recovery point is 18 cm. The left eye moves out at the break point, but no diplopia is reported

5.15.5 Interpretation

Children and adults should be able to converge to within about 7.5 cm and recovery should return within 10.5 cm (Rouse et al. 1999). An NPC larger than these figures suggests possible convergence insufficiency and should be investigated further. This investigation should include jump convergence (section 5.16), distance and near heterophoria (sections 5.7–5.10), near fusional reserves (section 5.12) and near fixation disparity (section 5.13). Given the high prevalence of accommodative insufficiency in children with convergence insufficiency (Rouse et al. 1999), tests of accommodation (sections 5.17–5.19) should also be conducted in these patients. The effect of any new refractive error or refractive change on these measurements should be assessed.

Instead of a failure of one eye to converge it is possible that diplopia will be reported and/or that both eyes are seen to no longer view the target because of over-convergence by one eye. This is rarely encountered but when is does arise it suggests that the patient may have an abnormally high AC/A ratio (section 5.11). This should be recorded and additional investigations should be carried out.

5.15.6 Most common errors

1. Measuring the *subjective* NPC only. This can lead to an incorrect finding of a remote NPC in older patients who can confuse blurring of the target with doubling and therefore report 'doubling' at their near point of accommodation, which is typically much further away than the NPC.

2. Carrying out the test once only; the test should be carried out at least twice to gain an impression of test repeatability.

3. Moving the target too rapidly or unsteadily.

4. Moving the target too slowly causing the patient, especially children, to lose interest.

5. Not encouraging the patient enough to keep the target single (particularly children).

6. Testing the eyes in upward or primary gaze instead of slightly downward gaze.

7. Carrying out the test in patients who have a heterotropia. Such patients will suppress the image in the deviating eye and may therefore never experience doubling of the target.

5.16 JUMP CONVERGENCE

The test involves assessing the quality of convergence as fixation jumps from a distant or mid-distant target to a near target. There are two versions of this test but the principle and procedures to be followed are identical in the two cases. In one case, the ability of the patient to quickly switch fixation between a distant (6 m/20 feet) and a near (e.g. 20 cm) target is assessed. In the other version, jump convergence is assessed between two relatively near targets (e.g. one at 60 cm, and the other at 20 cm).

5.16.1 Convergence ability

See section 5.15.1.

5.16.2 Advantages and disadvantages

Tests of jump convergence are not normally included in the diagnosis of convergence insufficiency, perhaps because it provides qualitative rather than quantitative data. However, the test has its advocates and the task carried out by the patient in the jump convergence test has the advantage that it more closely reflects typical near viewing situations where fixation is continually switching between near targets; it is seldom in the real world that we would encounter a target that moves slowly and predictably towards us along the midline as with the NPC task. Early research suggested poor jump convergence was more prevalent than a remote NPC and was more closely associated with symptoms (Pickwell & Hampshire 1981). The test is relatively easy to perform and can be used as an additional assessment in patients who show signs of convergence insufficiency, and in patients with symptoms that could suggest convergence problems who show a normal NPC. However, the test is limited by the qualitative nature of the results and is less well known than the NPC. Furthermore, it has not been subjected to the same research evaluation as the test of NPC.

5.16.3 Procedure

1. Seat the patient comfortably with their head erect and eyes in slightly downward gaze. The patient should wear their refractive correction for distance viewing. Sit directly in front of the patient so that both eyes can be viewed simultaneously, but so that distance fixation is not obscured.

2. Keep the room lights on. If necessary, position additional lighting to illuminate the patient's eyes and/or the target, thus avoiding shadows.

3. Indicate clearly to the patient both a distant single letter of a size one line larger than the patient's VA of the poorer eye (e.g. if the patient's VAs are 6/4 and 6/9, use a 6/12 letter as a target) and near (fixation rule) target. Position the near target about 20 cm in front of the patient. In another version of the test, the patient may be asked to switch fixation between a target at, say, 60 cm and another at, say, 20 cm.

4. Ask the patient to alternate fixation from the near target to the more distant target and back again.

5. Observe the eyes as they converge and diverge in order to gain an impression of the speed and accuracy in switching between the two target locations.

5.16.4 Recording

Record whether the jump convergence is smooth and fast or whether there are any jerky movements or an inability of one eye to converge adequately to the target. For example:

Jump convergence: smooth & fast;

Jump convergence: jerky, RE slower to converge.

5.16.5 Interpretation

Fast, smooth jump convergence should be observed to 10–15 cm. Poor, jerky jump convergence suggests possible convergence insufficiency and should be investigated further. As previously stated, the investigation for possible convergence insufficiency should include distance and near heterophoria (sections 5.7–5.10), near fusional reserves (section 5.12) and near fixation disparity (section 5.13) and the patient's accommodation (sections 5.17–5.19) should be fully assessed. The effect of any new refractive error or refractive change on these measurements should be determined. The near pupillary reflex should also be investigated.

5.17 PUSH-UP/PUSH-DOWN AMPLITUDE OF ACCOMMODATION

The amplitude of accommodation is the maximum amount of accommodation or focusing ability that the patient can exert in response to a near target. The near target is moved closer to the patient's eyes until it first blurs (the push-up amplitude) and then moved away from the eyes until it becomes clear (the push-down amplitude). An average of these two threshold values provides an indication of the amplitude of accommodation.

5.17.1 Amplitude of accommodation

Accommodation or focusing allows targets to be made clear over a large range of distances. The amplitude of accommodation measures the full range of accommodation: from the far point, where accommodation is fully relaxed, to the near point, with maximum accommodation exerted. If the far point is at infinity (as in the case of emmetropes and those wearing optimal refractive correction for distance vision), then measurement of the near point allows the amplitude of accommodation to be determined with ease. The amplitude is calculated simply by taking the inverse of the near point of accommodation, which is expressed in metres. For example, if the near point was 10 cm, the amplitude of accommodation is $1/0.10 = 10$ D. The amplitude of accommodation gradually falls with age, and causes patients over the age of about 45 years to have difficulty with near work and require reading glasses. Measurement of the amplitude of accommodation can help to identify the appropriate reading add required to alleviate the patient's near visual problems (section 4.22.3). The amplitude of accommodation becomes zero at age 55–60 (Charman 1989). If you obtain a measure for amplitude of accommodation in patients over 60 years of age, you are measuring their depth of focus and not accommodative amplitude.

5.17.2 Advantages and disadvantages

The push-up/push-down test is quick and easy to perform and assessment of the near point of clear vision relates to the typical symptom reported by early presbyopes. A combination of the push-up and push-down measurements is preferred as it provides a useful compromise between the slight overestimate of the push-up technique and the slight underestimate of the push-down technique (Rosenfield 1997). The most commonly used alternative involves using increasing amounts of minus spherical lens power until distance vision blurs ('Sheard's technique'). This method typically provides lower estimates of amplitude of accommodation than those provided by the push-up method (Kragha 1986) and it can only be satisfactorily measured using a phoropter. In addition, the minus lens method provides a less clinically relevant measure than the push-up technique, which provides a direct measurement of the near point of clear vision (Atchison et al. 1994).

5.17.3 Procedure

1. Explain the test to the patient: 'I am going to measure the focusing power of your eyes.'

2. The test is usually performed with the patient wearing their optimal distance correction, but can be performed with the patient's spectacles as a screening test. If the test is to be performed on early presbyopes they should wear a partial addition ($\approx$ + 1.00 for 45–55 years) to ensure they can see the stimulus at the end of the near-point rule. The clinician should sit directly in front of the patient to allow a simultaneous, unobstructed view of the two eyes. In young children with very high amplitudes, slight linear differences of the near point produce

large dioptric differences, and it is useful to add a −3.00 D lens to place the near point further from the spectacle plane. This also ensures that depth-of-focus errors are minimised (Atchison et al. 1994).

3. Direct additional lighting over the patient's shoulder to illuminate the reading card without shadows.

4. The test is usually performed monocularly (right and left) followed by a binocular measure of accommodation amplitude. The procedure is common for all viewing conditions. For monocular measures occlude one eye.

5. Indicate to the patient to view the smallest size text they can see on the near chart when positioned at about 40 cm (often N5, 0.4M, 20/20). The angular size of the text will increase as it is moved closer to the patient.

6. Move the target slowly towards the patient. Instruct the patient: 'Please look at this print. I am going to move it closer to you and I want you to tell me when it first becomes blurred.' Keep moving the target until the patient notices that the letters begin to blur.

7. At this first noticeable blur, ask the patient to try and clear the print. If they can, continue to move the print closer to the eye until the first sustained blur is reached and measure the distance to the spectacle plane.

8. From a point very slightly ($\approx$ 0.50 D) beyond the first blur position, gradually move the target away from the patient and ask them to indicate when it first becomes clear. Measure the distance to the spectacle plane.

9. The amplitude of accommodation can be determined by taking the dioptric average of these two values (push-up amplitude and push-down amplitude).

10. Add the effect of any additional lenses to the measured dioptric near point to obtain the true amplitude. For example, if a +1.00 DS lens was added and the measured amplitude was 4.50 D, the actual amplitude of accommodation is 3.50 D as the additional lens provided 1.00 D. If a −3.00 DS lens was added and the scale indicates

an amplitude of 7.50 D, the true amplitude is 10.50 D.

11. Repeat for the left eye.

12. Repeat binocularly.

13. If the measured amplitude differs significantly from known age-matched normal values, repeat the test to ensure that the abnormal finding is not an artefact of the procedure. In young adults, differences of less than 1.50 D between recorded and age-matched values, or between recordings on two separate occasions, are not usually clinically significant (Rosenfield & Cohen 1996).

5.17.4 Recording

Record the number of dioptres of accommodation for each eye. Examples:

Amps (push-up/push-down) RE 8.50 D, LE 8.50 D, BE 10.00 D

Amps (push-up) OD 4.00 D, OS 4.00 D, OU 5.00 D.

5.17.5 Interpretation

Push-up values for the amplitude of accommodation may be artificially raised due to the effect of depth of focus. As the print is brought closer to the patient, its angular size increases and, as a result, more and more defocus can exist before the patient becomes aware of it. This can be overcome by using increasingly smaller print as the near card is brought closer to the eyes (Atchison et al. 1994). It can also be limited by adding a -3.00 D lens in front of a younger patient's eyes, so that the measured near point is moved further away from the eyes. By combining the push-up finding with the push-down result (which tends to slightly underestimate the amplitude), this problem is minimised.

Normal values of monocular spectacle accommodation are shown in Table 5.5. If the measured amplitude is significantly (>1.50 D; Rosenfield & Cohen 1996) lower than the age-matched normal values, the patient may have accommodative insufficiency. Binocular values of the amplitude of accommodation are usually a little higher (1–2 D) than the monocular values as the convergence response

Table 5.5   Monocular expected accommodation levels as a function of age.

Age (years)	Accommodation (D)		
	Donders	Duane	Sheard
10	14.00	11.00	–
15	12.00	10.50	11.00
20	10.00	9.50	9.00
25	8.50	8.50	7.50
30	7.00	7.50	6.50
35	5.50	6.50	5.00
40	4.50	5.50	3.75
45	3.50	3.50	–
50	2.50	–	–
55	1.75	–	–

Duane–Hoffstetter formula for probable amplitude of accommodation:

Maximum amplitude = $25.0 - 0.40 \times$ age.

Average amplitude = $18.5 - 0.30 \times$ age.

Minimum amplitude = $15.0 - 0.25 \times$ age.

helps to induce additional accommodation (convergence accommodation). If amplitude of accommodation is reduced to a level below 5.00 D in a patient aged over 40 years wearing optimal distance correction but who has difficulty reading, the patient is presbyopic.

Anomalies of accommodation may be associated with a wide variety of conditions including various systemic and ocular medication (probably the most common cause), trauma, inflammatory disease, metabolic disorders such as diabetes and other systemic diseases (Rosenfield 1997). Reduced amplitudes of accommodation have also been reported in children with Down's syndrome (Woodhouse et al. 1993) and cerebral palsy (Leat 1996). Wick & Hall (1987) found that a battery of tests (amplitude, lead/lag of accommodation, accommodative facility and a cycloplegic refraction) was required to detect accommodative dysfunction, and that just because a patient had an adequate amplitude of accommodation, this did not mean that accommodative function was normal.

5.17.6 Most common errors

1. Not stressing to the patient to report the *first* signs of blur; it should be stressed that this is not the same as the point at which they can no longer read the text.

2. Not investigating whether, at the first reported blur, the patient can 'bring the print back into focus'.

3. Carrying out the test without optimal distance correction in place. This will have the effect of overestimating the amplitude in myopes and underestimating the accommodative amplitude in hyperopic individuals.

4. Moving the card too slowly and from too far away will tire the patient and can result in an artificially low score.

5.18 NOTT AND MEM DYNAMIC RETINOSCOPY

Nott and Monocular Estimation Method (MEM) dynamic retinoscopy provide an objective assessment of accomodative error to a near target.

5.18.1 Accommodative lag or lead

Accommodative lag and lead indicate whether a patient's accommodation level to a target is slightly less (lag) or slightly more (lead) than expected. This can be measured objectively using various dynamic retinoscopy techniques or subjectively using relative accommodation measurements or the binocular crossed-cylinder method. The latter two subjective measurements are more often used in the assessment of accommodation to help determine the tentative reading addition and are discussed elsewhere (section 4.22).

5.18.2 Advantages and disadvantages

Dynamic retinoscopy offers a quick, repeatable and valid means for establishing the accuracy of the patient's accommodation system (McLelland & Saunders 2003) and requires minimal extra equipment. Both dynamic retinoscopy tests provide results that are less variable than the crossed-cylinder or near duochrome techniques (Rosenfield et al. 1996). As with most clinical techniques, practice is required in order to develop proficiency in carrying out the tests, especially in relation to the short time in which to make retinoscopy judgements. One study has

suggested that the Nott technique provides more accurate estimates of the accommodative response (Rosenfield et al. 1996) as it does not require the introduction of supplementary lenses.

5.18.3 Nott dynamic retinoscopy procedure

1. The patient should wear their optimal distance refractive correction in the trial frame, or their existing spectacles if lens powers are not significantly different from the optimal refraction result. The phoropter should not be used for this test because of the risk of inducing proximal accommodation.

2. Explain the test to the patient: 'I am going to check the focusing ability of your eyes using this torch that will shine a light into your eye.'

3. The test should be carried out in conditions that approximate, in so far as possible, normal reading conditions and the card to be viewed by the patient needs to be located close to the patient's typical reading distance (e.g. 40 cm). The card should contain letters (or pictures for young children) in a position that permits you to perform retinoscopy close to the patient's visual axis. A near chart with a central aperture works well. The letters should be one line bigger than the binocular near visual acuity (typically N6, 0.5M, 20/30).

4. Dim or turn off the room lights but use additional lighting to illuminate the near chart.

5. Ask the patient to focus on the letters.

6. Perform retinoscopy on the right eye from 50 cm (typically 10 cm behind the near point card) along the horizontal meridian (with the streak vertical). Perform retinoscopy as quickly as possible as the retinoscope light will interfere with binocularity.

7. If neutrality is not observed at 50 cm, change the working distance (further away if 'with' movements are seen at 50 cm, and closer if 'against' movements are seen) until the neutral point is seen. Note the distance of your retinoscope when the neutral point is obtained.

8. Repeat the procedure on the left eye.

5.18.4 MEM dynamic retinoscopy procedure

1. Attach a MEM card or hold a fixation stick to the front of your retinoscope. The card should contain letters or pictures around a central aperture, through which retinoscopy is performed.

2. Dim or turn off the room lights and use additional lighting to illuminate the near chart.

3. Ask the patient to focus on the letters. To maintain appropriate fixation and accommodation you may need to ask children to read some of the letters out aloud or to name details in the picture.

4. Perform retinoscopy on the right eye from the patient's typical working distance (usually around 40 cm) along the horizontal meridian (with the streak vertical). Retinoscopy should be performed in the usual manner, but the lenses should only be placed in front of the patient's eyes for the least amount of time possible. This is to maintain binocularity, which is interrupted by the retinoscope's light. Try to ensure that the accommodative system does not change in response to any added lenses. To ensure the latter does not occur, you need to place the plus lens in front of the eye for 0.50 seconds or less.

5. Record the dioptric power of the lens that provides neutrality.

6. Repeat the procedure on the left eye.

5.18.5 Recording

For the Nott technique, record the dioptric difference between the near chart and the position of the retinoscope when neutrality is observed. If the neutrality point is behind the near chart position, then there is a lag of accommodation. If the neutrality point is in front of the near chart position, then there is accommodative lead. For example, if the near chart is at 40 cm and neutrality is observed at 57 cm, then the accommodative lag is $+2.50$ D

-1.75 D $= +0.75$ D. It is useful to learn corresponding distances and dioptric values, such as 80 cm (1.25 D), 67 cm (1.50 D), 57 cm (1.75 D), 50 cm (2.00 D), 44 cm (2.25 D) and 40 cm (2.50 D).

For the MEM technique, record the dioptric value of the lens that produces neutrality. Positive lenses indicate a lag of accommodation and negative lenses indicate a lead of accommodation.

5.18.6 Interpretation

Typically, the accommodative response to a target is slightly less than the accommodative stimulus. For example, a target positioned at 40 cm provides an accommodative stimulus of 2.50 D, but the normal accommodative response is slightly less, at about 2.00 D. The target remains clear due to depth of focus. Accommodative lags of 1.00 D or greater could be due to uncorrected (or insufficiently corrected) presbyopia and/or hyperopia, or it can indicate a lack of accommodative amplitude or reduced accommodative facility in a pre-presbyopic patient. The lack of an accommodative lag or an accommodative lead can indicate latent hyperopia, pseudomyopia or accommodative spasm. It is claimed that the MEM technique provides lags which are on average twice those found using the Nott method (Cacho et al. 1999) but most studies find results that are similar (reviewed in Rosenfield 1997).

5.19 ±2.00 DS FLIPPERS

±2.00 DS flippers, which consist of a pair of +2.00 D spheres, which can be flipped to a pair of −2.00 D spheres, are used to assess a patient's ability to rapidly change accommodation without changing vergence.

5.19.1 Accommodative facility

Accommodative facility is the ability of a patient to rapidly change accommodation. A reduced accommodative facility has been shown to be related to symptoms experienced in near viewing and it may exist even when other accommodative measures, such as the amplitude of accommodation (section 5.17), are at normal levels (Wick & Hall 1987).

5.19.2 Advantages and disadvantages

The test can be performed rapidly with minimal additional equipment. Measures of accommodative facility may be useful in diagnosing binocular vision problems in symptomatic patients whose phorias and visual acuities are normal (Gall & Wick 2003). It appears to have diagnostic value in that a reduced facility correlates with near symptoms and facility increases as symptoms are alleviated through treatment. Indeed, flippers can be part of the treatment. There is little justification for the use of the ±2.00 DS flippers other than that they are the power traditionally used. Indeed, it may be that what is required is a range of flipper powers that relate to the patient's amplitude of accommodation (Wick et al. 2002). For example, for a young patient with an amplitude of 12.00 D, the ±2.00 DS represent only a 33% range of the amplitude, whereas they represent a 67% range of the amplitude in an older patient with an amplitude of 6.00 D. Yothers et al. (2002) suggest using an amplitude-scaled test for adults, which uses a test distance that requires 45% of the amplitude of accommodation to be exerted and a lens flipper range that is 30% of the amplitude. For example, a patient with 7.00 D of accommodation would indicate the use of an approximate working distance of 32 cm (1/3.15, i.e. 45% of 7.00) and a flipper range of 2.10 (30% of 7.00) giving a flipper power of ±1.00 D.

5.19.3 Procedure

Many authors recommend measuring the binocular accommodative facility with a suppression check (typically using Polaroid glasses with the Bernell No. 9 vectogram). For appropriate comparison, the monocular measurements should be made with the same set-up except that one eye is now fully occluded. Alternatively, accommodative facility can be measured using standard near charts with binocular facility only measured if other tests indicate that the patient does not suppress at near. In this case, the 'clinical pass' values (section 5.19.5), which were obtained using the Polaroid system, cannot be used for comparison. Some authors just test binocularly first and only measure monocular facility if the binocular results are reduced. If the binocular facility is reduced, but monocular facility values

are within normal limits, then this suggests a binocular dysfunction not associated with accommodative facility.

1. If testing monocularly, occlude one eye. Keep the room lights on and if necessary, use localised lighting so that the patient's eyes can be easily seen without shadows.

2. Explain the measurement to the patient: 'I am now going to test how quickly your focusing muscles can work.'

3. Ask the patient to hold a near chart at the normal reading distance (40 cm is often used as standard). Ask them to look at a letter one line bigger than their binocular near visual acuity. This would typically be about N6 (0.4M, 20/30).

4. Explain the test to the patient: 'I want you to keep looking at the word/letter … I am going to place a lens in front of your eye that may make the word appear blurred. I want you to focus and make the print clear again as soon as you can. As soon as it becomes clear, say 'clear'. I will then flip another lens in front of the eye that may make the word appear blurred again. As before, I want you to refocus quickly and make the word clear again, and then say 'clear'. We will repeat this for 60 seconds.' Demonstrate the procedure to the patient so that they understand what is required of them before the test is started.

5. Start your watch as soon as you place the +2.00 D lens in the lens flippers (twirls) in front of the patient's right eye and ask them to tell you as soon as they get it clear by saying 'clear'.

6. As soon as the patient reports that the word is clear, quickly flip the lens flippers to the −2.00 lens and ask the patient to inform you as soon as the letters become clear again.

7. Count the number of times the patient utters 'clear' in 60 seconds. One cycle consists of clearing both the plus and the minus lenses.

8. Repeat for the left eye.

9. Repeat the test binocularly if the patient does not suppress at near. Some practitioners use a polaroid bar reader placed over the near chart

while the patient wears polaroid glasses. This provides a check on suppression because the patient will only be able to read half of the text if suppression is present.

5.19.4 Recording

Record the number of cycles/minute for each eye and then for the binocular viewing condition. One cycle consists of clearing both the plus and the minus lenses.

5.19.5 Interpretation

The normative data reported in the literature are variable, possibly because data were gathered across a range of ages but reported as a grand average or because they were collected from unselected samples (e.g. samples may have included patients with symptoms and accommodative or vergence dysfunctions). For these reasons, published normative data may be somewhat unreliable (Wick et al. 2002) and practitioners are encouraged to gather their own normative data for a range of age groups. Suggested 'clinical pass' criteria in young adults are 11 cycles/minute (monocular). The task becomes more difficult with the polaroid system, so that a clinical pass binocularly is 8 cycles/minute (Zellers et al. 1984). For children aged between 8 and 12 years, 'clinical pass' criteria are 7 cycles/minute (monocular) and 5 cycles/minute (binocular polaroids) (Scheiman et al. 1988).

5.19.6 Most common errors

1. Holding the flippers so that the patient cannot see the page.

2. Not allowing the patient to practise before starting the test.

3. Not turning the flippers fast enough so that the cycles/minute reflect the hand-speed of the examiner instead of a measure of accommodative facility.

4. Attempting to perform the test on a presbyopic patient.

5.20 WORTH 4-DOT TEST

This test checks for suppression by asking the patient to report the number and colour of dots they can see when looking through red–green goggles at four lights or dots of different colours. Two of the lights are green in colour and there is one red and one white light. The transmission characteristics of the red–green goggles are such that the eye wearing the red filter (usually the right eye) views the red lights and the eye viewing through the green filter (normally the left eye) will see the two green lights. Both eyes see the white light.

5.20.1 Assessment of suppression

A properly functioning motor system is a requirement for binocular vision, but it does not guarantee that binocular vision exists. Suppression testing provides an indication of whether the patient is capable of fusing the images from the right and left eyes. When the retinal images differ in size as in aniseikonia, or in clarity as in uncorrected anisometropia, amblyopia or unilateral eye disease, it is possible that the image from the two eyes are not fused because one eye is suppressed. An inability to appreciate diplopia in some of the motor system assessments, such as the near point of convergence (section 5.15), may already have suggested suppression. Simple assessments of suppression are also available on the Mallett unit (section 5.13) and with some stereopsis tests (sections 5.22 & 5.23). Binocular refraction techniques, such as the Turville infinity balance, can also provide an assessment of whether gross suppression exists (section 4.18).

5.20.2 Advantages and disadvantages

The Worth 4-dot test is widely available, relatively cheap, easy to use and can be used to assess fusion at distance and near. It provides a rather coarse indication of suppression in the sense that other tests may reveal the presence of suppression when the 4-dot test suggests that none is present. This is particularly true for near 4-dot testing because of the relatively large angular size of the lights when viewed at near compared to distance viewing. Conversely, the rivalry produced by the red–green goggles may lead to dissociation even in a patient with useful or normal binocular vision so that the test can suggest the existence of suppression when none is present under habitual viewing conditions. The major disadvantage of the test is that luminance of the red and green targets can vary widely between tests, as can the transmission characteristics of the red and green goggles, with the result that the test outcome can vary depending on whether the goggles are used in the standard format (red goggle in front of the right eye) or reversed (Simons & Elhatton 1994). Another disadvantage of the test is that a patient with constant strabismus and abnormal retinal correspondence may achieve a normal result. A positive test result does not therefore guarantee the presence of normal binocular vision.

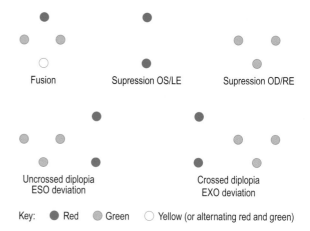

Fig. 5.11   Diagram illustrating the possible patient responses to the Worth 4-dot test.

5.20.3 Procedure

1. Explain the test to the patient: 'This test checks whether you are using both eyes at the same time to see.'

2. Place the red–green spectacles on the patient (over their spectacles if worn for that particular test distance). The eye with the red filter in front of it (usually the right eye) will see the red light and the eye with the green filter in front of it (usually the left eye) will see the green lights. Do not allow the patient to see the torch before putting the red–green spectacles on.
    a) For testing at 6 m: Ensure that the patient is wearing their distance spectacles/contact lenses.
    b) For testing at 40 cm: Hold the Worth 4-dot torch/flashlight at the patient's reading position, so that the patient looks slightly downward at it. In the case of presbyopic patients, ensure that the patient wears appropriate refractive correction for the near test distance. he torch is usually held with the red light at the top and white light at the bottom (Fig. 5.11).

3. Keeping the room lights on, now turn on the Worth 4-dot instrument.

4. Ask the patient: 'How many dots do you see?'

5. There are four possible responses (Fig. 5.11):
    a) '4 dots seen': This generally indicates that the patient has normal flat fusion. The response can be checked by asking 'How many red dots do you see? How many green ones?' Normally, patients will see one red, two green and one yellow dot. The white dot may appear yellow, or alternate between red and green due to retinal rivalry.
    b) '2 dots seen'. These will be the red and white, seen by the patient as two red dots. This indicates suppression of the eye with the green filter in front of it (usually the left). To detect alternating and/or intermittent suppression ask: 'Are the number of dots changing as you look at them?' If the number of dots seen is constant, check to see if fusion can be achieved by briefly occluding the non-suppressed eye.
    c) '3 dots seen'. These will be the two green dots and one white dot, seen by the patient as three green dots. This indicates suppression of the eye with the red filter in front of it (usually the right). To detect alternating and/or intermittent suppression ask: 'Are the number of dots changing as you look at them?' If the number of dots seen is constant, check to see if fusion can be achieved by briefly occluding the non-suppressed eye.

d) '5 dots seen': This indicates diplopia. The right eye (usually with the red filter) will see two red dots. The left eye (with the green filter) will see three green dots. Ask the patient to indicate where the red dots are in relation to the green ones. If the red dots (usually seen by the right eye) are to the right of the green dots, this indicates uncrossed diplopia and an eso deviation. If the red dots are to the left of the green dots, this indicates crossed diplopia and an exo deviation. If the red dots are below the green dots, this indicates a R/L deviation. If the red dots are above the green dots, this indicates a L/R deviation.

6. If suppression or diplopia is found, repeat the testing with the room lights off.

7. If suppression is found at distance but not at near, measure the extent of the suppression scotoma by moving the near target away from the patient and asking them to report when suppression occurs.

8. In patients who show suppression, it can be useful to repeat the test with the red–green goggles reversed to ensure an accurate assessment (Simons & Elhatton 1994).

Note: Children who cannot respond verbally can be asked to touch the dots to indicate the number seen, and 'touching four' indicates normal flat fusion. There is some evidence to indicate that although the test will reliably detect suppression in this way, it is unlikely to differentiate between normal fusion and alternating suppression (Lueder & Arnoldi 1996).

5.20.4 Recording

Record the normal perception of four dots at 6 m and 40 cm as:

'W 4-dot: fusion @ DV & NV' or similar.

If suppression is found, indicate which eye was being suppressed. Indicate whether suppression was found at both distance and/or near in both the light and dark. Indicate whether the condition was intermittent or constant.

If diplopia is found, indicate the direction of deviation suggested. Indicate whether diplopia was found at both distance and/or near in both the light and dark.

5.20.5 Interpretation

If a patient without strabismus sees all four dots on the test, they have normal 'flat' fusion. Flat fusion is binocular fusion that does not necessarily indicate stereopsis and is also called second-degree fusion. If a patient with strabismus sees four dots with the test, then this indicates that they have abnormal retinal correspondence (ARC). If the response is suppression of the right eye (i.e. the response is 2 green dots) or suppression of the left eye (i.e. the response is 3 red dots) then there is a suppression scotoma larger then the angular subtense of one of the four dots. The dots on the distance target have a smaller angular subtense than those on the near target. Because suppression is more common for targets imaged in central vision, suppression is therefore found more frequently for distance viewing than for near. The size of the suppression scotoma can be estimated by moving the near target further away from the patient than the standard 40 cm until they report suppression. The distance that the target is from the patient should be recorded. If the patient achieves fusion in the dark but not in the light, this indicates a shallower level of suppression as compared to the situation where suppression is present in both the dark and light room conditions.

5.20.6 Most common errors

1. Performing the test with the patient's vision unaided, or when they have poor visual acuity through their spectacles.

2. Assuming that the absence of suppression confirms the presence of stereopsis.

5.21 4$^\triangle$ BASE-OUT (BO) TEST

The 4$^\triangle$ base-out test is used as a test of suppression in the specific case of a suspected microtropia. It is used in combination with tests of visual acuity, refraction, eccentric fixation, abnormal retinal correspondence (ARC) and stereopsis to confirm a diagnosis of microtropia.

5.21.1 Assessment of microtropia

Microtropia may present as a primary condition or as a residual deviation after the treatment of a larger strabismus. It is characterised by a small strabismus that is not seen using the cover test, slight amblyopia (typically better than 6/12, 20/40), anisometropia, eccentric fixation, foveal suppression, ARC and reduced stereopsis. The lack of movement on the cover test is because the angle of the strabismus is equal, or similar, to the angle of eccentric fixation.

5.21.2 Advantages and disadvantages

The test requires little additional equipment and is quick and straightforward to perform. However, its repeatability is relatively poor and visually normal children can show atypical responses (Frantz et al. 1992).

5.21.3 Procedure

1. Seat the patient comfortably. Keep the room lights on and, if necessary, use additional lighting so that the patient's eyes can be easily seen without shadows. The test cannot be performed using a phoropter, and a trial frame with the optimal distance refractive correction (or the patient's spectacles) should be used.

2. Explain the measurement to the patient: 'I am going to perform a test that will help me diagnose the problem with your right/ left eye.'

3. Isolate a letter using the projector chart. The letter should be one line larger than the distance visual acuity of the amblyopic eye. Alternatively, use an isolated letter from a Sheridan–Gardner acuity test or similar. The target should be an isolated letter on a featureless background.

4. Ask the patient to keep looking at the letter, even if it appears to move.

5. Place the $4^\triangle$ BO prism over the eye with the better VA (Fig. 5.12b). The eye should make a swift movement inwards due to the prism. The fellow eye, which is likely to have slightly reduced VA (due to amblyopia and/or eccentric fixation if the patient has microtropia), should make a conjugate versional movement (i.e. in the same direction as the sound eye) due to Hering's law. If the eye with reduced VA does not have suppression it will then show a fusional vergence or refixation movement to avoid diplopia (i.e. it will move back to where it started). If the eye with reduced VA has suppression, then no refixation will be seen. You should repeat this several times to confirm your result.

6. Now place the $4^\triangle$ BO prism over the eye with reduced VA (Fig. 5.12a). In a microtropia (which is generally of the esotropic type) the $4^\triangle$ BO prism will merely shift the retinal image within the suppression scotoma of the amblyopic eye. In such a case, neither eye will move. You should repeat this several times to confirm your result.

5.21.4 Recording

Record 'positive' if there is no movement of the amblyopic eye with the $4^\triangle$ BO test. This indicates suppression. Record 'negative' if an appropriate eye movement was seen with the $4^\triangle$ BO test. For example, $4^\triangle$ BO test: positive LE (OS).

5.21.5 Interpretation

The $4^\triangle$ BO test is a useful test to help in the diagnosis of microtropia. However, it should be noted that visually normal children can show atypical responses (Frantz et al. 1992).

5.21.6 Most common errors

1. Making a decision on the test result on the basis of the first introduction of the prism.

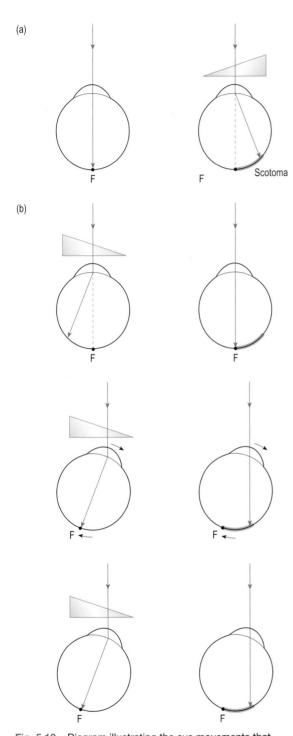

(a)

(b)

Scotoma

F   F

F   F

F   F

F   F

Fig. 5.12 Diagram illustrating the eye movements that should occur during a 4-prism dioptre test when the prism is placed in front of (a) a microtropic eye (there are no eye movements) and (b) the fellow normal eye. See preceding text for details.

5.22 TNO STEREO TEST

The TNO stereo test consists of stereograms in which the images presented to each eye have been superimposed and printed in complementary colours. The stereograms have no apparent depth until seen through a pair of red–green goggles. Video clips of the TNO and Frisby tests being used are available on the website 🖱.

5.22.1 Stereoacuity

The fundamental characteristic of binocular vision in humans is stereoscopic vision. The two eyes receive slightly disparate views of objects due to being separated horizontally by around 6 cm. This disparity can be used to signal the relative depth of objects. There are three main requirements for stereoscopic vision: a large binocular overlap of the visual fields, partial decussation of the afferent visual fibres and coordinated conjugate eye movements. Any obstacle to normal visual development early in life will be reflected in the level of stereoacuity attained. Stereoscopic vision is absent in patients with strabismus and is either poor or absent in patients with amblyopia. Stereopsis is a useful method for evaluating the level of binocular vision present in all patients but its ease of testing makes it particularly suitable for investigation of binocular vision in children (Heron et al. 1985).

5.22.2 Advantages and disadvantages

The advantage of the TNO test is that monocular cues are eliminated, unlike for the Titmus Fly test (section 5.23). The patient is required to describe the shape of the raised figure and since this shape is only seen if stereopsis is present there is no possibility of 'cheating' (Fig. 5.13). It may not be possible to perform this test with young children as they may not be happy to wear the red–green goggles, although children from the age of about 3 years can perform the test (Heron et al. 1985). For younger children (6 months to 4 years) it is best to use tests that do not require goggles to be worn such as Lang (5.23.7) or Frisby tests (5.22.7; Broadbent & Westall 1990). One disadvantage of the test is that the transmission characteristics of the red and green lenses

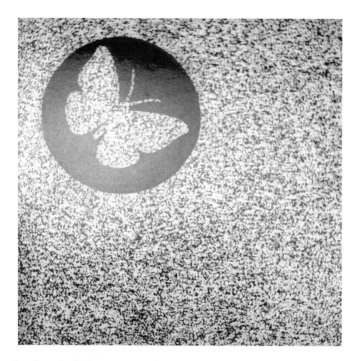

Fig. 5.13   The butterfly plate from the TNO stereo test. One butterfly is shown in the figure and is seen monocularly, the other butterfly can only be seen with stereopsis through the red and green goggles.

may lead to different contrast levels being experienced by the patient (Simons & Elhatton 1994). In some patients this can lead to a different test result depending upon which way the goggles are worn (i.e. red before right eye or green before right eye; Simons & Elhatton 1994).

5.22.3 Procedure

1. Explain the test to the patient: 'I am now going to test your 3-D vision.' Place the red–green goggles over the patient's habitual correction. For the bifocal wearer, the test should be properly positioned for near-point viewing.

2. Hold the booklet at about 40 cm, angled so that it is parallel to the plane of the patient's face.

3. Keep the room lights on. Additional lighting over the patient's shoulder can be used to illuminate the booklet if required.

4. For a general screening test, the first four plates are useful as the disparity is large and provides a qualitative assessment of

stereopsis. If the patient has a short attention span it is advisable to present Plate III alone as this gives a good early qualitative indication if stereopsis is present. Find out if the following images can be seen:

Plate I: In this plate there are two butterflies, one can be seen monocularly, whereas the other can only be seen if stereopsis is present (Fig. 5.13). Ask the patient: 'How many butterflies can you find on this page? Can you point to them?'
Plate II: There are four discs. Two may be seen without stereopsis. Ask the patient: 'How many circles? Which is the biggest?'.
Plate III: Four 'hidden' shapes (circle, square, triangle, and diamond) are arranged around a central cross that is visible without stereopsis. Ask the patient: 'Can you find a cross/square/triangle/circle/diamond? Can you point to it?' This plate is very useful with children, as they like to find and name shapes. You will need to remember the correct locations of the shapes in order to verify the accuracy of the responses.

Plate IV: This is a suppression test. There are three discs. When viewed through the goggles, one disc is seen with the right eye, one is seen by the left eye, and one seen binocularly. Ask the patient: 'How many circles can you see on this page? Can you point to them?'

To determine a quantitative measure of stereopsis proceed to plates V to VII.

5. Plates V to VII:
These plates present images that require stereoacuities from 480″ to 15″ (seconds of arc) to be present. For each stereo level, two discs with a sector missing are presented in different orientations. Using the demonstration on the left of the display, ask the patient: 'In each of these squares there is a cake with a piece missing. Can you find the cake and point to the piece that is missing?'

6. If the patient is hesitant about an answer, allow them plenty of time to view the test plate. If only one of the two tests for each stereo level is called correctly, allow them a second attempt at the incorrect one, but if called incorrectly again, or if the patient does not volunteer an answer, record the result as the previous correctly identified stereo level.

7. Record the patient's stereoacuity in seconds of arc using the information provided with the test. It is important to record the name of the test used (TNO, etc.), as performance on stereotests will vary.

8. In patients achieving a poor test result, it can be useful to repeat the test with the red–green goggles reversed to ensure an accurate assessment of stereoacuity (Simons & Elhatton 1994).

5.22.4 Recording

1. If the stereo shapes are identified in Plates I–III but not V–VII, record 'Gross Stereopsis; TNO plates I–III correct'.

2. If Plate IV result is abnormal, record which eye is being suppressed.

3. For Plates V–VII, record the stereoacuity as 'at least' the highest level where both responses were correct, e.g. 'TNO stereoacuity ≤15″'.

5.22.5 Interpretation

If stereoacuity is recorded as ≤40″ you can assume that any ocular misalignments cannot be larger than Panum's fusional area. It is clinically acceptable to assume that stereoacuity of less than 60″ is normal (Heron et al. 1985). Constant strabismus usually leads to a complete loss of stereoacuity and amblyopia and other causes of monocular vision loss typically lead to a dramatic reduction in stereoacuity. In addition, small amounts of blur (binocular or monocular) and/or aniseikonia can reduce stereoacuity so that a patient's optimal stereo threshold is only obtained with their optimal refractive correction, i.e. reduced stereopsis when viewing with the patient's existing spectacles could be due to refractive blur if the correction is not optimal. In addition, fixation disparity may lead to reductions in stereopsis (Saladin 2005).

5.22.6 Most common errors

1. Not checking on the accuracy of responses for Plates II and III due to unfamiliarity with the locations of the targets on the page.

2. Not allowing sufficient time for the patient to view the stereo figure.

3. Measuring stereopsis before the refraction with the patient's own spectacles, which may not be optimal.

4. Instructing the patient in a manner that leads the patient to the correct answers.

5.22.7 Alternative procedure: the Frisby test

The test presents a sheet of perspex on which are printed four squares that contain triangular-like shapes in a random pattern (Fig. 5.14). Three of the four squares have the shapes all printed on the same side of the perspex. Some of the shapes that make

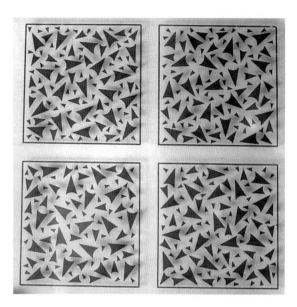

Fig. 5.14 One of the Frisby plates. The faint dark areas in the background are shadows produced by the photographic flash.

up the fourth square are printed in a circular pattern on the other side of the perspex sheet. No goggles are needed and the patient has to select the square that contains the circle in depth. The sheets of perspex are 1 mm, 3 mm and 6 mm thick and are presented at a range of fixation distances to achieve the necessary disparity. The test is usually shown first at 40 cm, which allows a best stereoacuity of 85" to be measured. In theory any disparity can be introduced by changing the fixation distance for each of the three plates. An auditory 'reward' for a correct answer is a useful modification of the test for younger children (Saunders et al. 1996). Monocular cues can be provided with movement of the plate or patient's head. It is therefore important that the plate is displayed squarely and the patient's head kept still to minimise parallax effects.

5.23 TITMUS FLY TEST

This is a popular clinical stereoacuity test that uses crossed polaroid filters to present slightly different aspects of the same object to each eye. The vectograph consists of two superimposed, similar

patterns that are polarised at right angles to each other. Some aspects of each pattern are identical, whilst for others, small crossed and uncrossed disparities are introduced (Heron et al. 1985). When the patterns are viewed with polaroid goggles the patterns are seen in depth if stereopsis is present. A video clip of the test being used is available on the website 🖼.

5.23.1 Stereoacuity

The fundamental characteristic of binocular vision in humans is stereoscopic vision. Stereopsis is a useful method for evaluating the level of binocular vision present in all patients but especially in Z children (Heron et al. 1985) because a poor level of stereopsis, or an absence of stereopsis, suggests a developmental anomaly of vision (e.g. strabismus, amblyopia) that needs to be fully investigated.

5.23.2 Advantages and disadvantages

The Titmus Fly is one of the most commonly encountered stereopsis tests and it is popular with children, although the fly can scare nervous or timid patients. The main disadvantage of this test is that it contains monocular cues (Hall 1982) which are particularly evident if the test is viewed without the polaroid goggles but are still present to some extent even when the goggles are worn. An intelligent patient could identify which is the odd one out monocularly by observing which of the circles is slightly displaced from the centre (see Fig. 5.15). This disadvantage can be overcome to some extent by asking the patient whether the target seen in depth lies in front or behind the other animals/circles. The target seen in depth is usually seen in front of the others, but by turning the book upside down the target seen in depth is behind the other animals/circles. It may not be possible to perform this test with young children as they may not be happy to wear the polaroid goggles, although children from the age of about 3 years (Heron et al. 1985) can usually be tested. For younger children (6 months to 4 years) it is best to use tests that do not require goggles to be worn such as Lang (5.23.7) or Frisby tests (5.22.7; Broadbent & Westall 1990).

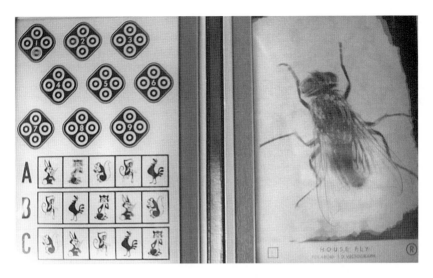

Fig. 5.15 The Titmus stereopsis test. Notice that monocular cues provide the correct answers for some of the tests (compare this to the TNO butterfly plate in Fig. 5.13)

5.23.3 Procedure

1. Explain the test to the patient: 'I am now going to test your 3-D vision.'

2. Ask the patient to hold the booklet at about 40 cm, angled so that it is parallel to the plane of the patient's face.

3. Keep the room lights on. Additional lighting over the patient's shoulder can be used to illuminate the booklet if necessary.

4. If you are measuring stereopsis in children, first show them the fly. Ask the patient to wear the polaroid goggles (you could refer to these as 'magic glasses' to younger children to make the test more of a game). Note the patient's reaction and ask them to pinch the wings of the fly. A positive test result is indicated if, in attempting to touch the wings, the child pinches the air a few centimetres above the chart.

5. Cartoon animals: Ask the patient to look at the top row of animals and tell you which is the odd one out. Then ask the patient why this one appears different to the others. If the patient volunteers that it is different because it is closer to them (or because it stands out) this is a strong indication that stereopsis is present. If there is any doubt that the patient may know the answer that was expected (e.g. sibling tested previously when the child was present), turn the test upside down and the figure that appeared in front should now appear behind. Repeat this for the two lower rows of animals.

6. Circle patterns (also known as the Wirt test): Starting at the top array of circles, ask the patient which one of the circles is the odd one out. Check the test card to ensure that they gave the correct answer and, as with the cartoon figures, ask why it appears different. Continue with this process until the patient cannot tell which is the unique circle or until they give a wrong answer. The stereo level measured with the test is the smallest disparity that could be correctly detected.

7. Record the result in seconds of arc.

5.23.4 Recording

1. If the patient's reaction and pinching of the fly's wings indicates they could see the fly in depth, record 'Gross Stereopsis (Titmus fly)'.

2. Record the stereoacuity as 'at least' the highest level where a response was correct, e.g. 'Titmus

Fly $\leq$ 40′. The disparities of the animals range from 400″ to 100″ and the disparities of the circles range from 800″ to 40″.

5.23.5 Interpretation

It is clinically acceptable for up stereoacuity to 60′′ to be considered normal (Heron et al. 1985). A lack of stereoacuity could be due to strabismus and reduced stereoacuity could be due to amblyopia or other causes of poor vision in one eye. Small amounts of blur (binocular or monocular) and/or aniseikonia can also reduce stereoacuity and if reduced stereopsis is found with the patient's existing spectacles, it is worth re-measuring with the correction found after subjective refraction if the prescription has changed.

5.23.6 Most common errors

1. Not allowing sufficient time for the patient to perceive the stereo figures.

2. Instructing the patient in such a manner that leads the patient to the answers (e.g. by asking 'which stands out?' rather than 'which one is different?'

3. Measuring stereopsis before the refraction with the patient's own spectacles, which may not be optimal.

5.23.7 Alternative procedure: Lang stereotest

This test was designed to simplify stereopsis screening in children. The test is a single card that can be held easily by the clinician or the patient. It only assesses gross stereopsis and provides targets of a moon arc (200 seconds), star (200 seconds), car (400 seconds) and an elephant (600 seconds). The star can also be seen monocularly to help attract the attention of young children. Pre-verbal children respond by reaching for the images and this action can be used to indicate that some stereopsis is present. A preferential-looking procedure can also be adopted in pre-verbal children: this involves comparing the child's fixation when the card is held in

the normal fashion as compared to when it is rotated by 90 degrees. This is a useful test to have available as it is easy to use, does not require goggles, provides valuable information and is relatively inexpensive (Manny et al. 1991). You need to be careful not to allow the test to be tilted as this can provide monocular cues.

5.24 CLASSIFICATION OF INCOMITANT HETEROTROPIA

This is a heterotropia in which the angle of deviation varies with direction of gaze. Video clips of the motility test being used to assess a variety of incomitant heterotropias are provided on the website ✍.

5.24.1 Congenital vs. acquired deviations

1. Congenital incomitant deviations are usually due to a developmental problem in the anatomy or functioning of one of the six extraocular muscles or their nerve supply.

2. Acquired incomitant deviations can occur due to conditions such as diabetes, hypertension, multiple sclerosis, thyrotoxicosis, temporal arteritis or tumour. These may be long-standing or of recent onset.

3. Recent-onset incomitancies can be the first sign of the underlying disease and it is therefore essential to determine if the condition is of recent onset or long-standing. Missing the signs of these conditions, particularly in children, is a significant cause of malpractice claims in the US (Classé & Rutstein 1995). Signs and symptoms that can differentiate between new and old ocular muscle palsies are shown in Table 5.6. Long-standing incomitancies tend to become more comitant as time passes.

5.24.2 Paralysis, paresis and mechanical restrictions

1. Paralysis: The action of one or a group of extraocular muscles is completely abolished.

Table 5.6 Signs and symptoms that can help to differentiate between an old and new ocular motor palsy.

Sign/symptom	Old	New
Diplopia	Rare	Almost always present
Onset	Generally unknown	Probably sudden
Ambylopia	Common	Rare
Trauma	Not usual	Common
Symptoms	Not usual	Common and extreme
Comitance	Spread of comitance may obscure original palsy	Always incomitant
Abnormal head posture	If present well established and difficult to alter	Can be marked but easy to alter. Covering paretic eye eliminates problem
Past-pointing	Absent	Present
Health	Not usually related	Current health may be a significant issue

2. Paresis: The action of a muscle is impaired but not abolished.

3. Mechanical restrictions: Incomitant deviations can also be caused by mechanical restrictions. An incomitancy caused by mechanical restriction continues to exhibit the same restricted movement when measured monocularly, whereas the movements of a paretic eye are more normal when measured monocularly.

5.24.3 Primary and secondary angle of deviation

The angle of deviation is largest when the eyes are turned in the direction of maximum action of the affected muscle. The size of the deviation can also vary with respect to the eye that is used to fixate.

1. The primary angle of deviation is observed when the non-affected eye fixates.

2. The secondary angle of deviation is observed when the affected eye fixates. The secondary angle is usually larger than the primary angle in a recently acquired incomitancy.

5.25 THE MOTILITY TEST (BROAD H TEST)

This test involves observing the patient's eyes as they move to follow a penlight or non-luminous target in a cross or H pattern to the edge of the binocular field from the primary position. The task of the practitioner is to determine whether there are one or more positions of gaze in which a misalignment of the patient's eyes can be observed and/or for which the patient reports doubling of the target. Video clips of the motility test being used to assess a variety of incomitant heterotropias are provided on the website.

5.25.1 Incomitant heterotropia

See section 5.24.

5.25.2 Advantages and disadvantages

This is the simplest method of evaluating a deviation in the nine diagnostic positions of gaze (Clement & Boylan 1987). It is relatively quick and easy to perform and requires no extra equipment. Assessment of versions (binocular eye movements in the same direction) are used as a screening technique, and the technique can be repeated monocularly (assessing ductions) if an incomitancy is detected to help differentiate between incomitant deviations due to paresis/paralysis and mechanical restrictions. The only disadvantages of the motility test are that it requires practice in terms of both dexterity (achieving smooth movements of the penlight) and interpretation of the results.

5.25.3 Procedure

1. Keep the room lights on and illuminate the eyes without shadows. Explain the test to the patient: 'This test checks whether all your eye muscles are working well together.'

2. Ask the patient to remove any spectacles. Spectacles can make observation of the eyes more difficult and the frame may hide the fixation target. In addition, in peripheral gaze, diplopia can be induced by the prismatic effect produced by anisometropic spectacles and the 'jack-in-the-box' effect of myopic spectacles, particularly with small, modern frames. Sit directly in front of the patient so that both eyes can be viewed simultaneously.

3. The target used is not critical as long as the patient can easily see it, although a penlight is particularly useful as it allows you to observe the corneal reflexes and it will indicate when the light has moved from the binocular field into the monocular field as one of the corneal reflexes will disappear. A picture on a fixation stick should be used when examining children.

4. Instruct the patient: 'Please watch my light and follow it with your eyes. Keep your head still. Tell me if the light appears double or blurred or if your eyes feel uncomfortable at any time'. Patients sometimes call a diplopic or overlapped image 'blurred', so that this is useful to include in your instructions.

5. Shine the penlight towards the patient from approximately 40 cm and move it in an arc with the patient's head as the centre. Move the penlight so that the patient's eyes follow to the edge of the binocular field. The loss of the corneal reflex will help to indicate that you have moved into the monocular field. Note that at the limits of movement, even normal muscles can feel uncomfortable and may even produce reports of diplopia/blur due to end-point nystagmus.

6. Move the penlight into the nine diagnostic positions of gaze by moving the target in a cross (Fig. 5.16) or broad H formation. Many

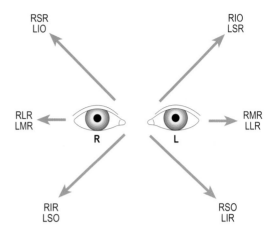

Fig. 5.16   The six cardinal diagnostic positions of gaze, showing the yoke muscles that principally maintain the eyes in these positions. Assessment of motility in the vertical midline is necessary for the diagnosis of conditions such as A and V patterns. The three diagnostic positions on the midline supplement the six positions of fixation demonstrated in the figure. IO, inferior oblique; IR, inferior rectus; LR, lateral rectus; MR, medial rectus; SO, superior oblique; SR, superior rectus.

clinicians have a preference for the manner in which the light is moved but either type of movement is acceptable (Clement & Boylan 1987). During downgaze, you may need to hold up the patient's eyelids to gain a useful view. You may need to transfer the target/penlight from your left to your right hand when switching between the patient's right and left visual fields.

7. Carefully look for any misalignment of the eyes in all positions of gaze (the corneal reflexes can help you in this). Also determine whether the movements of the eyes are smooth and accurate (see pursuit eye movements, section 5.26).

8. If the eye movements were smooth and accurate with no reported diplopia, the test is complete and the results can be recorded.

9. Note and record the position of the eyes when any of the following occur:
   a) The patient reports any diplopia or discomfort.
   b) Any underaction or overaction in one eye.
   c) Jerky or inaccurate pursuit eye movements.

d) The size of the palpebral apertures differs between the R and L eyes and varies as a function of the direction of gaze.

10. Locate the gaze direction that yields the greatest diplopia as this indicates the direction in which the greatest underaction occurs. This can be difficult for some patients as similar separations of the doubled images may be reported in different directions of gaze.

11. Establish whether the doubled images are horizontally, vertically or diagonally separated. Diagonal separation is found most commonly in cases where one or more of the oblique or vertical recti muscles are affected.

12. Cover each eye in turn to identify which eye is seeing which image. When the eyes are elevated, the eye that sees the higher image is seen by the paretic eye (red–green goggles can help in distinguishing the images). When the eyes are looking down, the eye seeing the lower image is seen by the paretic eye. Similarly, when the eyes are looking right or left, the paretic eye is the eye that sees the image that is further to the right or left, respectively. A cover test (section 5.5) performed in this direction of gaze can be used to confirm the diagnosis.

13. If an incomitancy is observed, repeat the testing monocularly (assessment of ductions) to help discriminate between paretic and mechanical incomitancy.

5.25.4 Recording

Where the ocular movements appear full and no diplopia is reported in any position, a normal result has been obtained. This is usually recorded using the acronym SAFE (or FESA). This indicates that the ocular motility movements were (S) Smooth, (A) Accurate, (F) Full and (E) Extensive. For a patient with strabismus, normal motility can be recorded as 'No incomitancy detected'. In a patient with strabismus in the primary position, it is likely that diplopia will not be reported by the patient in any direction of gaze. For this reason, in patients with strabismus in the primary position, it is objective (i.e. the practitioner's) judgements alone that will

decide whether the deviation is comitant or incomitant. In cases where you detect incomitancy, or diplopia is reported by the patient, record a cross/H-pattern to clearly indicate where diplopia was experienced or incomitancy noticed. Also, record any apparent underactions or overactions, clearly stating which eye and in which gaze direction this was observed. Increasingly, incomitancies are recorded using a 9-point scale (Vivian & Morris 1993). Using this system, overactions and underactions are recorded on a basic template in the primary field of action of each muscle. Underactions are recorded as negative numbers on a scale from −1 to −4, where −4 represents the greatest underaction. Similarly, overactions are recorded using positive numbers on a scale from +1 to +4, where +4 represents the greatest overaction. For example, underactions that are scored as −4 indicate that the eye is unable to move at all from the primary position into the field of action of that muscle and overactions of a horizontal rectus muscle are graded according to the amount of cornea covered by the canthus; in extreme overaction (+4), half of the cornea is concealed. This diagrammatic representation also provides a useful way of signalling the presence of a A- or V-pattern, restrictions of movements as well as other ocular movement abnormalities (e.g. up- and down-drifts, up- and down-shoots) (Vivian & Morris 1993).

If a head tilt is present it should be noted and the practitioner may find it useful to perform the motility in the head-straight and head-tilted conditions and compare the results. The movements observed during a motility test may conform to one of the so-called 'alphabet' patterns (von Noorden 2002). For example, if the deviation is significantly (>15 prism dioptres) more convergent (i.e. more eso, less exo) in upgaze than in downgaze, this is referred to as an A-pattern. Similarly, the term V-pattern describes a situation where the deviation is significantly more divergent (i.e. more exo, less eso) in upgaze than in downgaze. Note that incomitancies of this nature do not always conform strictly to the A and V patterns. For example, some patterns may be more correctly described as Y or inverted Y patterns.

5.25.5 Interpretation

To understand the actions of the extraocular muscles (EOMs) you must first understand their plane of action and how they work together. There are two types of binocular eye movements: versions, where the eyes move in the same direction (e.g. to the right) and vergences, where the eyes move in the opposite direction (e.g. convergence). For all versions and vergences, two muscles (the yoke muscles, one from each eye) move the eyes in the desired direction.

The actions of the medial and lateral recti are the easiest to explain:

- To look right, the right lateral rectus (RLR) and the left medial rectus (LMR) must contract. These are the yoke muscles that allow you to look right. These contracting muscles are called agonists. At the same time, the RMR and LLR, the antagonists, must relax.

- To look left the LLR and the RMR must contract.

- To converge, the RMR and LMR must contract.

- To diverge, the RLR and LLR must contract.

Clinically, it is relatively easy to examine the lateral and medial recti as all that is required is to get the patient's eyes to follow a target along the horizontal meridian. A movement to the patient's right will assess their RLR and LMR. A movement to the patient's left will assess their LLR and RMR. Any underaction or overaction of one compared to the other can be detected. An underaction could be caused by a mechanical restriction or muscle paresis/paralysis. An overaction will occur in the non-paretic eye if the paretic eye is fixating the target. This is because to be able to fixate the target the paretic muscle must receive more innervation than normal. Because of Hering's law of equal innervation, this means that the yoke muscle in the non-paretic eye will also receive this abnormally large innervation and this will produce an overaction. It should not be assumed that the non-paretic eye will always fixate. The paretic eye could be the eye with the best visual acuity or the dominant eye and therefore likely be the eye that fixates. Consider a patient with amblyopia in the left eye, who develops a muscle palsy in the right eye. The right eye is likely to fixate the target in motility testing and therefore overactions are likely to be seen in the left (non-paretic) eye.

The clinical interpretation of motility test results are more complicated when diplopia is experienced

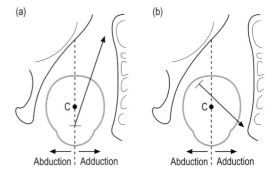

(a)   (b)

Abduction ┊ Adduction   Abduction ┊ Adduction

Fig. 5.17   The planes of action of the superior rectus (a) and superior oblique (b) muscles are shown passing medial to the centre of rotation of the eye (C).

on upwards or downwards gaze, because there are four muscles that help to elevate (the right superior rectus, RSR; left superior rectus, LSR; right inferior oblique, RIO and left inferior oblique, LIO) and depress the eyes (the right inferior rectus, RIR; left inferior rectus, LIR; right superior oblique, RSO and left superior oblique, LSO). All four elevators are used approximately equally in looking straight up and all four depressors are used approximately equally in looking straight down and so these positions provide little information regarding which muscle(s) is/are affected when attempting to assess an incomitancy. However, the elevator/depressor power varies as the eyes look up and right, up and left, down and right and down and left (Fig. 5.17) so that clinical determination of affected muscle(s) can be made. The muscle planes of the vertical recti muscles mean that when the eye is abducted (looking temporally) by 23°, the plane of action of the vertical recti muscles are in line with the line of sight and the centre of rotation of the eye (Fig. 5.17a). At this position, the SR acts purely as an elevator and its power as an elevator is at its maximum. Similarly, when an eye is abducted (looking temporally) by 23° the IR acts purely as a depressor and its power as an elevator is at its maximum. However, when an eye is adducted (looking nasally) the vertical recti muscles have little elevator or depressor power (Fig. 5.18).

The muscle planes of the superior oblique muscles (Fig. 5.17b) mean that when an eye is adducted (looking nasally) by about 51°, the plane of action of the SO and IO muscles are in line with the line of sight and the centre of rotation of the eye. At this position, the IO acts purely as an elevator and the SO

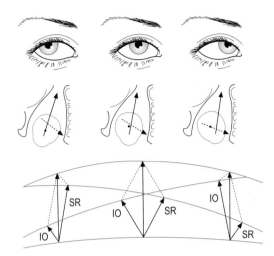

Fig. 5.18 The relative actions of the elevator muscles, the superior rectus (SR) and inferior oblique (IO). The lower diagram shows a vector analysis of the relative actions of these muscles as the eye moves across the upper motor field.

acts purely as a depressor and their power as elevators/depressors are at a maximum. When an eye is abducted (looking temporally) the oblique muscles have little elevator or depressor power (Fig. 5.18).

For these reasons, if you ask a patient to look out about 40° (approximately midway between 23° and 51°) to their right and then to look up, any restriction of movement upwards is the fault of the RSR or LIO. Similarly, if you ask a patient to look approximately 40° to their left and then to look up, any restriction of movement upwards is the fault of the LSR or RIO. If you ask a patient to look approximately 40° to their right and then to look down, any restriction of movement downwards is the fault of the RIR or LSO. If you ask a patient to look approximately 40° to their left and then to look down, any restriction of movement downwards is the fault of the LIR or RSO (Fig. 5.18). Note that 40° is an ideal angle to use when attempting to investigate the extraocular muscles that may be responsible for the incomitancy, but when performing the motility test, you should move the penlight beyond 40° and out to the edge of the binocular field.

Versions vs. ductions

Duction (monocular) testing (step 12) helps to differentiate between an incomitant deviation due to paresis/paralysis and one due to mechanical restriction.

With an incomitant deviation due to a paresis, the underaction seen during version (binocular) testing is less obvious during duction testing, and any overaction will not be seen monocularly. An underaction that is similar when tested monocularly and binocularly suggests a mechanical restriction and may require further testing using forced ductions. To aid or confirm a diagnosis of the underaction/restriction, to measure the extent of the deviation and to assess the degree of incomitancy, further tests are required such as the 9-point cover test (section 5.27).

5.25.6 Most common errors

1. Not using a penlight. This makes the detection of incomitant deviations more difficult. It is also more difficult to determine when the patient's eyes are at the edge of the binocular field.

2. Not asking the patient to report doubling, or not fully investigating reported doubling.

3. Relying too much on the patient to report doubling (i.e. not paying enough attention to symmetry of corneal reflexes).

4. Performing the test too quickly or too slowly.

5. Moving the target in a straight line rather than an arc, so that increasingly unequal angular demands are made of the two eyes as the target is moved into a peripheral position of gaze.

6. Not holding the top lid when viewing the eye movements in downgaze.

7. Misinterpreting a large intermittent squint as an incomitancy.

5.26 PURSUITS (AS PART OF MOTILITY TESTING)

The test involves observing the patient's eyes as they follow a moving target and determining their smoothness and accuracy.

5.26.1 Pursuit eye movements

Pursuits are conjugate eye movements that are used to maintain fixation of a target at the fovea, while the target is being moved. When a foveated target moves, the pursuit response begins after a latency of around 130 ms and the pursuit movements are at the same velocity as the target. Because of the latency, a small, catch-up saccade is seen initially to allow the moving target to be foveated. Assuming the target moves in a predictable fashion (constant speed and direction), it can then be followed using pursuit movements.

5.26.2 Advantages and disadvantages

A simple and repeatable assessment of pursuit eye movements can be made by direct observation of the patient's eyes as they follow a moving target (Maples & Ficklin 1988) and, as this task is performed during motility/broad H testing for incomitancy (section 5.25), the pursuit reflexes can be assessed at the same time. Alternatively, pursuit eye movements can be assessed separately. The main disadvantage of this examination relates to the fact that the information obtained is qualitative rather than quantitative. For this reason, the same test result may be interpreted in different ways by different practitioners.

5.26.3 Procedure

1. The procedure is the same as for motility testing.

2. Look for jerky pursuit movements, fixation losses or movements that are not at the same speed as the movement of the target.

3. The assessment can be repeated monocularly during duction testing if binocular problems are seen.

5.26.4 Recording

Pursuits can be recorded as part of motility test result (see section 5.25.4). If normal pursuit eye movements are seen, record 'smooth and accurate pursuits' or similar. If pursuits are abnormal, record the type of abnormality (e.g. 'jerky eye movements' or 'unable to maintain fixation') and indicate if one eye is more at fault than the other.

5.26.5 Interpretation

Pursuit eye movements should be smooth, conjugate and accurate, with minimal losses of fixation. Abnormal pursuit eye movements could indicate ocular motor nerve paresis, cerebellar disease or Parkinson's disease or they may be due to systemic medications, particularly antidepressants. In cases of abnormal pursuit eye movements, further evaluation of the visual system is warranted, e.g. visual fields, contrast sensitivity testing, etc. as referral may be necessary.

5.26.6 Most common errors

1. Moving the target at an inappropriate speed, or in a non-smooth fashion.

2. Misinterpreting the result due to lack of experience.

5.27 9-POINT COVER TEST OR OR 9-POINT MADDOX ROD/ MODIFIED THORINGTON

The test involves performing a cover test or Maddox rod or modified Thorington test in the nine principal positions of gaze.

5.27.1 Degree of incomitancy

To allow a more reliable diagnosis of which muscle(s) is/are affected, it is necessary to perform a test that dissociates the eyes and allows a comparison of primary and secondary angles in all positions of gaze (Thomson et al. 1990). A difference between the primary and secondary angles of deviation distinguishes a paralytic from a non-paralytic strabismus. The primary deviation is the deviation seen in the paretic eye when the fellow eye fixates. The secondary deviation is that seen in the fellow eye when the paretic eye fixates, and is always larger than the primary deviation. An overaction is likely to be seen in the non-paretic eye if the paretic eye is fixating the target. This is because to be able to fixate the target the paretic muscle must receive more innervation than normal. Because of Hering's law of equal innervation, this means that the yoke muscle in the non-paretic eye will also receive this abnormally large innervation and this will produce an overaction. The simplest example to take is a paresis in one of the horizontal muscles, such as the right medial rectus. If the left eye fixates, the primary deviation will be seen as an underaction of the right medial rectus and an exotropia of the right eye will be observed by the practitioner. If the right eye fixates, the right medial rectus must receive more innervation than normal to enable this fixation. Because of Hering's law of equal innervation, this means that the yoke muscle in the non-paretic eye, the left lateral rectus, will also receive this extra innervation and will produce an overaction (leading to an exotropia of the left eye).

5.27.2 Advantages and disadvantages

The 9 point cover test/Maddox rod/modified Thorington test requires no additional equipment and provides quantitative information about the size of the deviation in different positions of gaze. This can be useful when monitoring an incomitant deviation to determine if it is getting better or worse. The 9 point cover test has an advantage over the Maddox rod test in that it is an objective test and therefore it can be used in patients with suppression. An experienced practitioner will be able to carry out the procedure swiftly and smoothly. However, considerable practice is required. The results of the 9 point test can be supported by investigation with the Hess screen method, although this test is seldom available in primary eye care settings.

5.27.3 Procedure

1. Perform a near cover test (section 5.5) in each of the nine positions of gaze. An alternating cover test is more useful than the cover/uncover test as movements will be more obvious. Note that in the cover/uncover test, the deviation may differ depending on which eye is fixating. If quantitative measures are required, horizontal and vertical prism bars are needed in order to neutralise the vertical and horizontal deviations.

2. Alternatively, perform a Maddox rod (section 5.8) or modified Thorington test (section 5.7) in each of the nine positions of gaze. It may be necessary to hold the Maddox rod in free space to allow the line to be seen in peripheral gaze directions. At each gaze point, the line is presented horizontally and vertically in order to determine the vertical and horizontal deviation angles, respectively.

5.27.4 Interpretation

If the angle of deviation varies depending upon direction of gaze, this is conclusive evidence that an incomitancy exists. The gaze direction which produces the biggest deviation is likely to be the field of action of the affected muscle. Interpreting the results of the alternating cover test in a peripheral gaze direction can be difficult because it requires first-hand knowledge of not only the primary actions of each extraocular muscle but also their secondary and tertiary actions. By way of example, let us suppose that our patient has a paresis of the right superior rectus (RSR). When the patient is asked to look up and to their right, diplopia will be experienced. Even though the RSR is an elevating muscle, the diplopia reported by the patient will not be purely vertical; i.e. the dual images of the light will be diagonally separated. Since the paresis affects the right eye, let us consider that it is the right eye that had not been fixating the light (note: this is usually the case but there are circumstances in which the paretic eye can fixate). Since the RSR is responsible for elevating, adducting and intorting the eye, the right eye will be seen to be turned down and out relative to where it should be. The extorsion will be harder to appreciate. While the patient continues to look in this direction, the cover is placed over the left eye. The RSR now receives the extra innervation it needs to allow it to fixate the light and as a result the eye is seen to move up and in. A little intorsion may be observed but this is much less obvious than the diagonal movement that results from the combined upwards and inwards motion of the eye. When the cover is switched from the left to the right eye, the left eye will be seen to move in the opposite direction to the movement seen in the right eye. In other words, the left eye will move down and in. This is because the extra innervation to the RSR was accompanied by extra, but unnecessary innervation to the RSR's yoke muscle, the left inferior oblique (LIO). The LIO moves the eye upward and outwards, and it also responsible for extorting the eye. The extra innervation that was received by the LIO when it was behind the cover has now taken the eye too high and too far away from the nose to view the light. For this reason, to re-fixate, it is seen to move in a diagonal fashion, downwards and inwards, with perhaps a little intorsion evident.

5.27.5 Recording

Quantitative measures of the deviation angle (horizontal and vertical) are seldom needed in all directions of gaze. Indeed, the aim of these tests is to identify the likely source of the problem. Thus, the test result is normally recorded in a fashion which identifies the muscle(s) that is/are affected; e.g. 'bilateral super rectus underaction'.

If quantitative measures are required, both vertical and horizontal prisms are needed to neutralise the movements on alternating cover test and during the Maddox rod or modified Thorington test in the various gaze positions.

5.27.6 Most common errors

1. Not keeping the viewing distance fixed in the various positions of gaze.

2. Failing to ensure occlusion occurs in peripheral gaze directions (cover test).

3. Switching the cover too quickly and not allowing the eyes time to take up position when prompted to fixate (cover test).

4. Not repeating the Maddox rod or modified Thorington test with the rod in front of the left eye.

5.26.7 Additional technique: double Maddox rod

By placing a Maddox rod in front of one eye the extent of an incyclo- or excyclo-rotation of the eye can be quantitatively evaluated. When the rod is placed horizontally the streak should, of course, appear to be vertically oriented. If the streak does not appear vertical, this indicates the presence of cyclorotation and the rod orientation in the trial frame can be adjusted until the patient reports that the streak is vertical. The magnitude and direction of the rotation required to generate the impression of verticality is a measure of the nature and size of cyclorotation. The same procedure can be employed when a Maddox rod is placed before each eye. In this case a prism may be needed to dissociate the rods and the patient's task is to assess whether or not they appear parallel. This is known as the double Maddox rod test and it is useful in bilateral conditions in which an underaction or overaction of the elevating or depressing extraocular muscles is present or suspected. The patient's head should be in the primary position and the head should be held straight.

5.28 PARK'S 3-STEP TEST

The technique of assessing movements of the eyes as the head is tilted successively toward one shoulder and then toward the other was introduced by Hoffmann and Bielschowsky but has since come to be known as the Bielschowsky head tilt test (von Noorden 2002). The manner in which this test is normally used in the clinical setting is referred to as the Park's 3-step test.

5.28.1 Advantages and disadvantages

This test can provide useful information to help determine the affected muscle in cases of known or suspected incomitancy. The test is useful in cases of paresis of any of the cyclovertical muscles, but the results are more dramatic when the oblique muscles are affected compared to when the vertical rectus muscles are involved. No additional equipment is required to perform this test. It offers the additional advantages in that the test is objective, allowing the practitioner to observe and measure the magnitude of any deviations without subjective responses from the patient, making it suitable for use in young children. However, the test result can be affected by a number of factors including the paresis of more than one muscle and mechanical restrictions by previous surgery to the extraocular muscles. Furthermore, interpretation of results may be more difficult than in the case of the Hess screen test.

Table 5.7 Park's three-step method for identifying the paretic muscle when the deviation is vertical.

	Deviation has a vertical component							
1. Which is the hyper eye?	RE (OD) hyper				LE (OS) hyper			
2. Is the deviation greater on left or right gaze?	Left gaze		Right gaze		Left gaze		Right gaze	
3. Is the deviation greater on head tilt to the right or left?	Right	Left	Right	Left	Right	Left	Right	Left
Likely paretic muscle	RSO	LSR	LIO	RIR	LIR	RIO	RSR	LSO

LE (OS), left eye; LIO, left inferior oblique; LIR, left inferior rectus; LSO, left superior oblique; LSR, left superior rectus; RE (OD), right eye; RIO, right inferior oblique; RIR, right inferior rectus; RSO, rights superior oblique; RSR, right superior rectus.

5.28.2 Procedure

1. In order to carry out the Park's 3-step test, the practitioner should attempt to answer the following three questions:
   a) Which is the hyperdeviated eye in the primary position? The answer to this question may be obvious by simply viewing the patient or it may require the practitioner to carry out a cover/uncover test in the primary position (section 5.5).
   b) Is the hyperdeviation greater in right or left gaze?
   c) Is the hyperdeviation greater with head tilt to the right shoulder or to the left shoulder? This portion of the test is the Bielchowsky head tilt test.

5.28.3 Interpretation

Determine the muscle that the Park's 3-step test suggests is paretic by matching the test result to the information provided in Table 5.7. If, for example, the *right* eye is the hyperdeviated eye in the primary position (Answer to Question 1), the deviation is greater on *leftwards* gaze (Answer to Question 2), and greater when the head is tilted to the *right* (Answer to Question 3), the muscle implicated is the *Right Superior Oblique (RSO)* (Table 5.7).

It is easier to recall the result patterns associated with the oblique muscles being affected. In the case of superior oblique muscles, the answers to the three questions will be *right-left-right* when the Right Superior Oblique is affected, and *left-right-left* when

the Left Superior Oblique is affected. In the case of the inferior oblique muscles, the result will be *right-right-right* in the case of the Left Inferior Oblique and *left-left-left* for the Right Inferior Oblique.

5.28.4 Most common error

It is not necessary to use prisms in order to complete the test. However, if prisms are used to measure/neutralise the deviation, the base must be held with its base parallel to the palpebral fissure when the head is in the tilted position, rather than parallel with the floor. This is to ensure that the prism has the same relation to the eye as in the primary position (von Noorden 2002).

5.29 SACCADES

5.29.1 Saccadic eye movements

Saccadic eye movements are used to quickly redirect our eyes so that an object of interest falls on the fovea. They are conjugate eye movements in that the eyes move by the same amount and they are the fastest of all eye movements with velocities as high as 700 degrees per second. Saccades serve several distinct functions:

- They occur at a frequency of about 20/minute and are used to continually scan the environment.

- Reflexive saccades occur in response to new visual, auditory or tactile cues.

- Voluntary saccades can be made to commands ('look at the pen') and to imagined or remembered target locations.

- They are particularly important during reading.

- They can also be voluntarily suppressed for the maintenance of steady foveal fixation.

- They form the resetting part of nystagmus and return the eyes to foveal fixation following a vestibular or optokinetic slow-phase deviation.

Saccades originate in the left and right frontal eye fields (Broadmann's area 8) of the frontal lobes.

5.29.2 Advantages and disadvantages

A simple assessment of saccadic eye movements can be made by direct observation of the patient's eyes as they switch fixation from one target to another. No additional equipment is required and the test is very simple, quick and reasonably reliable (Maples & Ficklin 1988). A disadvantage of carrying out a dedicated test of saccades is that, if any abnormal pattern of saccadic eye movements does exist, it is likely to become apparent during other binocular vision testing. In addition, the information obtained is qualitative rather than quantitative. For this reason, the same test result may be interpreted in different ways by different practitioners.

5.29.3 Procedure

1. Seat the patient comfortably with their head erect and eyes in slightly downward gaze. Make sure the patient is wearing their near correction. Sit directly in front of the patient so that both eyes can be viewed simultaneously.

2. Keep the room lights on. Position additional lighting to illuminate the patient's eyes or the target (whichever is necessary) without shadows.

3. Explain the measurement to the patient: 'This test determines how well your eyes move to change their viewing position.'

4. Hold your right and left index fingers pointing upwards approximately 30° to 40° either side of the patient's midline and at a distance of 40 to 50 cm from a point midway between the eyes.

5. Instruct the patient: 'Please look at my right finger … Now at the other finger… and now the first finger again, etc.' Repeat for about five cycles.

6. Grade the saccadic movements into one of four categories:
   a) 4+ : Smooth and accurate.
   b) 3+ : Slight undershoot.
   c) 2+ : Gross undershooting, any overshooting or slight increased latency.
   d) 1+ : Inability to do the task or greatly increased latency.

7. The assessment should be repeated monocularly if binocular problems are present or if the test result is 2+ or 1+.

5.29.4 Recording

If normal saccadic eye movements are seen, record Saccades: 4+ or 3+, or 'smooth and accurate saccades' or similar. If saccadic eye movements are abnormal (2+ or 1+) record the type of abnormality and indicate whether one eye is more at fault than the other.

5.29.5 Interpretation

All saccadic eye movements should be fast (completed in less than 1 second), conjugate and accurate, with no overshoots requiring secondary compensatory eye movements. A small undershoot with a compensatory eye movement is normal. Dysmetria denotes inaccurate saccadic eye movements and includes hypometria (undershooting) or hypermetria (overshooting). Abnormal saccadic eye movements could indicate ocular motor nerve paresis, internuclear ophthalmoplegia, myasthenia gravis, cerebellar disease, Alzheimer's disease, Parkinson's disease, gross visual field defects (saccades are used to keep the target within an intact part of the visual field) or could be due to systemic medications, particularly antidepressants. In cases of abnormal saccadic eye movements, visual field assessment is warranted and referral may be necessary. It is worth remembering that disorders of saccadic, pursuit and fixational eye movements generally occur together.

5.29.6 Most common error

1. Misinterpreting the results due to lack of experience. For example, not realising that small undershoots are frequently seen.

5.30 BIBLIOGRAPHY AND FURTHER READING

Carlson, N.B. and Kurtz, D. (2004) *Clinical procedures for ocular examination*, 3rd edn. New York: McGraw-Hill.

Ciuffreda, K.J., Levi, D.M. and Selenow, A. (1991) *Amblyopia: basic and clinical aspects*. Boston: Butterworth-Heinemann.

Stidwell, D. (1998) *Orthoptic assessment and management*, 2nd edn. London: Blackwell Science.

5.31 REFERENCES

Atchison, D.A., Capper, E.J. and McCabe, K.L. (1994) Critical subjective measurement of amplitude of accommodation. *Optometry and Vision Science* 71, 699–706.

Brautaset, R.L. and Jennings, J.A. (1999) The influence of heterophoria measurements on subsequent associated phoria measurement in a refractive routine. *Ophthalmic and Physiological Optics* 19, 347–350.

Broadbent, H. and Westall, C. (1990) An evaluation of techniques for measuring stereopsis in infants and young children. *Ophthalmic and Physiological Optics* 10, 3–7.

Cacho, P.M., Garcia-Munoz, A., Garcia-Bernabeu, J.R. et al. (1999) Comparison between MEM and Nott dynamic retinoscopy. *Optometry and Vision Science* 76, 650–655.

Calvin, H., Rupnow, P. and Grosvenor, T. (1996) How good is the estimated cover test at predicting the von Graefe phoria measurement? *Optometry and Vision Science* 73, 701–706.

Casillas, E.C. and Rosenfield, M. (2006) Comparison of subjective heterophoria testing with a phoropter and trial frame. *Optometry and Vision Science* 83, 237–241.

Charman, W.N. (1989) The path to presbyopia: straight or crooked? *Ophthalmic and Physiological Optics* 9, 126–132.

Choi, R.Y. and Kushner, B.J. (1998) The accuracy of experienced strabismologists using the Hirschberg and Krimsky tests. *Ophthalmology* 105, 1301–1306.

Ciuffreda, K.J., Rosenfield, M. and Chen, H.W. (1997) The AC/A ratio, age and presbyopia. *Ophthalmic and Physiological Optics* 17, 307–315.

Classé, J.G. and Rutstein, R.P. (1995) Binocular vision anomalies: an emerging cause of malpractice claims. *Journal of the American Optometric Association* 66, 305–309.

Clement, R.A. and Boylan, C. (1987) Current concepts of the actions of the extraocular muscles and the interpretation of oculomotility tests. *Ophthalmic and Physiological Optics* 7, 341–344.

Evans, B.J.W. (2002) *Pickwell's Binocular vision anomalies*, 4th edn. Oxford: Butterworth-Heinemann.

Fogt, N., Baughman, B.J. and Good, G. (2000) The effect of experience on the detection of small eye movements. *Optometry and Vision Science* 77, 670–674.

Frantz, K.A., Cotter, S.A. and Wick, B. (1992) Re-evaluation of the four prism dioptre base-out test. *Optometry and Vision Science* 69, 777–786.

Freier, B.E. and Pickwell, L.D. (1983) Physiological exophoria. *Ophthalmic and Physiological Optics* 3, 267–272.

Gall, R. and Wick, B. (2003) The symptomatic patient with normal phorias at distance and near: what tests detect a binocular vision problem? *Optometry* 74, 309–322.

Gall, R., Wick, B. and Bedell, H. (1998) Vergence facility: establishing clinical utility. *Optometry and Vision Science* 75, 731–742.

Hall, C. (1982) The relationship between clinical stereotests. *Ophthalmic and Physiological Optics* 2, 133–143.

Heron, G., Dholakia, S., Collins, D.E. et al. (1985) Stereoscopic threshold in children and adults. *American Journal of Optometry and Physiological Optics* 62, 505–515.

Hung, G.K., Ciuffreda, K.J. and Rosenfield, M. (1996) Proximal contribution to a linear static model of accommodation and vergence. *Ophthalmic and Physiological Optics* **16**, 31–41.

Jampolsky, A., Flom, B. and Fried, A. (1957) Fixation disparity in relation to heterophoria. *American Journal of Ophthalmology* **43**, 97.

Jenkins, T.C.A., Pickwell, L.D. and Yekta, A.A. (1989) Criteria for decompensation in binocular vision. *Ophthalmic and Physiological Optics* **9**, 121–125.

Kaban, T., Smith, K., Beldavs, R. et al. (1995) The 20-prism-dioptre base-out test: an indicator of peripheral binocularity. *Canadian Journal of Ophthalmology* **30**, 247–250.

Kragha, I.K.O.K. (1986) Amplitude of accommodation: population and methodological differences. *Ophthalmic and Physiological Optics* **6**, 75–80.

Leat, S.J. (1996) Reduced accommodation in children with cerebral palsy. *Ophthalmic and Physiological Optics* **16**, 385–390.

Lueder, G.T. and Arnoldi, K. (1996) Does 'touching four' on the Worth 4-dot test indicate fusion in young children? A computer simulation. *Ophthalmology* **103**, 1237–1240.

Lyon, D.W., Goss, D.A., Horner, D. et al. (2005) Normative data for modified Thorington phorias and prism bar vergences from the Benton-IU study. *Optometry* **76**, 593–599.

McClelland, J.F., Saunders, K.J. (2003) The repeatability and validity of dynamic retinoscopy in assessing the accommodative response. *Ophthalmic and Physiological Optics* **23**, 243–250.

Mallett, R. (1988) Techniques of investigation of binocular vision anomalies. In: *Optometry* (eds K. Edwards and R. Llewellyn). London: Butterworths, pp. 238–269.

Manny, R.E., Martinez, A.T. and Fern, K.D. (1991) Testing stereopsis in the pre-school child: is it clinically useful? *Journal of Pediatric Ophthalmology and Strabismus* **28**, 223–231.

Maples, W.C. and Ficklin, T.W. (1988) Interrater and test-retest reliability of pursuits and saccades. *Journal of the American Optometric Association* **59**, 549–552.

Miller, J.M., Hall, H.L., Greivenkamp, J.E. et al. (1995) Quantification of the Bruckner test for strabismus. *Investigative Ophthalmology and Visual Science* **36**, 897–905.

Mohney, B.G. (2001) Common forms of childhood esotropia. *Ophthalmology* **108**, 805–809.

Mohney, B.G. and Huffaker, R.K. (2003) Common forms of childhood exotropia. *Ophthalmology* **111**, 2093–2096.

Mohney, B.G., Erie, J.C., Hodge, D.O. et al. (1998) Congenital esotropia in Olmsted County, Minnesota. *Ophthalmology* **105**, 846–850.

North, R.V. and Henson, D.B. (1981) Adaptation to prism induced heterophoria in subjects with abnormal binocular vision or asthenopia. *American Journal of Optometry and Physiological Optics* **58**, 746–752.

Pardhan, S. and Elliott, D.B. (1991) Clinical measurements of binocular summation and inhibition in patients with cataract. *Clinical Vision Science* **6**, 355–359.

Penisten, D.K., Hofstetter, H.W. and Goss, D.A. (2001) Reliability of rotary prism fusional vergence ranges. *Optometry* **72**, 117–122.

Pickwell, D. (1989) *Binocular vision anomalies*. Oxford: Butterworth-Heinemann.

Pickwell, L.D. and Hampshire, R. (1981) The significance of inadequate convergence. *Ophthalmic and Physiological Optics* **1**, 13–18.

Rainey, B.B., Schroeder, T.L., Goss, D.A. et al. (1998a) Reliability of and comparisons among three variations of the alternating cover test. *Ophthalmic and Physiological Optics* **18**, 430–437.

Rainey, B.B., Schroeder, T.L., Goss, D.A. et al. (1998b) Inter-examiner repeatability of heterophoria tests. *Optometry and Vision Science* **75**, 719–726.

Rosenfield, M. (1997) Accommodation. In: *The ocular examination: measurements and findings* (ed. K. Zadnik). Philadelphia: W.B. Saunders.

Rosenfield, M. and Cohen, A.S. (1996) Repeatability of clinical measurements of the amplitude of accommodation. *Ophthalmic and Physiological Optics* **16**, 247–249.

Rosenfield, M., Ciuffreda, K.J., Ong, E. et al. (1995) Vergence adaptation and the order of clinical vergence range testing. *Optometry and Vision Science* **72**, 219–223.

Rosenfield, M., Portello, J.K., Blustein, G.H. et al. (1996) Comparison of clinical techniques to assess the near accommodative response. *Optometry and Vision Science* **73**, 382–388.

Rosenfield, M., Rappon, J.M. and Carrel, M.F. (2000) Vergence adaptation and the clinical AC/A ratio. *Ophthalmic and Physiological Optics* **20**, 207–211.

Rouse, M.W., Borsting, E., Hyman, L. et al. (1999) Frequency of convergence insufficiency among fifth and sixth graders. The Convergence Insufficiency and Reading Study (CIRS) group. *Optometry and Vision Science* **76**, 643–649.

Rouse, M.W., Borsting, E. and Deland, P.N. (2002) Reliability of binocular vision measurements used in the classification of convergence insufficiency. *Optometry and Vision Science* **79**, 254–264.

Saladin, J.J. (2005) Stereopsis from a performance perspective. *Optometry and Vision Science* **82**, 186–205.

Saunders, K.J., Woodhouse, J.M. and Westall, C.A. (1996) The modified Frisby stereotest. *Journal of Pediatric Ophthalmology and Strabismus* **33**, 323–327.

Scheiman, M. and Wick, B. (2002) *Clinical management of binocular vision*, 2nd edn. Philadelphia: J.B. Lippincott.

Scheiman, M., Herzberg, H., Frantz, K. et al. (1988) Normative study of accommodative facility in elementary schoolchildren. *American Journal of Optometry and Physiological Optics* **65**, 127–134.

Schor, C.M. and Horner, D. (1989) Adaptive disorders of accommodation and vergence in binocular dysfunction. *Ophthalmic and Physiological Optics* **9**: 264–268.

Schor, C.M. and Narayan, V. (1982) Graphical analysis of prism adaptation, convergence accommodation, and accommodative convergence. *American Journal of Optometry and Physiological Optics* **59**, 774–784.

Sheedy, J.E. and Saladin, J.J. (1977) Phoria, vergence, and fixation disparity in oculomotor problems. *American Journal of Optometry and Physiological Optics* **52**, 474–481.

Sheedy, J.E. and Saladin, J.J. (1978) Association of symptoms with measures of oculomotor deficiencies. *American Journal of Optometry and Physiological Optics* **55**, 670–676.

Siderov, J., Chiu, S.C. and Waugh, S.J. (2001) Differences in the near point of convergence with target type. *Ophthalmic and Physiological Optics* **21**, 356–360.

Simons, K., Elhatton, K. (1994) Artifacts in fusion and stereoscopic testing based on red/green dichoptic image separation. *Journal of Pediatric Ophthalmology and Strabismus* **31**, 290–297.

Stidwell, D. (1997) Epidemiology of strabismus. *Ophthalmic and Physiological Optics* **17**, 536–539.

Thomson, W.D., Desai, N. and Russell-Eggitt, I. (1990) A new system for the measurement of ocular motility using a personal computer. *Ophthalmic and Physiological Optics* **10**, 137–143.

Vivian, A.J. and Morris, R.J. (1993) Diagrammatic representation of strabismus. *Eye* **7**, 565–571.

von Noorden, G.K. (2002) *Binocular vision and ocular motility: Theory and management of strabismus*. London: C.V. Mosby.

Walline, J.J., Mutti, D.O., Zadnik, K. et al. (1998) Development of phoria in children. *Optometry and Vision Science* **75**, 605–610.

Wick, B. and Hall, P. (1987) Relation among accommodative facility, lag and amplitude in elementary schoolchildren. *American Journal of Optometry and Physiological Optics* **64**, 593–598.

Wick, B., Yothers, T.L., Jiang, B.C. et al. (2002) Clinical testing of accommodative facility: Part 1. A critical appraisal of the literature. *Optometry* **73**, 11–23.

Woodhouse, J.M., Meades, J.S., Leat, S.J. et al. (1993) Reduced accommodation in children with Downs's syndrome. *Investigative Ophthalmology and Visual Science* **42**, 2382–2387.

Yekta, A.A., Pickwell, L.D. and Jenkins, T.C.A. (1989) Binocular vision, age and symptoms. *Ophthalmic and Physiological Optics* **9**, 115–120.

Yothers, T., Wick, B. and Morse, S.E. (2002) Clinical testing of accommodative facility: Part II. Development of an amplitude-scaled test. *Optometry* **73**, 91–102.

Zellers, J.A., Alpert, T.L. and Rouse, M.W. (1984) A review of the literature and a normative study of accommodative facility. *Journal of the American Optometric Association* **55**, 31–37.

6

OCULAR HEALTH ASSESSMENT

C. LISA PROKOPICH, PATRICIA HRYNCHAK AND DAVID B. ELLIOTT

6.1 RELEVANT CASE HISTORY INFORMATION

6.1.1 Symptoms

Blurred vision, asthenopia, headache and diplopia are most commonly caused by ametropia and decompensated heterophoria, but can be caused by diseases of the oculovisual system. In particular, symptoms of *sudden* vision loss suggest likely ocular disease rather than ametropia, although such symptoms can also be due to gradual monocular vision loss that was suddenly noticed. Gradual vision loss in elderly patients can often indicate age-related cataract and/or maculopathy. A myriad of other symptoms can also accompany diseases of the oculovisual system and these include ocular discomfort, itching, redness, tearing, discharge, pain, soreness, tenderness, haloes around lights, flashes, floaters, spots before the eyes, glare, photophobia, loss of peripheral vision, etc. It is also important to note that some diseases, such as primary open-angle glaucoma, are symptomless until the late stages.

6.1.2 Ocular history

A history of previous ocular disease and treatment can indicate what signs should be detected during your subsequent investigations (e.g. keratic precipitates after iritis, a lens implant and posterior capsular remnants after cataract surgery) and a detailed ocular history can save significant unecessary investigation. In addition, a history of certain recurring diseases, such as trichiasis, corneal erosion and blepharitis, can make subsequent diagnoses easier.

6.1.3 Family ocular and medical history

There are many eye diseases that are hereditary and a positive family history indicates that there is a greater chance that the patient will also have the particular hereditary condition. Common familial eye diseases include age-related cataract and both primary open-angle and closed-angle glaucoma and common familial systemic diseases include diabetes mellitus and hypertension.

6.1.4 General health and medications

Some systemic diseases, such as diabetes mellitus and hypertension, are well known to cause complications in the eye. In addition, some systemic medications can have adverse ocular effects and these should be investigated, particularly if the patient has been taking the medication for a long period and/or at high dose. For example, it is well known that beta-blockers prescribed for systemic hypertension can cause dry eyes and oral corticosteroids can cause posterior subcapsular cataracts.

6.2 RELEVANT VISUAL FUNCTION INFORMATION

Tests of visual function that are used in a standard eye examination such as visual acuity, or those that are occasionally used as screening tests, such as visual field or more rarely contrast sensitivity, may highlight possible ocular disease which must then be investigated. In some cases, the use of some tests of visual function is indicated after ocular disease is suspected or diagnosed. For example, the photo-stress recovery time test (section 3.8) is indicated when subtle maculopathies are suspected.

6.2.1 Visual acuity

Optimal visual acuity measurements (sections 3.2 and 3.3) that are different in the two eyes or are reduced compared to age-matched normal values indicate some ocular abnormality and must be explained. A pinhole visual acuity test should be used to make sure that the reduced visual acuity is not due to an incorrect determination of the refractive correction.

6.2.2 Visual fields

Visual field screening (sections 3.11–3.14) can be used to detect eye disease in patients without signs or symptoms. In addition, visual field analysis (section 3.15) can be used to help in the differential diagnosis and monitoring of eye disease.

6.2.3 Contrast sensitivity, glare testing and colour vision

Reductions in contrast sensitivity and colour vision and increases in disability glare can indicate ocular disease, even when visual acuity is normal. Both contrast sensitivity (section 3.10) and colour vision (sections 3.19–3.21) can be reduced in patients with optic neuritis and multiple sclerosis and in diabetics with little or no background retinopathy. Disability glare (section 3.9) can be significantly increased in patients with minimal capsular opacification and posterior subcapsular cataract.

6.3 RELEVANT BINOCULAR VISION INFORMATION

Recent-onset incomitant heterotropias can be the first sign of the underlying ocular or systemic disease including diabetes, hypertension, multiple sclerosis, thyrotoxicosis, and temporal arteritis and it is therefore essential to determine if the condition is of recent onset or long-standing. Missing the signs of these conditions, particularly in children, is a significant cause of malpractice claims in the US (Classé & Rutstein 1995). Signs and symptoms that can differentiate between new and old ocular muscle palsy are shown in Table 5.6 and incomitant heterotropias are discussed in section 5.24.

6.4 VARIATIONS IN APPEARANCE OF THE NORMAL EYE IN YOUNG ADULTS

The vast majority of patients examined in primary eye care have normal, healthy eyes. This section presents information about some of the subtle variations that occur in the normal eye and section 6.5 presents changes that commonly occur with normal ageing. To discriminate between ocular disease and the normal eye, it is essential to know the many presentations that a normal eye can make and a collection of photographs of these normal variations is presented in the book and on the website 🐾 to supplement the information provided in atlases of ocular disease. The text regarding variations in appearance of the normal eye provided on the website 🐾 is an updated version of that presented here. The variations in younger adult eyes are mainly caused by differences in ocular size and pigmentation and the occasional presence of embryological anomalies or remnants. Several of the photographs shown here, and others on the website, are courtesy of Dr. Konrad Pesudovs (Flinders University, Adelaide).

6.4.1 Eyelids

Epicanthus: Bilateral inner canthal nasal folds that are very common in oriental races and common in Caucasian infants, where they can make the child appear strabismic.

6.4.2 Cornea and conjunctivae

Pigment spots: Can be seen beneath the conjunctiva at the point of scleral canal emissaries, particularly arteries, in heavily pigmented eyes.

Palisades of Vogt: Limbal epithelial folds that run radially. They are more easily seen in heavily pigmented eyes.

Congenital conjunctival melanosis: Flat, pigmented areas of conjunctiva, typically near the limbus, seen in heavily pigmented eyes.

Concretions: Typically asymptomatic, small (1–3 mm), yellow-white calcium lesions found in the palpebral conjunctiva of the upper and lower eyelid (Haicl & Jankova 2006). They can be found in young adults, but are more common in elderly patients. The majority are superficial, hard and single (Haicl & Jankova 2006). About 6% of concretions can cause symptoms, likely due to corneal irritation.

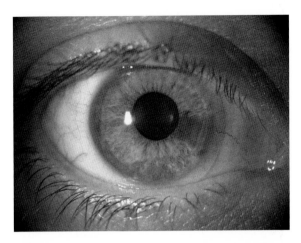

Fig. 6.1   A wedge-shaped section of hyperpigmentation (heterochromia). (Please see colour plate section)

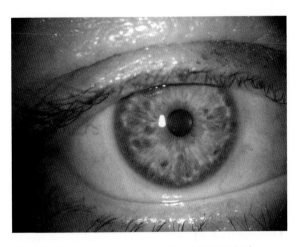

Fig. 6.2   Iris naevi. (Please see colour plate section)

Pinguecula: A degenerative thickening of the bulbar conjunctiva, particularly nasal. It is seen in younger adult patients exposed to UV, wind and dust, although it is very common in the elderly (Panchapakesan et al. 1998).

6.4.3 Iris

Pigment changes in the iris: Little or no pigment gives 'blue eyes'. With increasing amounts of pigment, the iris is seen as green, hazel or brown. Variations in pigment can produce wedge-shaped sections of hyper- or hypopigmentation (heterochromia, Fig. 6.1) in one or both eyes. Hyperpigmented spots (naevi or 'iris freckles', Fig. 6.2) are

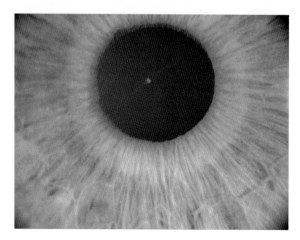

Fig. 6.3   Persistent pupillary membrane. (Please see colour plate section)

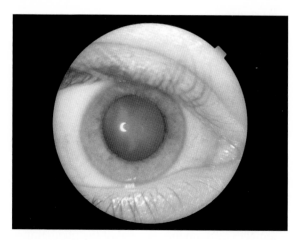

Fig. 6.4   A Mittendorf dot. (Please see colour plate section)

common, but should be monitored using photography for changes due to the slight risk of malignant melanoma.

Persistant pupillary membrane: Strands of the embryonic pupillary membrane that remain into adulthood. One end of the strand inserts into the iris colarette and the other is either attached to the anterior lens capsule or floats in the anterior chamber (Fig. 6.3).

6.4.4 Crystalline lens

Mittendorf dot: Seen as a small black dot in fundal retro-illumination (Fig. 6.4) and a white dot on the posterior capsular surface in direct illumination. It is a remnant of the attachment of the hyaloid canal to the posterior lens surface. The hyaloid artery runs from the ophthalmic artery at the optic disc to the crystalline lens where it spreads over the lens in a capillary net.

Zones of discontinuity: These zones are lens fibre layers of different refractive index in the continually growing lens cortex that lead to increased light scatter at the interfaces (Koretz et al. 1994; Fig. 6.5).

Y-sutures: The lens is formed by fibres that arch over the lens equator and join with other fibres to form branching suture lines which take on an upright 'Y' appearance anteriorly and an inverted 'Y' appearance posteriorly in the fetal lens (Fig. 6.5). As the lens continues to grow, the suture patterns

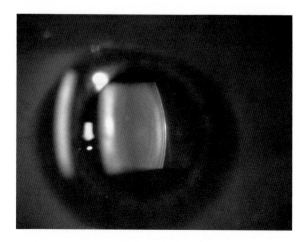

Fig. 6.5   Zones of discontinuity and a Y-suture in a posterior lens section. (Please see colour plate section)

become more complex (Kuszak et al. 1994) and more difficult to see.

6.4.5 Vitreous

Vitreous floaters: The vitreous of younger patients is typically clear, although the large eyes of young myopes are more likely to have vitreous floaters due to vitreous liquefaction. Vitreous floaters cast a shadow on the retina and are most obvious to the patient in bright light conditions and when the patient is looking at white walls, snow, etc. Patients typically report seeing black flecks floating in their vision.

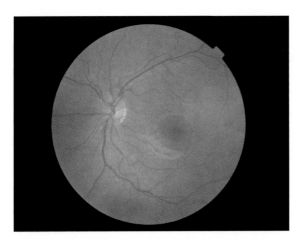

Fig. 6.6 Small optic disc with minimal cupping and a visible nerve fibre layer of a young emmetropic Caucasian patient. Some reflections can be seen in a broken ring outside the macular region. (Please see colour plate section)

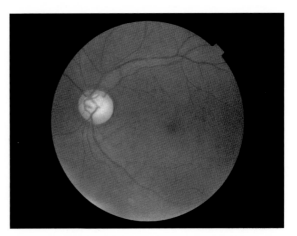

Fig. 6.8 Large optic disc and large cupping (CD ratio ≈0.60) and a visible nerve fibre layer of a young emmetropic Afro-Caribbean patient. The inferior edge of the photograph shows some light scatter from the edge of the undilated pupil. (Please see colour plate section)

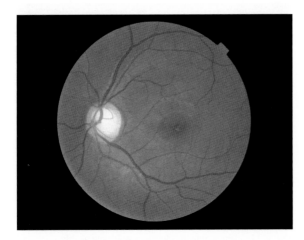

Fig. 6.7 Large optic disc and large cupping (CD ratio ≈ 0.60), a visible nerve fibre layer and macular pigmentation of a young, slightly myopic Asian patient. Some reflections can be seen in a broken ring outside the macular region and beside some of the main blood vessels. (Please see colour plate section)

6.4.6 Optic nerve head

Size and shape: The optic nerve head or disc comes in a variety of shapes and sizes (Figs 6.6 and 6.7). Discs have been shown to be smaller in Caucasians, and progressively larger in Mexicans, Asians and African North Americans (Jonas et al.

1999; Figs 6.6, 6.7 and 6.8). Disc size is larger in myopes beyond −8D and smaller in hyperopes greater than +4D (Jonas 2005). Oval discs are often found with corneal astigmatism and the direction of the longest optic disc diameter can indicate the axis of astigmatism (Jonas et al. 1997).

Optic cupping: The central proportion of the nerve head usually contains a depression called the 'cup'. This is often an area of pallor due to the absence of axons. However, in some cases the cup can extend beyond the area of pallor, so that this should not be used as an indicator of cup size during 2-D evaluations such as provided by direct ophthalmoscopy. The physiological cup-to-disc ratio is normally less than 0.60, but is relative to the size of the disc; that is, small cupping should be seen in a small-sized disc (Fig. 6.6) and large cupping is expected in large discs (Figs 6.7 and 6.8). For this reason, a medium cup in a small disc may be as indicative of glaucoma as a large cup in a medium-sized disc, highlighting the importance of assessing disc size. A large physiological cup (>0.6) can also be seen in highly myopic patients. Accurate measurement of the optic disc size is not required in a primary eye care exam, but some attempt should be made to categorise the disc as small, average or large. Note that the measured optic disc size will differ depending on the condensing lens and slit lamp used (Ansari-Shahrezaei et al. 2001). Note

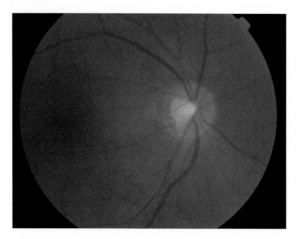

Fig. 6.9   Magnified view of a deep cup with visible lamina cribrosa (CD ratio ≈ 0.25), a choroidal crescent, visible nerve fibre layer and cilio-retinal artery of a young myopic Caucasian patient. (Please see colour plate section)

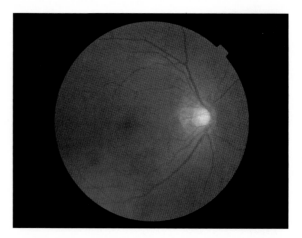

Fig. 6.10   Tilted disc with the nasal side raised and blood vessels nasally displaced. There is a temporal choroidal crescent, slightly tessellated fundus and visible nerve fibre layer. The fundus of the other eye was a mirror image of this one. (Please see colour plate section)

that the CD ratio is generally determined to be larger when the optic disc is examined stereoscopically with indirect ophthalmoscopy than when examined monocularly with direct ophthalmoscopy (Varma et al. 1992). The optic nerve head and cups of the two eyes are typically mirror images of each other and differential diagnosis of many optic nerve head anomalies is provided by an inter-eye comparison.

6.4.7 Other variations of the optic nerve head

Lamina cribrosa: Seen in about 30% of eyes as grey dots at the bottom of the optic cup (Healey & Mitchell 2004; Figs 6.9 and 6.13). It is a sieve-like connective and glial tissue that is continuous with the scleral canal. It is more visible in larger discs and larger cups (Healey & Mitchell 2004).

Nerve fibre layer striations: These are brightest at the superior and inferior poles, where the nerve fibre layer is thickest and are best seen in young patients, particularly those with heavily pigmented fundi (Figs 6.7 to 6.10).

Tilted discs: The tilt can be seen with the 3-D view of fundus biomicroscopy. With direct ophthalmoscopy it is seen as an oval disc whose edges cannot be focused at the same time. They are often

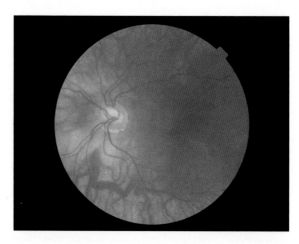

Fig. 6.11   Tilted disc syndrome and highly visible choroidal blood vessels in a young, highly myopic and astigmatic Caucasian patient. The disc is tilted inferior nasally with situs inversus. (Please see colour plate section)

caused by the optic nerve being inserted into the globe at a more acute angle and are then typically bilateral and elevated nasally, tilting downwards temporally and often have a temporal scleral and/or choroidal crescent (Fig. 6.10).

In the tilted disc syndrome, discs are more commonly tilted inferior nasally with a nasal staphyloma and *situs inversus*, where the temporal blood vessels first course towards the nasal retina before sharply changing course (Fig. 6.11). These are

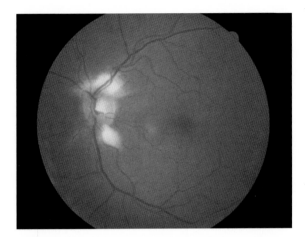

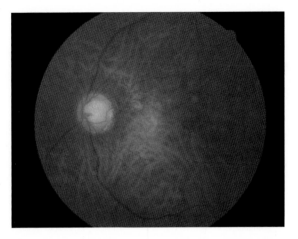

Fig. 6.12   Myelinated nerve fibres. There is a purplish reflection between the macula and disc and the inferior edge of the photograph shows some light scatter from the edge of the undilated pupil. (Please see colour plate section)

Fig. 6.13   A tigroid fundus with a large optic disc and cup (CD ≈ 0.55), visible lamina cribrosa and choroidal crescent in a young myopic patient. (Please see colour plate section)

thought to be caused by an incomplete closure of the embryonic fetal fissure, similar to the aetiology of a coloboma. The tilted disc syndrome is strongly associated with astigmatism and, to a lesser extent, high myopia.

Peripapillary atrophy (PPA):   PPA can be categorised into zones alpha and beta (Jonas & Budde 2000). Zone beta PPA is the central zone of atrophy, adjacent to the disc and is found in about 15% of normal eyes and is more common in glaucoma. The RPE and choriocapillaris are lost and all that is visible are the large choroidal vessels and sclera. Zone alpha is the outer zone of PPA with irregular hyper- and hypopigmented areas in the RPE, either on their own or surrounding zone beta PPA. It is very commonly seen in normal eyes. PPA is most commonly found at the temporal edge of the disc.

Myelinated nerve fibres: Found in up to 1% of patients and represents myelin sheathing of the optic nerve fibres that extends beyond the lamina cribrosa (Fig. 6.12) and presents a superficial, white, feathery opacification. Typically benign, although may cause visual field loss at threshold.

Drusen of the disc: A familial, typically bilateral condition, found in up to 1% of patients, which gets more obvious with age. In children, they may not be seen and the disc appears swollen. They are golden, autofluorescent, glowing, calcific globular deposits that sit in front of the lamina cribrosa.

Unfortunately, they are not benign and can shear blood vessels and/or nerve fibres, leading to haemorrhages and progressive visual field loss.

6.4.8 Fundus pigmentation

Fundus colour: The colour of the fundus is determined by the choroidal blood supply and the amount of pigmentation in the choroid and overlying retinal pigment epithelium (RPE). Fundus pigmentation typically mimics skin pigmentation. Compare the Asian and Afro-Caribbean fundi in Figures 6.7 and 6.8 to the Caucasian fundus in Figure 6.6. With a lightly pigmented or thin RPE, the choroidal vessels and choroidal pigmentation can be seen (Figs 6.11 and 6.13).

Macula: The macula lutea area contains a yellow-brown pigment, although the amount is highly variable between individuals, and is most obvious in highly pigmented eyes (Figs 6.7, 6.12 and 6.14). A bright reflex may be seen at the foveola in younger patients, as the ophthalmoscope light is reflected back from the foveal pit.

Tesselated or tigroid fundus: A thin RPE allows the red choroidal vessels and heavily pigmented choroid to be seen and can give a tiger stripe appearance (Figs 6.10 and 6.13). It is more commonly seen with the thin retina of myopic patients (Tekiele & Semes 2002).

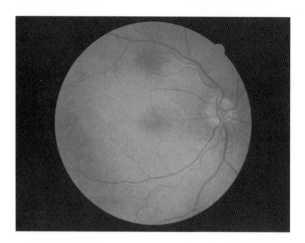

Fig. 6.14   A choroidal naevus, ≈ 1 DD in size, about 3 DD from the disc between 10 and 11 o'clock. The disc is small and flat. (Please see colour plate section)

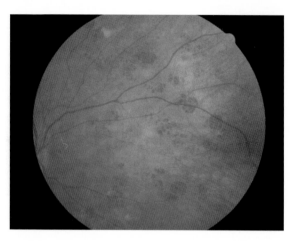

Fig. 6.15   Bear tracks in the peripheral retina. (Please see colour plate section)

Choroidal naevus: A commonly found localised area of choroidal pigmentation, also known as a benign choroidal melanoma. They have a prevalence up to 30%, although they can be easily missed with the direct ophthalmoscope and its limited field of view. They appear grey as your view of a choroidal naevus is filtered through the RPE and sensory retina (Fig. 6.14). Naevi can be flat or raised, with drusen often appearing on the surface with age. They vary in size, although the vast majority are less than 2 disc diameters. A choroidal naevus larger than 5 DD may be malignant and should be referred for further investigation. All naevi should be routinely monitored, preferably using photography, as they can rarely transform into a malignant melanoma. They can be described to patients as a freckle on the back of their eye.

RPE window defect: A fairly common, benign, yellow-white, well-circumcribed dot or circle in the fundus caused by the absence of melanin in the RPE in a localised area. It is typically not associated with surrounding RPE hyperplasia as would be seen with a chorioretinitis. It is easily differentiated from the red-brown retinal hole, which often has a surrounding cuff of retinal oedema or RPE hyperplasia. RPE window defects can enlarge with age, but this is of no concern.

Congenital hypertrophy of the retinal pigment epithelium (CHRPE): These patches of pigment are typically darker than naevi with sharply defined edges, often with a depigmented halo just inside the border. The latter are sometimes called halo naevi. They can be large and isolated or small and grouped together, when they are known as 'bear tracks' (Fig. 6.15). With age, the central pigment can be lost (sun burst effect). CHRPEs can be a marker for familial adenomatous polyposis (FAP), a hereditary bowel disorder which can commonly progress to colon cancer, so that the patient's general physician should be informed of their presence (e.g. Iwama et al. 1990).

6.4.9 Retinal blood vessels

Arteries versus veins: The retinal veins are typically dark red-purple and the retinal arteries are about two-thirds the thickness and a brighter red, with a slight reflex along the centre of the vessel. The arterioles and venules should have a smooth course and cross at oblique angles without nipping or compressing the venule.

Venous pulsation: Present in most adult eyes and most obvious at the point of entry of the central retinal vein into the optic nerve.

Cilio-retinal artery: Found in about 15–20% of normal eyes as an artery that hooks out of the temporal edge of the disc and runs towards the macula (Fig. 6.9). Its shape gives it the nickname of the 'shepherd's crook'. It is derived from the short posterior ciliary system or choriocapillaris rather than

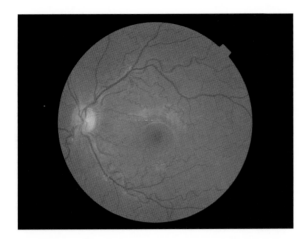

Fig. 6.16 Very tortuous retinal arteries and visible macular pigment in a young Caucasian patient. Some reflections can be seen in a broken ring outside the macular region, just above the ring and beside some of the blood vessels. (Please see colour plate section)

the central retinal artery and it becomes most relevant after a central retinal artery occlusion, when it saves the retina around its distribution. Of course, the cilio-retinal artery can itself become occluded.

Congenital vascular tortuosity: Most commonly bilateral and involving both arteries and veins and all quadrants (Fig. 6.16). Acquired tortuosity, particularly of veins, is less common than the congenital condition, but should be considered as it is connected with a variety of ocular and systemic diseases. For this reason, eyes with very tortuous vessels should ideally be photographed and monitored.

6.4.10 Peripheral fundus

The posterior pole is bordered by the superior and inferior temporal vascular arcades and includes the macula and optic nerve head. The midperiphery extends anteriorly from the vascular arcades to the equator, which is defined by the posterior border of the vortex vein ampullae. The periphery extends anteriorly from the equator to the ora serrata, which is 4 to 5 DD beyond the equator, at the termination of the choroid and retina.

Vortex vein ampullae: The ampullae are the dilated sacs of the vortex veins, which receive blood from the tributaries of the vortex system, and are red-orange octopus- or spider-shaped, often surrounded by pigment. The ampullae are found at the equator, with at least one per quadrant, typically in the four oblique meridians, and up to 10 in each eye. They are most easily seen in a lightly pigmented eye.

Ciliary nerves and arteries: Two long posterior ciliary nerves bisect the superior and inferior fundus at the 3 and 9 o'clock positions in the fundus periphery and 10–20 short posterior ciliary nerves can be seen away from the horizontal meridian. They appear as faint, yellow-white short lines, often with pigmented borders. The long posterior ciliary arteries run below the corresponding ciliary nerve in the temporal retina and above it in the nasal retina. The short posterior ciliary arteries may have pigmented margins.

Peripheral cystoid degeneration: The most prevalent of the benign peripheral retinal conditions whose extent increases with age. The cystoid area appears as a hazy grey area of thickened retina near to the ora serrata that can extend to the equator. Red dots may appear with the cystoid degeneration and strands in the vitreous may appear above it.

Paving stone degeneration: This primary chorioretinal atrophy, with depigmented areas surrounded by RPE hyperplasia, is found in about 25% of patients over 20. If the lesions coalesce, the underlying choroidal vessels may be seen. It is often bilateral with about 75% of lesions being found in the inferior nasal quadrant. It is thought to be caused by occlusion of some of the peripheral choriocapillaris vessels.

6.4.11 Myopic eyes

The majority of myopia is due to an increased axial length and myopic eyes are big eyes. Pathological myopia is well recognised, but non-pathological myopic eyes also show typical changes.

Anterior angle: The anterior angle is typically deeper in myopes.

Vitreous floaters: The vitreous is more liquefied and degenerative the higher the myopia. This means that there is a higher prevalence of vitreous floaters and a greater likelihood of posterior vitreous detachment at an earlier age.

Myopic crescents: If the RPE is pulled away from the disc in long myopic eyes, a crescent-shaped section of the choroid (choroidal blood vessels and pigment) can be seen (Fig. 6.13). If both the RPE and choroid are pulled away from the disc, a white scleral crescent can be seen. These crescents are typically seen along the temporal edge (Tekiele & Semes 2002).

Optic nerve head: The optic disc is typically larger in high myopia (greater than −8 D; Jonas 2005) often with a larger cup-to-disc ratio (Fig. 6.13).

Peripheral retina: The retina of the large myopic eye is relatively thin. This leads to a greater prevalence of tessellated fundi (Fig. 6.13), visible choroidal vessels (Fig. 6.11) and lattice degeneration (Tekiele & Semes 2002).

6.5 VARIATIONS IN APPEARANCE OF THE NORMAL ELDERLY EYE

Although the research literature provides ample information about the prevalence of eye disease in the elderly, there is little information regarding the prevalence of benign changes. To discriminate between ocular disease and the normal eye, it is essential to know the many presentations that a normal eye can make and a collection of photographs of these normal variations is presented in the book and on the website 🖱 to supplement the information provided in atlases of ocular disease. The text regarding variations in appearance of the normal eye provided on the website 🖱 is an updated version of that presented here.

6.5.1 Eyelids

There is progressive loss of tone and bulk of the eyelids with age, leading to decreased lid tension (this is probably why with-the-rule astigmatism disappears with age), dermatochalasis, ectropion and ptosis.

Dermatochalasis: Benign, bilateral drooping of upper lid tissue over the septum or lid margin with age (Fig. 6.17). Cosmetic surgery is sometimes requested.

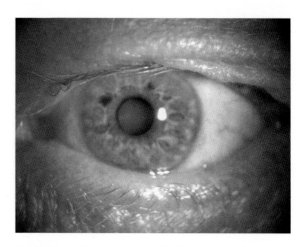

Fig. 6.17   Early dermatochalasis. (Please see colour plate section)

Ectropion: A common complaint, especially in the oldest elderly patients (over 80; Mitchell et al. 2001). The eyelid is often turned outward due to loose lids so that the inferior lid margin or puncta are not in contact with the eye. The patient may complain of epiphora or be symptomless.

Papilloma: The most common benign lesion of the eyelid and often known as a 'skin tag'. They are avascular, epithelial lesions of variable size, shape and colour (amelanotic to black) with a roughened surface reflecting the redundant epithelial cell growth (Fig. 6.24). Over time, they grow and become attached to the eyelid surface by a stalk (pedunculated), so that the papilloma can be moved back and forth. Commonly found on the eyelids of elderly patients and with little change in size once it has developed. You should reassure the patient and monitor the lesion, ideally using photography (Kersten et al. 1997). Papillomas can be removed for cosmetic reasons.

Sebaceous cysts: Common, benign, yellowish, 'cheesy' cyst of variable size (typically 2–5 mm). Superficial cysts are covered by a thin layer of epithelial cells. Multiple small sebaceous cysts are often called milia. Subcutaneous or deep sebaceous cysts are larger (variable, but up to 20 mm) and slightly movable and covered by normal skin. They are caused by blockages to the sebaceous glands, with the blocked pore subsequently becoming filled with the oily sebum (Fig. 6.18). You should reassure the patient and photograph the cyst, which can be removed for cosmetic reasons.

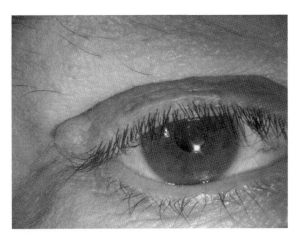

Fig. 6.18 Subcutaneous sebaceous cyst. (Please see colour plate section)

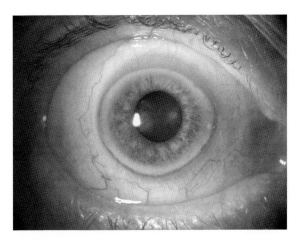

Fig. 6.20 Complete corneal arcus and cortical cataract viewed in direct diffuse illumination. The patient was able to maintain an unusually large palpebral aperture for the photograph. (Please see colour plate section)

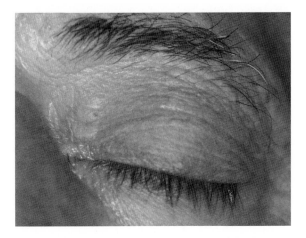

Fig. 6.19 Xanthelasma. (Please see colour plate section)

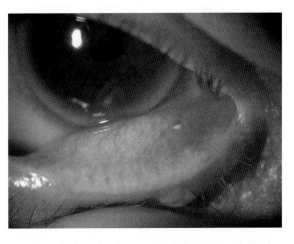

Fig. 6.21 Solitary hard concretion in the lower palpebral conjunctiva. (Please see colour plate section)

Xanthelasma: Bilateral, light brown-yellow, flat triangular lipid masses with a nasal base, typically found on the inner eyelids of elderly patients and especially females (Fig. 6.19). They usually have a familial aetiology, but can be linked with atherosclerosis and high cholesterol and this should be investigated. They often recur if removed, so the patient should be warned of this if considering cosmetic removal.

6.5.2 Cornea and conjunctivae

Corneal sensitivity reduces with age and there are corneal endothelial changes of decreased cell density and increased polymegathism and pleomorphism. Although there appears to be no loss of tear voume with age, the tear film is less stable. In addition, several drugs tend to reduce tear production and many are increasingly used with age. Other common corneal and conjunctival changes include:

Corneal arcus (arcus senilis): A commonly found greyish-white ring or part ring occurring in the periphery of corneas of older patients that is separated from the limbus by a thin ring of clear cornea (Figs 6.20 and 6.21). It is caused by lipid deposits in the corneal stroma.

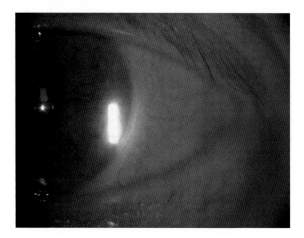

Fig. 6.22   Limbal girdle of Vogt seen in indirect illumination. (Please see colour plate section)

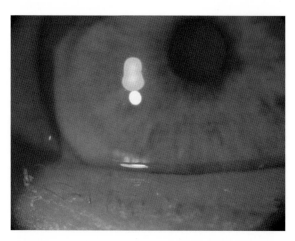

Fig. 6.23   A Hudson–Stähli line. (Please see colour plate section)

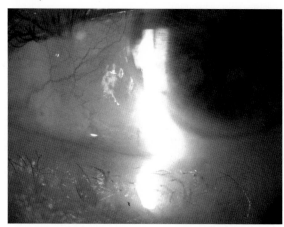

Fig. 6.24   A pinguecula seen to the left of the slit-beam in indirect illumination. A small papilloma is also visible on the lower lid. (Please see colour plate section)

Concretions: Typically asymptomatic, small (1–3 mm), yellow-white calcium lesions found in the palpebral conjunctiva of the upper and lower eyelid (Haicl & Jankova 2006). They can be found in young adults, but are more common in elderly patients. The majority are superficial, hard and single (Haicl & Jankova 2006; Fig. 6.21). About 6% of concretions can cause symptoms, probably due to corneal irritation.

Limbal girdle of Vogt: Common, bilateral degenerative condition producing a narrow band of white, crystal-like opacities along the nasal or temporal limbus, typically found in elderly female eyes (Fig. 6.22).

Hudson–Stähli line: Common, orange-brown iron deposition line found where the lid margins meet when blinking (Fig. 6.23). The line can be continuous or segmented and the prevalence typically matches the age of the patient, with 50% at age 50, 75% at age 75, etc. Many Hudson–Stähli lines are faint and are best seen with cobalt blue or ultra-violet light.

Pinguecula: A degenerative thickening of the bulbar conjunctiva, particularly nasal (Fig. 6.24). Although it is seen in younger adult patients exposed to UV, wind and dust, it is very common in the elderly (Panchapakesan et al. 1998). They can lift the lids away from the surrounding conjunctiva, leading to a local area of drying and hyperaemia.

6.5.3 Iris

Iris: The crypts disappear, especially near the pupil and the pupillary ruff appears eroded.

Pupil: As novice retinoscopists and ophthalmoscopists will readily confirm, the pupil gets smaller with age.

6.5.4 Crystalline lens

The lens continues to grow and thicken with age, leading to a gradual reduction in the anterior

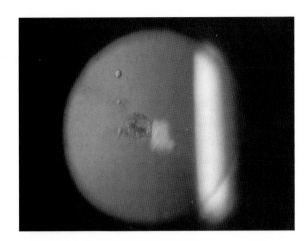

Fig. 6.25   A small posterior subcapsular cataract and several vacuoles seen in fundal retro-illumination. (Please see colour plate section)

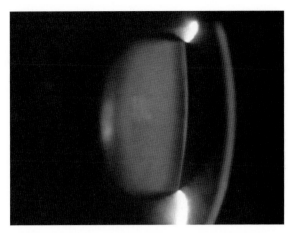

Fig. 6.26   Nuclear cataract seen by optical section. The blurred blue arc to the right is the out-of-focus cornea. (Please see colour plate section)

chamber. There is increased light scatter due to an increased number of cortical layers and the production of large aggregates in the lens nucleus. Chromophores that absorb blue wavelength light also increase with age, leading to increased lens yellowing. In addition, the prevalence of cataract increases substantially, with cataract causing a visual acuity of worse than 6/9 rising from approximately 5% in the 55–64 age group to over 40% in the over 75s (Klein et al. 1992). There are three main types of age-related cataract: cortical, nuclear and posterior subcapsular and around 30% of eyes have mixed cataract, i.e. more than one morphological type. Posterior subcapsular (PSC) cataracts are most worthy of note as they can hide behind the Purkinje images (cornea and lens reflexes) and be missed. Clinicians have been successfully sued for missing PSC cataracts in patients with no symptoms at the time of the eye examination but who subsequently had holidays ruined due to poor vision in a brighter, sunnier climate. If you have any suspicion of a PSC cataract, the patient's pupils must be dilated to allow a better view of the posterior lens.

Posterior subcapsular (PSC) cataract: Posterior subcapsular (PSC) cataract presents at the back of the lens just in front of the posterior capsule (Fig. 6.25). In the age-related vacuolar type of PSC cataract, localised reductions in refractive index and vacuoles are found in the early stages. Later, there is a posterior migration of epithelial cells from the lens equator. These converge onto the posterior pole,

forming the balloon or bladder cells of Wedl, and produce a new basement membrane (Eshagian 1982). Large particle scattering is increased by the many organelles in the epithelial cells and the new membrane. PSC cataracts can cause a dramatic reduction in vision because they are generally centrally positioned within the pupillary area. These opacities can also present earlier than the other morphological types, at about age 55 years. PSC cataracts can be associated with other ocular and systemic disease, such as retinitis pigmentosa and diabetes (Eshagian 1982) and are found as a side effect of systemic drugs such as oral corticosteroids.

Nuclear cataracts: These present as a homogenous increase in light scatter in the lens nucleus and can be associated with an increased yellowing or brunescence, which is indicative of blue wavelength-dependent light absorption (Fig. 6.26). These changes also occur to a lesser degree with normal ageing. Nuclear cataracts can produce a marked myopic shift, which is known as index myopia.

Cortical cataract: These are cuneiform or wedge-shaped opacities found in the anterior and/or posterior lens cortex and often hidden behind the iris (Fig. 6.27). Cortical cataracts are most often found in the inferionasal part of the lens, which may reflect ultra-violet radiation involvement in their aetiology. They are often associated with water clefts, which are optically clear wedges that can be

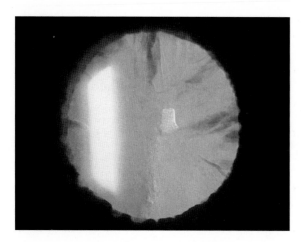

Fig. 6.27   Cortical cataract seen in fundal retro-illumination. (Please see colour plate section)

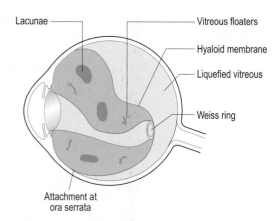

Fig. 6.29   The changes to the vitreous that occur with age.

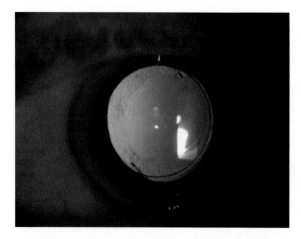

Fig. 6.28   An intraocular implant with peripheral posterior capsular remnants in a dilated pupil seen in fundal retro-illumination. (Please see colour plate section)

seen with slit-lamp biomicroscopy. Opacification is due to the scattering of light when it meets irregular interfaces between regions of different refractive index. Vision is only affected if the cortical spokes enter the pupillary area. Cortical cataracts can cause significant astigmatic changes.

Intraocular lenses and posterior capsular remnants: Given the very high prevalence of cataract surgery in the developed world, primary eye care clinicians will often examine a pseudophakic patient with an intraocular lens and some posterior capsular remnants (Fig. 6.28). If these remnants

encroach on the pupillary area and cause visual problems, referral for YAG laser capsulotomy should be suggested.

6.5.5 Vitreous

With ageing, liquefaction and syneresis (shrinkage) occur and this leads to an increase in vitreous floaters and posterior vitreous detachment (PVD).

Vitreous floaters: Vitreous floaters cast a shadow on the retina and are most obvious to the patient in bright light conditions and when the patient is looking at white walls, snow, etc. Patients typically report seeing black flecks floating in their vision. Some patients mistake them for flies or spiders moving out of the corner of their eye and are very relieved when these symptoms are explained.

Posterior vitreous detachments: PVDs are common after the age of 50, with the prevalence being similar to the patient's age, with even greater prevalence after cataract surgery. PVDs from the retina can be complete or incomplete and with or without collapse of the vitreous gel, with the most common being a complete detachment from the sensory retina with collapse of the gel (Fig. 6.29). Symptoms are classically a sudden onset of flashes of light, due to tugging on the vitreo-retinal adhesion, and floaters. If the vitreous detaches from the optic nerve head, it can be seen as a ring-like vitreous floater or Weiss ring (Fig. 6.30). The flashes of light are commonly reported as lightning streaks in

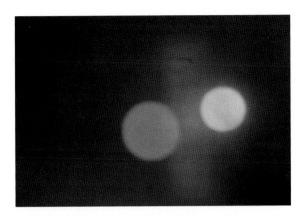

Fig. 6.30   A Weiss ring photographed using fundus biomicroscopy. (Please see colour plate section)

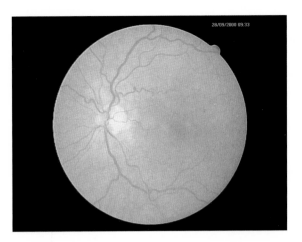

Fig. 6.31   Venous nipping of the inferior temporal vein, several 90 degree crossings, drusen temporal to the disc and some pigmentary changes at the macula. The contrast of the fundus view is slightly reduced, probably due to light scatter from early cataract. (Please see colour plate section)

peripheral vision. Retinal tears are associated with about 8% of cases of symptomatic PVD and must be investigated. They typically lead to symptoms of a shower of small floaters and signs of pigment granules (from the RPE) in the anterior vitreous (Shafer's sign), vitreous haemorrhage and the tear itself.

6.5.6 Fundus and macula

Naevus: Drusen often appear on the naevus surface with age.

Congenital hypertrophy of the retinal pigment epithelium (CHRPE):   With age, the central pigment can be lost (sun burst effect).

Macular pigmentary changes: Pigmentary changes occur at the macula with age, with increased disorganisation of the RPE and areas of depigmentation and pigment clumping (Figs 6.31–6.33). These changes need not cause losses of visual function, but can progress to early age-related maculopathy.

Drusen: Small, circular yellow or yellow-white dots, commonly seen around the macula (Figs 6.32 and 6.33), disc (Fig. 6.31) and more peripherally (Fig. 6.31). They consist of deposits lying between Bruch's membrane and the basement membrane of the retinal pigment epithelium. Drusen can be hard (smaller with sharp edges) or soft (larger with indistinct edges). The soft drusen are more of a

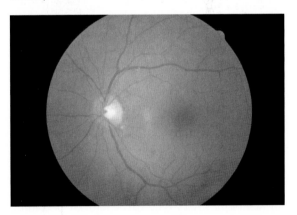

Fig. 6.32   Zone beta PPA, several 90 degree crossings and drusen in the macular area. Some choroidal vessels are visible. (Please see colour plate section)

concern as they indicate a compromised RPE that may lead to the development of dry or wet age-related maculopathy.

6.5.7 Retinal blood vessels

Changes to the retinal blood vessels can occur with normal ageing or can indicate early signs of hypertensive retinopathy (Hurcomb et al. 2001). The more significant the changes at an early age, the

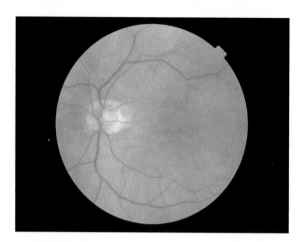

Fig. 6.33 Venous nipping of both temporal veins, several 90 degree crossings and drusen at the macula. There are two reflections, one between the macula and disc and one above the disc, and the edge of the photograph shows some light scatter from the edge of the undilated pupil. (Please see colour plate section)

more likely the changes are early hypertensive changes.

Age-related blood vessel changes: Arteriolar narrowing and hardening of the arteries occurs with increasing age and can cause a slight broadening of the reflex on the arterioles (Fig. 6.33).

Artery–vein crossing changes: Arteriosclerotic changes can lead to changes to the veins at artery–vein crossings, with 90-degree crossings (Figs 6.31–6.33) and nipping of the vein on the distal side of the artery (Figs 6.31 and 6.33), becoming increasingly common. The change to 90-degree crossings can give the veins a more tortuous appearance (Fig. 6.31).

6.5.8 Peripheral fundus

Peripheral pigmentary or tapetochoroidal degeneration: A granular pigment appearance between the equator and ora serrata that occurs in about 20% of patients after the age of 40 and becoming more prominent with age. It often has a honeycomb appearance and is associated with peripheral drusen. If the pigment takes on a reticular or bone spicule appearance, differential diagnosis with retinitis pigmentosa is required. It is a

degnerative condition of the RPE, possibly associated with vascular compromise.

Paving stone degeneration: This primary chorioretinal atrophy, with depigmented areas surrounded by RPE hyperplasia, is found in about 25% of patients over 20 but increases with age.

6.6 SLIT-LAMP BIOMICROSCOPY EXAMINATION

A slit-lamp biomicroscope consists of a compound binocular microscope and an illumination system, which are typically linked on a common pivot so that the illumination and viewing systems are focused in the same plane. The instrument was developed by Professor Allvar Gullstrand (1862–1930), who received the Nobel Prize in Medicine/Physiology for his work in geometrical optics in 1911.

6.6.1 Examination of the anterior segment and ocular adnexa

The purpose of this examination is to detect abnormalities or anomalies of the anterior segment of the eye and adnexa including the eyelids, eyelashes, conjunctiva, tear layer, cornea, anterior chamber, iris, crystalline lens and anterior vitreous. This procedure should be performed routinely during all full oculovisual assessments, during all contact lens assessments and during problem-specific assessments involving the anterior segment or adnexa. It should also be performed before and after any procedure that touches the eye such as tonometry and gonioscopy to determine the presence and severity of any iatrogenic damage. A slit-lamp is also required as part of the examination of the internal structures of the eye with fundus biomicroscopy and gonioscopy.

6.6.2 Advantages and disadvantages

Slit-lamp biomicroscopy examination is greatly preferred over direct ophthalmoscopy, penlight and loupe or Burton lamp assessment as it provides much greater resolution, depth of field and control of illumination, as well as higher illumination and

Table 6.1 Filters available on most slit-lamp biomicroscopes.

Filter	Typical symbol	Use
Cobalt blue	Blue filled circle	Enhances the view of fluorescein dye in the tear film of the eye. Typically used for fluorescein staining and Goldmann tonometry.
Red free	Green filled circle	Used to enhance the view of blood vessels and haemorrhages
Neutral density	Circle with hashed lines	Decreases maximum brightness for photosensitive patients
Heat absorbing	Built into most slit-lamps	Decreases patient discomfort
Grey	Circle with thick line	Decreases maximum brightness for photosensitive patients
Yellow filter	Yellow filled circle Located in the observation system	For good contrast enhancement when using fluorescein and the cobalt blue filter
Diffuser	May be a flip-up filter placed on the illumination source	Used for general overall observations of the eye and adnexa

more variable and greater magnification (from about 10× to 40×). Involuntary eye movements limit the clarity of highly magnified images and therefore limit the value of increasing the magnification beyond 40×. The quality of the image can be limited by the slit-lamp model that you have available. The more basic slit-lamp models typically have less resolution and/or depth of field, a smaller range of magnification and illumination and may not allow decoupling of the illumination and viewing systems. Resolution is improved in higher-level models by maximising the optical quality of the lenses, using multi-aspheric lens designs and using anti-reflection coatings. Disadvantages include that slit-lamp examination can produce discomfort in some photophobic patients due to the high illumination.

6.6.3 Procedure

Familiarity with the adjustment controls of the slit-lamp is required. The positions of the controls differ for different models but all slit-lamps have similar features. It should be possible to change the width and height of the beam, rotate the beam, change the angle between the light source and the viewing system, add filters over the light source (Table 6.1), change the magnification (this may involve changing the eyepieces to a stronger power), change the intensity of the illumination, adjust the height of the microscope and focus the microscope with the joystick. With most instruments it is possible to break the linkage between the illumination and viewing systems (decoupling), which allows focus on a point other than that being illuminated.

Brands of slit-lamps differ in their illumination and their observation systems. The Haag–Streit-type slit-lamps have a tower illumination system with the bulb above a mirror. This system has the advantage of being able to be decoupled in the vertical meridian, which is helpful when the slit-lamp is used for gonioscopy or fundus examination. Magnification is provided in one of three ways, a flip magnification system (the most basic with magnification typically provided at 10× and 16×), a rotating barrel or zoom continuous magnification. The range of powers for the latter are often from 10 to 40×. Slit-lamps also differ in the degree of convergence of the microscope. An optimal convergence of 10–15 degrees will provide greater binocular overlap of the images and less eyestrain.

1. If one is available, place the focusing rod in the appropriate holder, with the flat surface towards the viewing system. Normally, you will perform biomicroscope examination

without spectacles, as the field of view is greater the closer your eyes are to the slit-lamp eyepieces. If you have a high cylinder in your spectacle correction, you may need to wear your correction to obtain adequate resolution. To focus the eyepieces, first switch on the illumination system to produce a slit-image on the focusing rod. Look through one eyepiece and turn it fully counterclockwise (plus direction) then, while viewing the focusing rod, turn the eyepiece clockwise until the slit-image on the rod is first in sharp focus. Repeat the procedure for the other eyepiece. The eyepiece should be set at approximately zero if you are an emmetrope or wearing your correction and set to your mean sphere if you are uncorrected. More minus might be required in younger practitioners due to proximal accommodation. Once you have each eyepiece focused, adjust the distance between the eyepieces so that the image is centred in the field of view of each eye. You should see a single clear image.

2. Seat the patient comfortably on a stable chair without rollers, and ask the patient to remove any spectacles. Explain the procedure in lay terms to your patient: 'I am going to use this special microscope to carefully examine the front of your eyes.'

3. Adjust the height of the biomicroscope table so that the patient may lean forward comfortably and place their chin in the chin rest and forehead against the forehead rest. Adjust the chin rest so that the patient's eyes are at an appropriate height to provide a large enough vertical range to allow adequate examination of the adnexa. Many biomicroscopes have an eye alignment marker on a supporting beam of the headrest that should be level with the patient's outer canthus. If the patient is obese, an exaggerated bend at their waist will often allow satisfactory positioning.

4. Dim the room lights and ask the patient to look at your ear (your right ear for the patient's right eye and your left ear for the patient's left eye) or the instrument's fixation device so that the patient's gaze is in the primary position.

5. Use one hand to control the joystick (focusing and lateral/vertical movement) and the other to control the magnification and illumination and to manipulate the patient's eyelids.

6. There are several types of illumination that can be used alternately or in combination to thoroughly examine the anterior segment and adnexa. A general procedure for an anterior segment examination is to use direct illumination and a parallelepiped and/or diffuse illumination and is described below. This is followed by descriptions of additional techniques with examples of when they might be used. Students should practise these techniques regularly at first and subsequently use them when the patient's signs and symptoms dictate.

6. **Diffuse illumination:** Provides an overall assessment of the anterior segment and immediate adnexa under low magnification ($\approx$10$\times$, Figs 6.1, 6.2, 6.17–6.20). Adjust the illumination to a wide beam and place a diffusing filter in front of it. Examine the components of the anterior segment and adnexa in a systematic fashion as described below.

7. **Direct illumination using a parallelepiped:** Use low to moderate magnification ($\approx$10 $\times$) as magnification that is too high will result in missing obvious, moderately sized abnormalities. Set the illumination system at approximately 45° from the microscope position on the temporal side and use a beam width of approximately 2 mm. An illuminated block of corneal tissue in the shape of a parallelogram should be visible (Fig. 6.34). A beam that is too narrow will make it difficult to detect abnormalities. Assess each of the structures described below in a systematic manner using the following procedure: Focus on the temporal tissue first with the illumination coming from the temporal side. Move the slit-lamp laterally across the tissue until the centre is reached, maintaining good focus at all times. Then sweep the illumination system across to the nasal side, taking care not to bump into the patient's nose, and examine the nasal tissue. This scanning procedure may

(a)

(b)

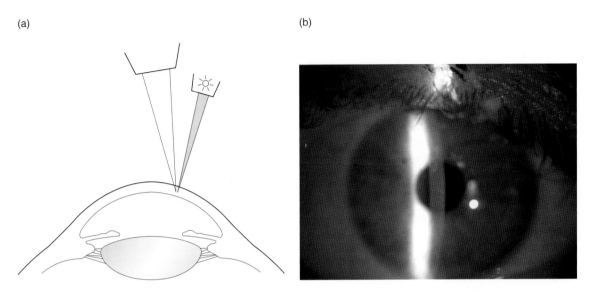

Fig. 6.34a   Diagram illustrating the position of the illuminating and viewing systems when using direct illumination.
Fig. 6.34b   A parallelepiped section of the cornea showing an old abrasion above the corneal apex.

be repeated several times to examine all areas of the tissue concerned.

a) Eyelids and lashes: Examine the superior temporal eyelid and lashes first using the scanning procedure described above. This can be easier with the patient's eyes closed. Examine the inferior lid and lashes in the same manner, while also examining lid apposition to the eye and meibomian gland appearance (see sections 6.7 and 6.8 for dry eye tests). Assess the lid for anomalies/abnormalities including an abnormal lid position (e.g. ptosis, entropion, ectropion), redness, inflammation, ulcers and growths. Inspect the lashes for colour (e.g. white), areas where the lashes are missing or misdirected and the presence of scales.

b) Conjunctivae: Ask the patient to look upwards while you pull the lower eyelid gently downward to expose the lower fornix for examination. Examine both the bulbar and palpebral conjunctiva using the scanning process described above. Next ask the patient to look downwards and gently pull up the upper eyelid, thereby exposing the superior bulbar conjunctiva for examination. Finally, ask the patient to look in right and then left gaze to allow examination of the entire conjunctiva and the caruncle.

c) Cornea and tear film: Use the scanning process described above to examine the cornea in three sweeps: inferior, central and superior. Examine the inferior cornea by having the patient look up and the superior cornea by having the patient look down and holding up the upper eyelid. With increasing experience you will be able to look at both the area illuminated (direct illumination, Fig. 6.34) and the area just outside the area of illumination (indirect illumination, Figs 6.22 and 6.35). It can be useful to assess the tear film after a blink. You can increase the width of the section of stroma seen by increasing the angle between the microscope and illumination system. You can obtain greater detail by increasing the magnification.

d) Assessment of the tear meniscus: The height of the tear meniscus can be determined by decreasing the height of the slit-lamp beam to one millimetre and then judging the relative height of the meniscus at the lower lid margin as a proportion of the beam height.

e) Iris: Examine the iris by moving the joystick towards the patient. The iris should come into focus. Use the scanning process described above to examine the iris with direct illumination. Take note of the depth of the anterior chamber.

f) Lens: To examine the lens properly the pupil must be dilated. Once dilated the lens can be examined in direct illumination with a parallelepiped or an optic section. For a non-dilated pupil the illumination

angle must be reduced until an optical section of the lens is just seen. This may be as small as 15° for an elderly patient with a small pupil. Sweeps of both the anterior lens (Fig. 6.26) and posterior lens (Fig. 6.5) should be made. Direct illumination is less useful for cortical cataracts as it can show large amounts of light scatter due to backward light scatter and reflections that do not cause vision loss. Retroillumination from the fundus (as described below) is more useful in evaluating posterior subcapsular cataract and cortical opacities (Figs 6.25 and 6.27). The depth of focus with

(b)

(a)

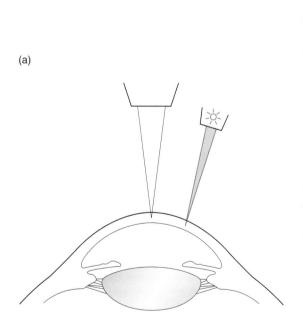
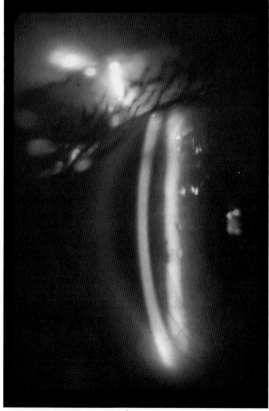

Fig. 6.35a Diagram illustrating the position of the illuminating and viewing systems when using indirect illumination. Alternatively, indirect illumination can be used without decoupling the illumination and viewing systems, by looking outside the illuminated area when the system is coupled and set up to view using direct illumination as in Figure 6.34a.
Fig. 6.35b Ghost vessels seen in indirect illumination (Courtesy of David Williams, Professor emeritus, University of Waterloo).

retroillumination of the lens is typically not sufficient to provide an assessment of both the anterior and posterior lens at the same time, so that separate assessments are required, particularly with higher magnification.

g) Anterior vitreous: Moving the joystick further towards the patient allows viewing of the anterior vitreous with a parallelepiped when the pupil is dilated. To look for anterior vitreous floaters

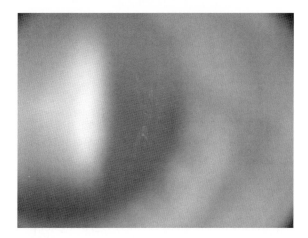

Fig. 6.36 Vitreous floaters seen in the anterior vitreous by direct illumination.

(Fig. 6.36), it can be useful to ask the patient to look up, look down and then straight ahead, so that the opacities become visible as they float through the field of view (see website 🖱).

6.6.4 'Specialised' slit-lamp techniques

If an abnormality/anomaly is suspected from the case history or detected during a routine slit-lamp examination of the anterior eye, one or more of the following illumination techniques may be useful in the assessment process. With experience, many or all techniques are used in fast succession. The slit lamp magnification can be varied to examine the anomaly more carefully noting its exact size, shape, appearance, depth and location. Additional photographs and short video-clips using these techniques are provided on the website 🖱.

1. Sclerotic scatter

1. This can be set up by directing a 1–2mm slit from 45–60° on the temporal side onto the temporal limbus. The light is totally internally reflected in a healthy cornea and only escapes at other parts of the limbus creating a glowing halo of light (Fig. 6.37). An

(a)

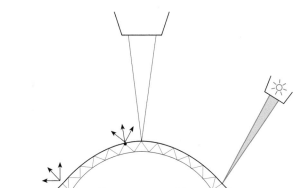

(b)

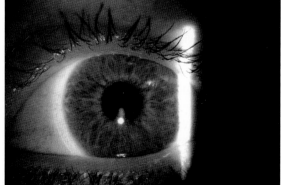

Fig. 6.37a Diagram illustrating the position of the illuminating and viewing systems when using the sclerotic scatter technique.

Fig. 6.37b Sclerotic scatter showing an S-shape of contact lens deposits.

abnormality scattering light within the cornea is observed as a white area against the black pupil. Only relatively large amounts of light scatter can be viewed with the naked eye and therefore it is preferable to view sclerotic scatter using the slit-lamp viewing system. As the technique involves observing the cornea while the illumination is directed at the limbus, the illumination and viewing systems of the slit-lamp must be decoupled.

2. Turn off the room lights to keep the surrounding light levels as low as possible so as to observe subtle amounts of light scatter.

3. Keep the slit-lamp coupled, set the magnification at about 10× and use a 1–2mm slit at about 45°. Focus the central cornea by ensuring the particles in the tear film are focused. Asking the patient to blink will move the tear film debris, making them easier to find. Lock the slit-lamp position to ensure the viewing system remains focused on the central cornea.

4. Decouple the slit-lamp and move the illumination system onto the temporal limbus so that a halo of light is seen around the whole limbus. Shorten the length of the slit so that it is all in contact with the limbus. Any extra slit length will produce light scatter from the sclera that could reduce the visibility of subtle defects.

5. Scan the cornea for areas of light scatter. Iatrogenic damage due to novice contact tonometry or gonioscopy use, foreign bodies, scars and central corneal clouding due to rigid contact lens wear can all be observed with this technique.

2. Optical section of the cornea

This is a type of direct illumination (where the illumination and viewing systems are sharply focused on the same area) in which the illumination beam is narrowed to allow a judgement of depth of any abnormalities within the cornea (Fig. 6.38). For example, it can be used to judge the depth of a foreign body in the cornea.

1. Set the illumination system at approximately 45° from the microscope using low to moderate magnification (≈10×).

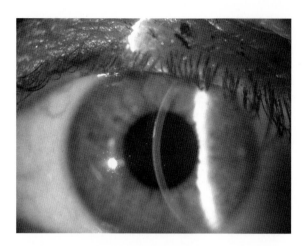

Fig. 6.38   A corneal section indicating that the corneal abrasion shown in Figure 6.34 is in the corneal epithelium.

2. If the area of the cornea you wish to view is temporal, place the illumination on the temporal side and if it is nasal, place it on the nasal side.

3. Narrow the beam to the narrowest possible width and sharply focus on the cornea using the joystick. As you have greatly narrowed the beam, you need to increase the slit-lamp illumination.

4. A section or slice of the cornea should now be visible (Fig. 6.38). The epithelium will be on the temporal side of the image if the illumination system is temporal to the viewing system with the endothelium on the nasal side.

5. The section of stroma can be broadened by increasing the angle between the microscope and illumination system.

6. Once the object of interest is identified, increase the magnification to obtain greater detail.

3. Optical section of the lens

The technique is similar to that described above except that the slit-lamp is focused on the lens. This assessment is best done after dilating the pupil. If the lens is to be assessed without dilating the pupil, the angle between the illumination source and the viewing system needs to be greatly reduced. This technique is the only accurate way of detecting and assessing nuclear cataract and can differentiate

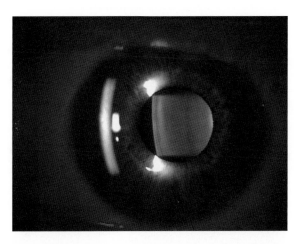

Fig. 6.39   An optical section of the lens anterior cortex (on the left side within the pupil) and lens nucleus (central). The posterior cortex is blurred and on the right side of the pupil. The blurred arc to the left is the out-of-focus cornea.

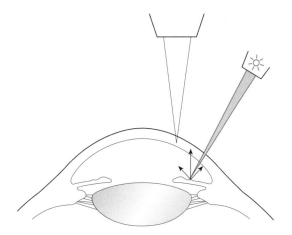

Fig. 6.40   Diagram illustrating the position of the illuminating and viewing systems when using retro-illumination from the iris.

anterior and posterior subcapsular cataracts. Posterior subcapsular cataracts typically have a much greater effect on visual disability.

1. For a well-dilated pupil, set the illumination system at approximately 45° from the microscope using low to moderate magnification ($\approx 10\times$). This is the standard angle for grading nuclear cataract using an optical section with the lens opacities classifications system (LOCS III).

2. For a non-dilated pupil, reduce the illumination angle until an optical section of the lens is just seen. This may be as small as 15° for an elderly patient with a small pupil.

3. Narrow the beam to the narrowest possible width and sharply focus on the lens by moving the joystick towards the patient after the cornea has come into focus. As you have greatly narrowed the beam, you need to increase the slit-lamp illumination.

4. A section or slice of the lens should now be visible. The anterior lens will be on the temporal side of the image if the illumination system is temporal to the viewing system with the posterior lens being blurred and on the nasal side (Fig. 6.39).

5. To view the posterior lens in optical section, the joystick needs to be moved further forward

and the angle of the illumination system may need to be reduced further (Fig. 6.5).

4. Indirect illumination

This technique (Fig. 6.35) is used to view areas that become bleached with excessive light using direct illumination, such as fine blood vessels at the limbus and microcysts. It is also used to look for iris features such as the outer rim of the iris sphincter.

1. Use a 1–2 mm parallelepiped, low to moderate magnification ($\approx 10\times$) and set the illumination system at 45° from the microscope.

2. Rather than focus on the illuminated area (direct illumination), simply direct your gaze just outside the area that is illuminated (indirect illumination). Subtle abnormalities can be seen using light scattered by the cornea away from the main area of illumination.

3. Increase the magnification as required.

4. The technique can also be used after decoupling the illumination and viewing systems.

5. Retro-illumination from the iris

This technique (Fig. 6.40) is used in the examination of corneal vessels, epithelial oedema and small

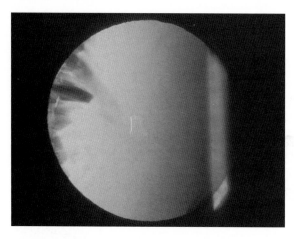

Fig. 6.41 A cortical cataract seen in retro-illumination from the fundus.

scars on the cornea with light reflected from the iris. Opaque features appear dark against a light background.

1. Use a 1–2 mm parallelepiped with low magnification and set the illumination system to an angle of about 45°.

2. If it is possible to view the abnormality in direct illumination, bring it into focus and then lock the joystick position.

3. Decouple the illumination and viewing systems, direct the light onto the iris and view the structure against the light reflected from the iris. The magnification can be varied as necessary.

6. Retro-illumination from the fundus

This is a commonly used technique to examine iris disorders and cataracts using light reflected from the fundus. Cataracts are seen as dark opacities against the red background glow from the fundus (Figs 6.25 and 6.27). It is a useful technique for examination of cortical and posterior subcapsular cataracts (Fig. 6.41). Retro-illumination can also be used to detect iris abnormalities such as peripheral iridotomies and loss of pigment (iris transillumination, Fig. 6.42). In this case, the red glow of the fundus is seen through holes or slits in the iris.

1. Use a 1–2 mm parallelepiped with low magnification and set the illumination system to an angle of 0°. Adjust the beam height to the height of the pupil.

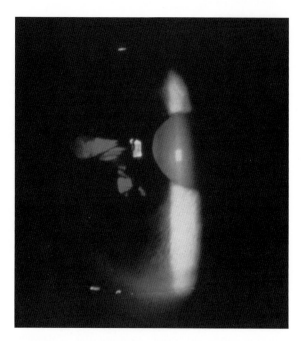

Fig. 6.42 Iris transillumination. Loss of localised iris pigment is shown by the red fundal glow appearing through parts of the iris when light is shone through the pupil (Courtesy of David Williams, Professor emeritus, University of Waterloo).

2. Focus on the iris or lens as appropriate.

3. You will only be able to focus the anterior or posterior part of the lens at any one time. You can gain an approximate focus on the anterior lens by focusing the iris. To focus the posterior lens you will need to push the joystick forwards towards the patient from this position. Note that cortical opacities can be found in both the anterior and posterior cortex. Posterior subcapsular cataracts will be seen only in the posterior plane of the lens. Observe any illumination coming through the iris.

4. To gain a retro-illumination image of the lens with an undilated small pupil, you may need to decouple the instrument slightly and alter the angle of illumination by a small amount.

7. Specular reflection

This technique is used to examine the endothelium (for polymegethism and pleomorphism), the

(a)

(b)

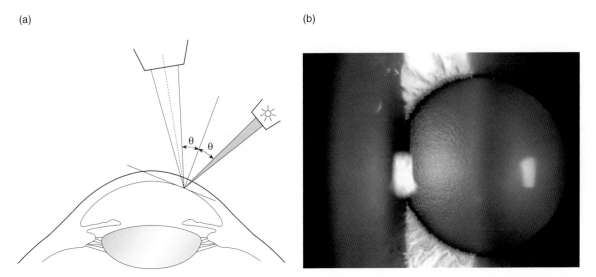

Fig. 6.43a   Diagram illustrating the position of the illuminating and viewing systems when using specular reflection to view the corneal endothelium.

Fig. 6.43b   Specular reflection from the anterior surface of the lens showing its orange peel appearance.

precorneal tear film and variations in contour of the epithelium.

When learning this technique, it is best to start by attempting to obtain an image of the anterior lens surface by specular reflection (Fig. 6.43b). It has the same appearance as an orange peel.

1. Set the illumination system at approximately 30° to 45° from the microscope, using a moderately wide 2–3 mm parallelepiped. Look through the eyepieces and focus the parallelepiped on the anterior lens.

2. Change the angle of illumination until a bright reflection is seen from the lens surface. This occurs when the angle of incidence equals the angle of reflection from the lens (Fig. 6.43a). This can also be obtained by moving the illumination/microscope system laterally until the angle of incidence equals the angle of reflection.

3. View the orange peel appearance of the anterior lens (Fig. 6.43b, note that the colour is white, not orange!) to the side of the bright reflex.

4. To examine the tear film and epithelium, set the illumination system at approximately 45° to 60° from the microscope, using a moderately wide 2–3 mm parallelepiped.

Look through the eyepieces and focus the parallelepiped on the cornea. The tear film can be used to help this focusing as it is easily identified by noting the particles floating within it. In this regard it can be useful to ask the patient to blink.

5. Change the angle of illumination until a bright reflection is seen from the precorneal tear film. This occurs when the angle of incidence equals the angle of reflection from the cornea. This can also be obtained by moving the illumination/microscope system laterally until the angle of incidence equals the angle of reflection.

6. To examine the endothelium set the magnification to about 25× with a fairly wide 2–3 mm parallelepiped and initially focus on the tear film.

7. Alter the illumination angle and/or lateral position of the slit-lamp until the bright corneal reflexes (Purkinje images) fall on top of the corneal section. There should be two reflexes: on the epithelial side of the corneal section there should be a bright white reflex from the epithelium and on the endothelial side a less bright, slightly yellowed reflex from the endothelium.

8. Increase the magnification to about 40× and move the focus slightly forward to focus on the endothelium. If you then look to the side of the bright endothelial slightly yellowed reflex (nasal or temporal to the reflex depending on the position of the illumination system), the duller picture of the endothelial hexagonal cells will be in view.

8. Slit-lamp examination with fluorescein

Fluorescein dye is often used to assess the integrity of the corneal epithelium as it stains epithelial defects (Wilson et al. 1995). The dye absorbs blue light and emits green. It can also be used to detect corneal perforation (Seidel's test – aqueous flowing out from the wound amidst the fluorescein).

1. Wet the tip of a fluorescein strip with sterile saline solution. Be careful not to contaminate the saline by touching the strip to the tip of the bottle. Shake excess fluid from the strip over a sink.

2. Ask the patient to look up and touch the strip to the inferior bulbar conjunctiva, being careful not to touch the cornea. The strip can also be touched to the upper bulbar conjunctiva, but this has the disadvantage that if the patient blinks or attempts to blink, the eye will rotate upwards (Bell's phenomenon) and the strip may scratch the superior cornea. Ask the patient to blink several times to allow the fluorescein to spread across the cornea. Remove any excess fluorescein using a tissue and be careful not to spill the dye on the patient's clothes as a stain will result.

3. With the patient at the biomicroscope, observe the cornea with cobalt blue light and medium magnification. When you are using the cobalt blue filter, you will need to increase the illumination. A Kodak Wratten number 12 yellow gelatin filter held in front of the biomicroscope viewing system will facilitate the view by filtering out the reflected blue light (compare photographs with and without the fitter on the website 🐭). Newer slit-lamps have this filter as a built-in option over the observation system. Observations should be made within 10 min of instillation of the dye

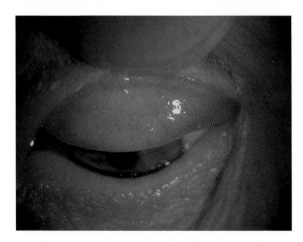

Fig. 6.44   The superior palpebral conjunctiva viewed after lid eversion.

or intercellular diffusion surrounding a lesion may mask its exact nature.

4. Soft contact lens wearers can replace their lenses after a biomicroscopic investigation using fluorescein as long as the dye is irrigated out of the eye using saline prior to lens reinsertion. Otherwise irrigation is not necessary. An alternative is to use Fluorexon which is a high molecular weight fluorescein that will not penetrate into a soft contact lens.

9. Eyelid eversion

This technique is used to examine the inferior and superior palpebral conjunctivae, particularly in contact lens wear and when looking for allergic conjunctival changes, papillae, and foreign bodies.

1. Ask the patient to look down and grasp the superior eyelashes.

2. Press gently on the superior margin of the tarsal plate using a cotton swab (or the index finger of the other hand), and at the same time pull the eyelashes upwards. This technique will evert the eyelid to permit viewing of the superior palpebral conjunctiva (Fig. 6.44) using a parallelepiped.

3. To re-evert the eyelid, hold the eyelashes and ask the patient to look up and gently pull the eyelashes away from the eye.

4. To evert the lower eyelid, pull the eyelid down and press under the eyelid margin while moving your finger upwards. The eyelid will evert over your finger.

10. Double eyelid eversion

This technique is used to find small foreign bodies in the superior fornix. Care should be taken to minimally irritate the palpebral conjunctiva.

1. Sterilise a small to medium-sized paperclip by soaking for 10 minutes in alcohol.

2. Bend the paperclip so that the two ends are apart at approximately 30 degrees.

3. Instil anaesthetic and fluorescein into the eye.

4. With the patient at the slit-lamp single-evert the upper eyelid. Place the longer end of the paperclip under the everted eyelid and gently pull the eyelid away from the globe.

5. Observe for any small foreign bodies using the cobalt blue filter on the slitlamp.

11. Conical beam

This technique is used to look for flare (i.e. protein) or floating cells in the anterior chamber (by using more magnification and a longer beam).

1. Turn off all the room lights and close your own eyes too for a few seconds to start to dark-adapt.

2. Set the illumination system at approximately 45° from the microscope using moderate magnification ($\approx$16$\times$).

3. Narrow the height and width of the beam to obtain a conical beam. A 1 mm wide and 3 mm long beam is generally used. Move the beam to the centre of the pupil and focus in the anterior chamber midway between the anterior surface of the crystalline lens and the posterior surface of the cornea.

4. Rock the illumination system gently from side to side and look for flare and cells. Cells are a sign of active inflammation and should be counted in the grading process. Aqueous flare is the result of leakage of protein through damaged iris blood vessels and is graded by the degree of obscuration of the iris details.

12. Meibomian gland evaluation

Meibomian gland dysfunction is considered to be the major cause of evaporative dry eye (Albietz 2000). A decrease of meibomian oil causes increased tear evaporation and ocular surface damage due to increased osmolarity (Yokoi et al. 1999). To assess the meibomian glands:

1. With the patient at the biomicroscope, use white light and medium magnification to inspect the lower eyelid margins.

2. Look for capping of the meibomian gland orifices (yellow mounds), notching of the eyelid margins (indentations) and frothing of the tears on the eyelid margins.

3. Pull the lower eyelid down and look for concretions (section 6.5.2, Fig. 6.21) in the palpebral conjunctiva.

4. Inform the patient that you are going to press on his or her eyelid and that they will feel some pressure. With mild pressure, press on the eyelid margins near the eyelashes and watch the meibomian gland orifices. Clear fluid should be expressed.

5. Capping of the orifices, a cheesy secretion on expression and frothing of the eyelid margins indicates meibomian gland dysfunction. Concretions can be associated with this condition. This can lead to excessive evaporation of the aqueous component of the tears and treating this aspect is often a component of dry eye management as aqueous deficiency and excessive tear evaporation often coexist.

6. Another method of assessing the meibomian gland function is to determine the position of the *Marx line* which is a clear line running along the lower lid margin after fluorescein is instilled into the eye. In normal eyes, this line is located on the conjuctival side of the meibomian gland orifices and in meibomian gland dysfunction it is located on the cutaneous side of the orifices. (Yamaguchi et al. 2006).

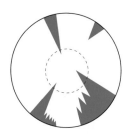
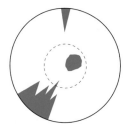

Fig. 6.45   Recording of cataract.

6.6.5 Recording

Normal appearance: If no abnormalities are detected, record 'clear' if the tissue is transparent, such as the cornea and lens. Otherwise record 'No abnormalities detected' (NAD) or 'Within normal limits' (WNL) or equivalent.

Anomalies/abnormalities: Record the size, shape, appearance and location of any abnormalities/anomalies using a diagram and a written description as well as digital imaging if available. In addition, observations such as fluorescein staining, corneal oedema, tarsal plate abnormalities (papillae, follicles), injection and vascularisation should be graded on a scale of 0 to 4+, with 0 being absence of a response, 1+ being trace response, 2+ being mild response, 3+ being moderate response and 4+ being severe response.

Cataracts: Unless digital imaging is available, record cortical and subcapsular cataracts by drawing them (Fig. 6.45). The undilated pupil can be recorded as a dashed line on this diagram. If there are cortical opacities in both the anterior and posterior cortex, both should be recorded. Nuclear yellowing and opacification can be graded on a scale of 0 to 4+ with 0 being absence of opacity and 4+ being the most severe form of opacity. For more precise grading, a cataract grading system such as the LOCS III system should be used (Chylack et al. 1993). In this type of system the cataract is graded on a decimal scale against standardised colour photographs.

Cells and flare: Cells are graded according to the number observed, with 5–10 cells 1+, 11–20 cells 2+, 21–50 cells 3+ and >50 cells 4+. Aqueous flare is graded from 0–4+ depending upon the visibility of the iris detail: faint to just detectable 1+,

moderate to iris details clear 2+, marked to iris details hazy 3+, intense with severe fibrinous exudates 4+.

Contact lens complications: Contact lens complications can be graded by using the Centre for Contact Lens Research Unit (CCLRU) or the Efron grading scales. These are standardised images of common complications at different levels of severity that aid in assessing the condition observed. The CCLRU scale uses photographs and the Efron scale uses images painted by ophthalmic artists (Efron et al. 2001). Grading scales can be a useful adjunct to practitioners in gauging the severity and monitoring the progression of ocular complications of contact lens wear.

6.6.6 Interpretation

A good understanding of the normal anatomy and physiology of the anterior segment and adnexa as well as the normal changes with age is required. Variations in normal appearance of the anterior segment and changes with age are briefly discussed in sections 6.4 and 6.5 respectively.

6.6.7 Most common errors

1. Not positioning the slit-lamp so that the patient is leaning forward into the chin rest. This often results in the patient not being able to maintain their forehead against the headrest, resulting in the image going in and out of focus.

2. Not focusing the eyepieces to compensate for your refractive error.

3. Not keeping the eyepieces clean.

4. Not reducing the room illumination for the procedure.

5. Not examining the superior cornea by having the patient look down and raising the upper eyelid.

6. Using an optic section with high magnification during the initial phases of the assessment.

6.7 TEAR BREAK-UP TIME

Tear break-up time (TBUT) is used to assess the stability of the tear film between blinks. Dry spots appear in the tear film that are thought to form by evaporation and retraction of the tear film after each blink and by diffusion of the superficial lipid through the aqueous layer to the mucin surface. TBUT is the standard assessment of tear film stability, but non-invasive tear break-up time and tear thinning time are becoming popular with some practitioners.

6.7.1 Dry eye assessment

Dry eye is a disorder of the tear film caused by tear deficiency or excessive tear evaporation. The features include a set of characteristic symptoms, ocular surface damage, reduced tear film stability and tear hyperosmolarity. Up to 25% of patients presenting to optometric offices have some level of dry eye symptoms. Causes of dry eye include meibomian gland dysfunction, atrophy or fibrosis of the lacrimal tissue (as in keratoconjunctivitis sicca) and medication use (e.g. beta-blockers, antihistamines, antidepressants, oral contraceptives, anticholinergics, acne medications, barbiturates and alcohol). The incidence of dry eye is also increased following refractive laser surgery (Ang et al. 2001) and nearly half of contact lens wearers report symptoms of dryness (Nichols et al. 2000). The National Eye Institute/industry workshop on clinical trials in dry eye lists the criteria for dry eye diagnosis as symptom assessment, interpalpebral surface damage, tear instability and tear hyperosmolarity. Although tear hyperosmolarity is mentioned as part of the criteria for diagnosis, it is currently impractical to measure in the clinical setting (Korb 2000).

Symptoms by case history, fluorescein staining (section 6.6.4), fluorescein tear break-up time and phenol red thread testing of tear quantity (section 6.8) are standard tools for the assessment of dry eye. Common practice amongst optometrists and ophthalmologists is to use symptoms and at least one other test in the clinical diagnosis of dry eye (Nichols et al. 2000). The symptoms of dry eye commonly include: irritation, dryness, foreign body sensation, burning, gritty sensation, transient blurring of vision, stinging pain, epiphora and contact lens intolerance. Less commonly mentioned symptoms include haloes around lights (especially at night), excessive tearing, stringy mucus discharge, redness, photophobia, itching and asthenopia. Patients often report closing their eyes to obtain some relief. Reading for long periods (or performing other concentrated visual tasks) reduces the blink rate significantly and can produce symptoms in some patients and exacerbate them in others. Environmental factors such as wind, air conditioning, airline travel and winter months, can produce similar effects on symptoms. Lifestyle causes of dry eye include smoking, high caffeine intake and a diet low in omega-3 fatty acids (Moss et al. 2000).

6.7.2 Advantages and disadvantages

Tear break-up time (TBUT) is fast, easy to perform and comfortable for the patient. It requires equipment that is standard to optometric practice such as a biomicroscope with a cobalt blue filter and sodium fluorescein. The main disadvantage of the technique is that it is intrinsically invasive. In addition, a localised corneal surface abnormality will typically produce a break-up of the tear film in that location and can suggest a falsely low TBUT. However, although a wide variability of the TBUT is present in normal individuals, a low TBUT has sufficient specificity to screen patients for evidence of tear film instability.

6.7.3 Procedure

Topical anaesthetics should not be used prior to TBUT measurement, as this may cause a spuriously fast TBUT.

1. With the patient at the biomicroscope, instil fluorescein into the tear film and ask the patient to blink several times.

2. Examine the tear film with a wide 2–3 mm parallelepiped and low magnification. Switch to the cobalt blue filter on the slit-lamp. The tear film should appear as a fine green film due to the fluorescein.

3. Ask the patient to hold their eyes open without blinking.

4. From the time of the blink, time how long it takes in seconds, before dark spots or streaks appear in the even green tear film after a blink. The use of the Kodak Wratten yellow filter number 12 held over the observation system is helpful for this evaluation.

5. If the patient blinks before 10 seconds have passed then the measurement cannot be made and the procedure must be re-started.

6. Repeat the measurement at least once and take an average.

7. If the tear film breaks up immediately and consistently in the same location there may be an epithelial basement membrane defect in that location on the cornea. The TBUT should be repeated, not considering this defect, to get an indication of tear film stability.

Non-invasive TBUT and tear thinning time: a non-invasive TBUT (NIBUT) or tear thinning time can be measured without disturbing the tear film.

1. Dry spots or a loss of transparency in the tear film are observed using diffuse, low-luminance, heat-filtered white light and moderate magnification. A grid or concentric ring pattern is projected onto the cornea and the patient is asked to blink. The time from the blink until the ring pattern becomes distorted provides a measure of the NIBUT. The tearscope is a commercially available test for measuring NIBUT (Bron 2001).

2. A similar test, the time elapsed after a blink to the first distortion of keratometer mires, has been called tear-thinning time (Little & Bruce 1994). Tear thinning occurs before break-up.

6.7.4 Recording

The TBUT or NIBUT value should be recorded in seconds for each eye individually. Indicate the method that was used to determine this value. For example, NIBUT with grid pattern, 10 *seconds* RE (OD), 12 *seconds* LE (OS).

6.7.5 Interpretation

The normal TBUT is between 15 and 45 seconds and a break-up time of less than 10 seconds is indicative of an unstable tear film. Normal TBUTs are sometimes limited by the patient's ability to keep their eyes open and not blink. Normal NIBUT in Caucasians is considered to be 10 seconds or more (Fukuda & Wang 2000).

6.7.6 Most common errors

1. Performing TBUT with a fluorescein/anaesthetic combination.

2. Spilling fluorescein on the patient's lids or clothes.

3. Touching the cornea with a fluorescein strip.

4. Holding the lid, which will reduce the TBUT.

5. Not rinsing out the fluorescein before reinserting soft contact lenses.

6.7.7 Additional tests: Rose Bengal and Lissamine green staining

Ocular surface damage caused by dry eye can be assessed using various vital dyes such as fluorescein (section 6.6.4, No.8), Rose Bengal and Lissamine green. Each dye has different properties such that it stains epithelial defects (fluorescein; Wilson et al. 1995), interacts with an impaired mucin layer on the epithelial surface (Rose Bengal) or stains dead and devitalised cells (Lissamine green). Fluorescein is used for the standard assessment for ocular surface damage, with Rose Bengal and Lissamine green reserved for more severe dry eye cases. Surface damage on both the cornea and conjunctiva is revealed with fluorescein staining (Wilson et al. 1995), which has a characteristic distribution confined to the interpalpebral area of the ocular surface. In severe dry eye the staining may extend to the unexposed surface of the globe, particularly the upper bulbar conjunctiva. Rose Bengal causes significant ocular discomfort (perhaps necessitating the use of topical anaesthesia) and it can be difficult differentiating its red stain from the underlying hue in patients with inflamed red eyes.

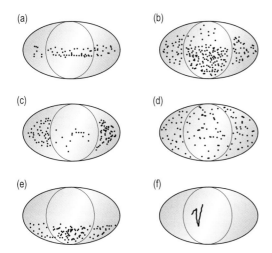

Fig. 6.46 Characteristic fluorescein staining patterns. (a) Band superficial punctate staining (SPS) due to conditions such as mild dry eye or exposure of the region. (b) More severe band SPS, possible in severe dry eye. (c) Rose Bengal staining in dry eye. (d) Diffuse SPS due to conditions such as adenoviral and staphylococcal keratoconjunctivitis and reactions to diagnostic or therapeutic eyedrops. (e) Inferior SPS due to conditions such as staphylococcal blepharoconjunctivitis and exposure of the region. (f) Foreign body or trichiasis (particularly when in the inferior cornea) tracks.

Rose Bengal can be photoactivated by ultraviolet radiation which can cause further toxicity, especially in dry eye patients with heavy staining (Bron et al. 2003), although liberal irrigation can mitigate this effect. In aqueous tear deficiency, Rose Bengal stains the interpalpebral conjunctiva, appearing in a triangular shape with the base in the limbus. In keratoconjunctivitis sicca resulting from lacrimal gland dysfunction, the exposed conjunctiva stains more than the cornea. In early disease the nasal bulbar conjunctiva stains, then the temporal and inferior cornea and, in advanced disease, the entire cornea. Lissamine green stains dead and devitalised cells green but is not toxic to healthy cells. Lissamine green gives comparable results to Rose Bengal but does not cause as much ocular discomfort especially in those patients with positive findings (Kim 2000). As with Rose Bengal, the staining is dose-dependent, therefore if a very small amount is used the staining will be very minimal (Bron et al. 2003). The staining areas on the cornea and the conjunctiva should be both described and drawn on a diagram of the anterior segment. The staining should be classified and differentiated from other causes (Fig. 6.46).

6.8 PHENOL RED THREAD AND SCHIRMER TESTS

6.8.1 Tear flow/volume tests to help classify dry eye disease

Dry eye can be classified as evaporative, in which excessive evaporation exists, or tear-deficient, in which there is a deficiency of aqueous tear secretion (Bron 2001). Evaporative dry eye can be assessed with meibomian gland evaluation (section 6.5.4, No. 10) and the evaluation of lid and blink dynamics, including the presence of ectropion or other lid anomalies causing poor lid closure (lagophthalmos). Tear-deficient dry eye (caused by Sjögren's syndrome or non-autoimmune conditions; Albietz 2000, Bron 2001), can be detected using tear flow/volume tests, such as the assessment of the tear meniscus (section 6.6.3, 7d) and the Schirmer and phenol red thread tests. These conditions are not mutually exclusive, however, as meibomian gland dysfunction is present in 70% of patients with tear-deficient dry eye (Bron 2001). Tear interferometry and laser meibometry are starting to be used to assess the quality and quantity of the tear lipid layer but are not yet in common clinical use (Yokoi & Komuro 2004). The simple assessment of the tear meniscus (section 6.6.3, 7d) can be combined with either the phenol red thread or Schirmer test for the assessment of tear flow/volume (Albietz 2000).

6.8.2 Advantages and disadvantages

The phenol red thread test is used clinically and is very easy to perform. Patients generally tolerate it well as only a soft thread is touched to the lid and the results are obtained in 15 seconds per eye. Due to the relatively quick assessment, it is useful for examining the tear volume before and after insertion of lacrimal occlusive devices. An average measurement of less than 11 mm in 15 seconds is considered diagnostic of aqueous deficient dry eye (Albietz 2000). Typically, 10–20 mm is considered borderline and greater than 20 mm is typically normal. The Schirmer tear test uses a 5 by 35 mm strip of filter paper to measure basic and reflex tear secretion when used without anaesthetic. In theory, it measures only basic secretion when used with anaesthetic. In practice, however, while anaesthetic reduces the amount of reflex secretion, it does not eliminate it completely. Environmental conditions such as temperature or humidity affect the reliability of the test. The Schirmer test is used in severe dry eye patients (Bron 2001) and as part of the definition of Sjögren's syndrome (Manthorpe 2006). However, research has suggested that it is neither reliable nor valid (e.g. Cho 1993). In addition, the test is poorly tolerated by patients as a relatively large, heavy paper strip is used and has to remain in contact with the tear film for 5 minutes. Poor correlation coefficients have been found between Schirmer and phenol red thread testing and with symptoms of dry eyes (Saleh et al. 2006) and with other tests of dry eye (Nichols et al. 2004). However, corneal sensitivity may vary in some patients with dry eye, so that a poor correlation may be expected. In addition, the phenol red thread and Schirmer testing were performed after fluorescein instillation (Nichols et al. 2004), which is not ideal.

6.8.3 Procedure

All available tests of tear volume may stimulate some degree of reflex tearing and should be undertaken prior to manipulation of the eyelids or to instillation of any fluid or dye into the tear film.

Phenol red thread tear test

1. Remove the threads by gently peeling the plastic film covering from the unsealed end of the aluminium sheet. The folded 3 mm end of the thread should be bent open at an angle that allows for easy placement onto the palpebral conjunctiva with forceps. The thread is placed at a point approximately one-third of the distance from the lateral canthus of the lower eyelid with the eye in the primary position. The lower eyelid is pulled down slightly and the folded 3 mm portion of the thread is placed on the palpebral conjunctival junction. Timing begins as soon as the thread touches the tear layer.

2. Each eye is tested with the eyes open for 15 seconds. During the test the patient is instructed to look straight ahead and blink

normally. Care should be taken to ensure that the thread does not come into contact with the cornea during the test. When the 15 seconds have elapsed the lower eyelid is gently pulled down and the thread gently removed with an upward motion. The entire length of the red portion of the thread is measured in mm from the very tip regardless of the fold.

3. Since tear volume can vary, reliability can be improved by repeating the test on different days. It may also be helpful to ask the patient if they could feel the thread during testing, as it could be indicative of a reflex tearing component to the measurement.

Schirmer tear test

1. Gently dry the outside of the closed lids. Bend the round wick end of the test strips at the notch approximately 120° before opening the sterile pouch. Peel back the pouch and remove the strips. Only handle the strips by the non-wick ends to avoid contamination.

2. Have the patient look up and gently pull the lower eyelid down and temporally. Place the bent hooked end of the strip at the junction of the temporal and central third of the lower eyelid margin. The strip should not touch the cornea when the eyelid is released. Release the eyelid and have the patient continue to look up, blinking normally. The patient can close his or her eyes if this is more comfortable but should not squeeze the eyes shut. Both eyes should be measured at the same time.

3. Note the time of insertion. Remove the strip after 5 minutes or when it is completely wet, whichever comes first. Measure the wetted portion of the strip from the notch towards the flat end in mm. Record this value.

4. The Schirmer II test is a test of reflex tear secretion and is rarely used. It is performed by irritating the nasal mucosa with a cotton-tipped applicator prior to inserting the filter paper. Clinically, asking the patient if he or she is 'able to cry' is usually a good indication of the reflex tearing ability and is preferred.

6.8.4 Recording

Record the distance in mm, and the test used for each eye. For example:

Schirmer: RE 8 mm; LE 5 mm.
Phenol red thread: OD 12 mm; OS 15 mm.

6.8.5 Interpretation

For the phenol red thread test, a measurement of <10 mm wetting represents true dryness, while 10 to 20 mm wetting is considered borderline, and >20 mm is generally considered normal. For the Schirmer test, a measurement of 10–15 mm or more without anaesthesia is regarded as normal tear production. A value of less than 5 mm is very suggestive of a true dry eye state. Several measurements should be made on repeated visits and averaged to obtain as accurate a result as possible.

6.8.6 Most common errors

1. Performing the test after manipulation of the lids, instillation of diagnostic drugs or dyes, or applanation tonometry.

2. Not considering the patient's ocular surface sensitivity (corneal and/or conjunctival) in the interpretation of the results.

3. Contaminating the strip with your fingers prior to insertion.

4. Using Schirmer testing to evaluate mild to moderate dry eye. It is most useful in the diagnosis of Sjögren's syndrome.

6.9 DIAGNOSTIC LACRIMAL OCCLUSION

Patients must be evaluated for the suitability for use of (semi-)permanent lacrimal occlusive therapy (punctal or intracanalicular plugs) prior to initiation of therapy. These plugs are relatively expensive and reversal of the occlusion may be difficult in some cases if patient selection was inappropriate and excess tearing or complications occur.

Temporary collagen plug occlusion is a relatively inexpensive diagnostic test performed with dissolvable implants in the drainage system to allow for the measure of suitability for therapeutic occlusion options. Diagnostic collagen plugs imbibe water and expand in the canaliculus to approximately twice their diameter, then proceed to dissolve in 4–7 days. After approximately one week, the patient is asked to return and subjective and objective assessments of dry eye are compared pre- and post-insertion of the plugs.

6.9.1 Therapeutic lacrimal occlusion

Dry eye and exposure keratitis are the most common ocular surface diseases encountered in optometric practice. Therapeutic management includes the use of aggressive artificial tears, anti-inflammatory therapies and lacrimal occlusive therapy. Occlusion of the lacrimal drainage system allows the reduced volume of tears to be preserved and the hyperosmolarity of the tears to be normalised. The consequence is not only improved ocular lubrication, but also enhanced comfort and healing of the ocular surface, as well as decreased risk of serious complications such as ocular infections (e.g. Nava-Castaneda et al. 2003). Lacrimal occlusion can also be useful for the patient with marginal dry eye who wishes to continue wearing contact lenses (Slusser & Lowther 1998), as well as for short-term occlusion during the healing process after ocular surgeries such as LASIK (Ang et al. 2001). Lacrimal occlusion has also been shown to enhance contact time of topically applied treatments such as anti-glaucoma medications.

6.9.2 Advantages and disadvantages

Temporary collagen plug occlusion is a relatively inexpensive diagnostic test performed with dissolvable implants in the drainage system to allow for the measure of suitability for therapeutic occlusion options. More than one trial of collagen implants may be required to prove to the clinician and/or patient that (semi-)permanent plugs will be a useful therapeutic option for their particular case. For example, patients with poor corneal sensitivity from nerve damage or chronic ocular surface disease may be unable to detect an improvement in comfort during the course of the collagen trial, and therefore may feel that long-term occlusion options will not be helpful for them. In those cases, the objective signs are more helpful in determining suitability and therefore repeated trials may be considered to monitor the corneal and conjunctival health to determine if occlusion is advisable. It is also generally true that a single collagen plug (even the largest size that can fit into the punctal opening) is often insufficient to appropriately occlude a canaliculus and therefore may generate a false negative trial. This is because the diameter of the canaliculus may be unrelated to the size of the punctum and a single plug may migrate out of the system before it has had the opportunity to imbibe water and occlude the drainage. Similarly, some clinicians occlude only the inferior canaliculi for the diagnostic test. While this may be appropriate in some circumstances, it is also more likely to generate a false negative diagnostic test. Full occlusion, even if it generates some degree of epiphora, is generally preferred and is short-lived. Measurement of tear thinning time suggests that superior plug insertion may not be necessary and that occlusion of the lower punctum is sufficient, although occlusion of both prolonged the preservation of tear volume (Farrell et al. 2003).

6.9.3 Procedure

Evaluate the patient carefully for dry eye and ocular surface disease (sections 6.7 and 6.8). Ask the patient whether they have any allergy (or opposition) to (bovine) collagen, silicone or other materials or anaesthetics. Discuss the procedure, any sensations the patient might experience during the procedure, and any potential adverse effects. Obtain informed consent. A video clip of the technique is shown on the website 🖱.

1. Disinfect jeweller forceps.

2. Inspect the puncta and choose the largest implant size that seems likely to fit into the punctal opening without punctal dilation. The 0.40 mm size is the most commonly used. Choosing a plug size that is too small (e.g. the 0.3 mm size) will often result in a false negative trial due to the plugs migrating straight through the system.

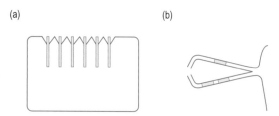

Fig. 6.47 Diagrammatic representation of (a) a set of six collagen plugs in their foam packaging, (b) hydrated collagen plugs in the canaliculi.

3. It is not generally advised to dilate the punctum prior to inserting the collagen plugs due to the possibility of the plugs refluxing back up and out of the puncta. However, in the case of very small puncta or when a first trial was not positive and the clinician feels that increasing the plug size might be helpful, careful dilation and insertion of larger plugs should be considered.

4. Seat the patient comfortably at the slit lamp biomicroscope or in an examination chair capable of reclining. In the latter case, a loupe may be used for magnification.

5. Anaesthesia of the puncta and ocular surface is not recommended as it reduces the ability of the patient to detect an immediate improvement in ocular surface symptoms. The procedure is generally well tolerated by patients when good technique is employed. The exception is a blepharospastic patient who cannot either fixate or remain still.

6. Open the sterile packet and grasp a single implant from the foam packet (Fig. 6.47a), preferably very close to the end of the plug and with it oriented approximately perpendicular to the forceps. This can be undertaken either using the biomicroscope magnification or outside the slit-lamp.

7. Inferior plug insertion: Inferior plug insertion is generally easier than superior. Instruct the patient to look upwards and temporally. Pull the lower eyelid away from the globe only enough to expose the punctum. Pulling the lid down and away too much will bend or kink the canaliculus.

8. Place the implant partially into the opening vertically following the anatomy of the vertical canaliculus. Pull *laterally* on the eyelid to straighten out the vertical and horizontal portions of the canaliculus. With the canaliculus straightened, advance the plug as far as possible, preferably almost all the way in. Release the forceps. While maintaining lateral positioning of the eyelid, close the tips of the forceps and gently push the rest of the implant into the opening until it disappears below the punctal ring. No part of the plug should be visible at the punctal opening.

9. Generally, use two implants in the inferior and one in the superior canaliculus to effectively occlude the system for diagnostic purposes (Fig. 6.47b). Single collagen implants may flush or reflux out of the system before they expand. Three implants in a canaliculus minimises the likelihood of the plugs refluxing out or flushing through.

10. Superior plug insertion: Instruct the patient to look downwards and temporally for the upper plug insertion. Using the thumb of the opposite hand to the forceps, press in towards the globe on the upper nasal lid. The upper punctum should evert from the eye. Again, try not to kink the canaliculus. Insertion proceeds as per the inferior plug insertion described above.

11. Repeat the phenol red thread test (section 6.8) after the patient has settled for a few minutes after plug insertion.

12. Ask the patient to keep a diary of symptoms over the next 5–10 days, and arrange a follow-up appointment in 7–10 days. If symptoms and tear film and ocular surface evaluations suggest that (semi-) permanent occlusion is appropriate, discuss the various options for therapeutic occlusion.

6.9.4 Recording

Record the type and number of plugs inserted into each canaliculus, and the symptoms, ocular lubricant used and the results of all dry eye assessment tests before and after their use. The results of the phenol red thread tear volume test (section 6.8) before and just after insertion of the plugs are of particular importance to determine if occlusion has been achieved. Consider adding additional plugs per canaliculus (up to three) if the phenol red thread results are not increased from the pre-plug values.

6.9.5 Interpretation

If a positive response is obtained with collagen plugs, a more long-lasting type of occlusion is indicated. Options include punctum or intracanalicular (semi-)permanent implants made of silicone, as well as newer intracanalicular options including thermosensitive polymers and hydrogel materials, all of which have relative benefits. Further collagen plug options now available claim to last up to 3 or even 6 months. These longer-lasting collagen plugs may be a good option in the treatment of conditions that are expected to show improvement, such as dry eye post-LASIK (Ang et al. 2001). When one of these options is indicated, a plug is generally inserted in the inferior punctum/ canaliculus first. If occlusion is not sufficient to relieve symptoms to an acceptable level and ocular signs remain, occlusion of the superior canaliculi may be considered. Before placing (semi-)permanent implants in the superior system, perform a second diagnostic test in the superior canaliculus with collagen plugs. If this procedure also shows benefit in either symptoms or ocular surface signs, consider a more long-lasting occlusion method for the superior puncta or canaliculi. If bothersome epiphora is reported during the second diagnostic test, superior occlusion is not advised.

6.9.6 Most common errors

1. Failure to use an adequate size or sufficient number of collagen implants to produce a positive response.

2. Dilating the puncta unnecessarily. This may cause subsequent plug reflux back out of the system before they can imbibe water and lodge in the canaliculi. Dilation of the puncta

may be necessary, however, if the punctal openings are too small to take a reasonable sized collagen plug or in the event of a presumed false negative first trial.

6.10 JONES 1 AND 2 AND ASSOCIATED TESTS

The Jones 1 and 2 tests and the associated tests of dye disappearance and dilation and irrigation are assessment tools for the lacrimal drainage system. The dye disappearance test and/or the Jones 1 test help to determine whether there is a stenosis or blockage of the nasolacrimal system. If they suggest a stenosis or blockage, then dilation and irrigation (D&I) of the system is indicated. Contraindications for dilation and irrigation include symptoms and signs of canaliculitis and dacryocystitis (including regurgitation of discharge from the punctum). Lacrimal sac palpation may help to determine if dilation and irrigation of the system is contraindicated. D&I itself may dislodge a concretion or mucous plug that has blocked the canaliculus. In this respect it is a therapeutic procedure. However, it is also a diagnostic procedure in that it helps to determine if the system is patent. Jones 2 testing is rarely recommended and is considered only if dilation and irrigation is unsuccessful and if differentiation of the site of the blockage is important (i.e. if the blockage is an upper system blockage (e.g. canaliculi) or a lower system blockage (e.g. lacrimal sac or duct)).

6.10.1 Nasolacrimal stenosis or blockage

Many patients complain of excess tearing. True nasolacrimal system obstruction (epiphora) must be differentiated from reflex tearing associated with conditions such as dry eye. Obstruction may occur anywhere in the pathway from the ocular surface to the nose (Fig. 6.48). The most common locations include the punctum, the vertical or horizontal canaliculus, the common canaliculus and the nasolacrimal duct. The latter two listed are more likely to cause significant tearing as they affect overall drainage, whereas a single punctum or canaliculus will reduce outflow through one of the two channels

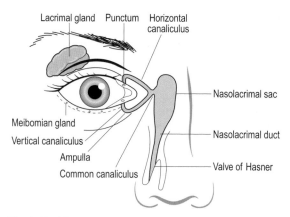

Fig. 6.48 The anatomy of the nasolacrimal system.

but will not impede it completely. If nasolacrimal system obstruction is suspected, an assessment of the lacrimal drainage system is required.

6.10.2 Advantages and disadvantages

The Jones 1 and dye disappearance testing allow the clinician to observe the patient while the dye is on the ocular surface. The blink dynamics (including completeness of lid closure and blink frequency) and tear drainage (dye disappearance or overflow) can be observed. Jones 1 is frequently noted to have false results; that is, no dye is recovered in the nose yet the clinician is suspicious that the system is patent. In this case, the observations of the patient can corroborate or refute the Jones 1 results and help to determine if dilation and irrigation is indicated. Though dilation and irrigation is considered to be well tolerated by patients and a relatively easy procedure to master, it is generally agreed that procedures should not be undertaken on patients if there is no clear indication or expected outcome.

Jones 2 testing is more difficult to perform than traditional dilation and irrigation as the patient's head must be dropped forward instead of reclined back in order that the effluent from the irrigation may be collected. This poses challenges for the clinician to irrigate the nasolacrimal system with impeded access and view of the lacrimal anatomy. Many clinicians feel that the differentiation between an upper and lower system blockage may be academic. This is because referral must be considered with a blockage in either the upper system (lacrimal anatomy) or the lower system (nasal anatomy) in a symptomatic patient. Generally, the referral is made to a surgical ophthalmologist with experience in the lacrimal system and dacryocytorhinostomy procedures. Alternatively, if a problem is suspected in the lower system, especially with a history of nasal trauma or chronic sinus problems, consideration can be given to referral to an ear, nose and throat specialist.

Generally, the procedures are well tolerated. The clinician must be careful to follow the anatomical structure of the patient's canaliculus or discomfort will be noted with advancement of the dilator and/or cannula. Specifically, if any instrument is advanced more than 2 mm into the vertical canaliculus, the lids must be pulled laterally to straighten the vertical and horizontal canaliculi, and the instrument must be angled towards the location of the common canaliculus at the nasal canthus. Small puncta pose a greater challenge as these need to be dilated more vigorously in order to allow for the entry of the 23-gauge cannula. Similarly, some patients have rapid closure of the puncta after dilation such that the irrigation cannula cannot be inserted. The puncta in such patients also may require repeated and slightly more vigorous dilation. The clinician may consider reapplying the pledget soaked with anaesthetic to the punctum after repeated attempts and when the patient is noting discomfort. The patient should be counselled not to jump forward when fluid is noted in the back of the throat. A swallowing reflex will be noted and some patients react by straightening their head forward. Finally, a bad taste is noted by some patients when the saline is irrigated through. A lozenge or candy usually helps to eliminate this taste promptly.

6.10.3 Procedures

For all procedures:

1. Try to assess if the tearing is due to a nasolacrimal obstruction or eyelid abnormality such as ectropion or entropion or due to paradoxical reflex tearing from a dry eye or other ocular surface problem (intermittent tearing). Ask about any history of facial trauma and/or nasal surgery.

2. Explain the procedure and obtain informed consent. Encourage the patient to blink normally and not to squeeze the eyes during the procedure(s).

3. Ask the patient to blow their nose and clean it thoroughly with tissues.

Fluorescein dye disappearance test

1. Instil equal amounts of fluorescein in each eye and observe the patient for 5 minutes.

2. Compare the relative heights of the tear meniscus at the inferior margin of each eye and the degree of fluorescein spilling over the patient's eyelids.

3. Do not allow the patient to blot the fluorescein as this might draw an excessive amount of fluorescein and tears out of the conjunctival sac. Wipe away any excess fluorescein dye which has spilled onto the patient's cheek to avoid unnecessarily staining the skin.

Jones 1 or primary dye test

1. Moisten two to four fluorescein strips with sterile saline and touch to the inferior nasal palpebral conjunctiva, introducing a large amount of dye and fluid into the conjunctival sac. False negative test results are more likely if insufficient dye is applied (Tucker & Codere 1994).

2. Allow the patient to blink normally for 5 minutes. Again, ensure that fluorescein dye does not remain in contact with the facial skin long enough to dry.

3. Note that the dye disappearance test may be undertaken simultaneously with the Jones 1 test by observing the dye distribution and disappearance characteristics.

4. Instruct the patient to occlude the nostril on the unaffected side (if tearing problem is unilateral) or one nostril at a time (if tearing problem is bilateral) and blow into a white tissue.

5. Inspect the tissue for fluorescein using a Burton lamp or the cobalt blue light on the slit-lamp biomicroscope.

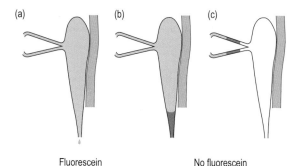

(a)   (b)   (c)

Fluorescein   No fluorescein

Fig. 6.49 Jones 1 test. (a) Fluorescein is recovered, indicating that the system is patent. (b) and (c) The absence of fluorescein indicates a blockage or stenosis in the system and the need for dilation and irrigation; (b) shows a lower system blockage and (c) an upper system blockage.

6. If no fluorescein is detected and especially if the dye was noted to have cleared from the eye other than over the lids onto the face, a false result may have been noted. Consider repeating the test or ask the patient to roll a sterile swab about 1 cm into the nose against the inferior turbinate. Check the swab for fluorescein with the cobalt blue light.

7. If *fluorescein is recovered* (Fig. 6.49a) no further tests are required as the nasolacrimal system is patent. Reflex tearing from dry eye and other causes should be reconsidered. D&I may still be considered if it is thought that there may be a partial blockage that might be relieved with irrigation.

8. If *no fluorescein is recovered* (Fig. 6.49b,c), there is either some degree of blockage of the drainage, a failure of the lacrimal pump mechanism, or a false negative result was obtained.

9. Consider dilating the punctum on the affected side and repeating steps (1) to (5). If fluorescein is now recovered, the source of the poor drainage was likely stenosis of the punctum.

Dilation and irrigation (D&I)

D&I is generally undertaken if no fluorescein is recovered with the Jones 1 test.

1. Prepare the instruments with appropriate disinfection of internal and external surfaces.

   Attach a reinforced 23 gauge cannula to a 3, 5, or 10 cc syringe.

2. Fill the syringe with 3 to 5 cc sterile saline. Push most of the saline through the cannula to thoroughly rinse the disinfectant, reserving approximately 1 cc for irrigation.

Dilation

3. Anaesthetise the superior and inferior puncta with a cotton-tipped applicator soaked with anaesthetic (e.g. proparacaine). Have the patient open his or her eyes. Pull the lower eyelid out of apposition with the globe and place the soaked pledget firmly on the inferior punctum. Have the patient close his or her eyes for several minutes over the soaked bud such that both puncta come into contact with the applicator.

4. Recline the patient slightly in the chair, and direct their gaze out and away from the canaliculus being dilated/irrigated. For example, have the patient look superior temporally to irrigate the inferior system. Use a magnifying lens (loupe) if necessary.

5. Pull the inferior eyelid away from the globe and place a long-tapered dilator vertically into the inferior punctal opening (<2 mm).

6. If the punctum is tight around the dilator, gently roll the dilator back and forth between your fingers to begin to dilate the punctum.

7. Once the dilator is inserted 1–2 mm, advance the dilator a little further while pulling laterally on the eyelid to straighten out the canaliculus. Continue to roll the dilator back and forth while directing the tip of the dilator nasally towards the location of the opening into the common canaliculus. Whitening of the punctal ring indicates expansion of the opening. Do not force the dilator too deeply into the canaliculus and retract if resistance is encountered or the patient experiences significant discomfort or a sharp pain.

8. If the punctum is not sufficiently enlarged or closes down before the cannula can be inserted, dilate again with the long tapered dilator and gently advance it further, again

respecting the anatomy and the patient's comfort.

9. The primary dye test (Jones 1) may be repeated after only punctal dilation; however, generally the clinician will proceed to irrigation.

Irrigation

10. Insert the cannula immediately after dilating the punctum. If the punctum cannot be opened sufficiently to insert the cannula, consider a smaller gauge cannula or a wider dilation of the punctum.

11. Pull the eyelid slightly away from the globe and insert the cannula 1–2 mm vertically then pull the eyelid taut laterally to continue 1 to 4 mm into the horizontal canaliculus, as with the dilator. If the cannula meets with gentle resistance, this is termed 'soft stop', and the cannula should not be advanced further as an obstruction exists in the canaliculus. The 'hard stop' position indicates that the cannula has come into contact with the nasal bone. This can only be achieved with a sufficiently long cannula to transverse the canaliculi and the lacrimal sac (>10 mm advancement).

12. Reach up with the thumb of the hand *not* holding the cannula/syringe. While watching carefully that the position of the cannula is maintained (i.e. that it is not inadvertently advanced further into the canaliculus), apply pressure to the plunger to introduce a small amount of saline (approximately 0.5 cc) into the system. Never force the fluid if resistance is encountered. If resistance is encountered, first withdraw the cannula and test that the cannula/syringe combination itself is not obstructed by pushing fluid through the syringe and cannula. Reintroduce the cannula.

13. Once a small amount of saline is introduced, the patient is asked to report when it is detected in the throat, at which time pressure on the plunger of the syringe is stopped and the cannula carefully withdrawn (go to step 15). Keep talking to the patient throughout the procedure to ensure that they remain still until the cannula is withdrawn safely.

14. If saline regurgitates from the canaliculus being irrigated, it is likely that this canaliculus is obstructed or stenosed.

15. If saline regurgitates from the contravertical punctum, a common canaliculus blockage should be suspected. Hold a sterile cotton-tipped applicator firmly on that punctum and try to irrigate again. Carefully withdraw the cannula.

16. Offer the patient a mint or lozenge as the saline can have an unpleasant taste for some patients.

Jones 2 test

1. Perform the Jones 2 test immediately following the Jones 1 test, after fluorescein has been instilled into the eye.

2. Incline the patient approximately 30 degrees.

3. Perform an irrigation of the nasolacrimal system and collect the effluent in a basin or tissue.

4. Inspect the effluent under blue light for the presence of fluorescein or other discharge.

6.10.4 Recording

Fluorescein dye disappearance: Record if the meniscus height is equal in each eye and if dye runs down over the patient's cheek or disappears into the nasolacrimal drainage system. Relative speed of disappearance between the eyes is also relevant. Take note of the completeness of the blink, including apposition of the puncta, and the lid position.

Jones 1: Record whether or not dye was recovered on each side. Note that some sources label the presence or recovery of dye as 'positive' and absence of dye as 'negative', so that a 'positive Jones 1 test' means that the system is patent. This is opposite to the usual convention of a positive test result being one that indicates a problem, so it is best to record whether or not dye is recovered in each test in order to avoid confusion, e.g. dye recovered in left nostril (left nasolacrimal system patent).

Dilation & Irrigation: Record whether or not the patient tasted salt or felt the solution in the throat. Also note if saline was regurgitated from the same canaliculus or from the contravertical canaliculus, e.g. saline detected in the throat after irrigation of left inferior canaliculus *or* saline regurgitation out of the same (inferior) canaliculus when irrigation attempted *or* saline regurgitation out of superior canaliculus when inferior canaliculus irrigated.

Jones 2: Record the presence or absence of fluorescein after the patient has expectorated into the basin or blown into a tissue. There are two possibilities:
  No dye recovered in effluent suggestive of an upper system blockage *or* dye recovered in effluent suggestive of a lower system blockage.

6.10.5 Interpretation

Fluorescein dye disappearance: Normally, the relative heights of the tear meniscus are equal in each eye and dye can be recovered from the nose when significant amounts are instilled into the eye. This indicates drainage system patency. If the heights are noted to be unequal, it implies that the eye with the larger meniscus may have impaired tear drainage. It is less likely that there is a unilateral poor meniscus due to dry eye or unilateral pseudoepiphora from reflex tearing from the dry eye. Most often the difference is representative of a difference in the drainage system patency between the two sides.

Jones 1: If fluorescein is recovered, no further tests are required as the nasolacrimal system is patent. However, some clinicians may consider dilation/irrigating if they feel there is a chance to dislodge a partial obstruction. If no dye is recovered, this indicates either a partial or full blockage in the system, a failure of the lacrimal pump mechanism, or it could be a false positive result. Insufficient fluorescein is the most likely cause of a false positive result (Tucker & Codere 1994). If mucopurulent effluent is recovered, canaliculitis or dacryocystitis should be suspected and irrigation should not be attempted during an active infection/inflammation phase.

Dilation & Irrigation: Normally fluid should exit from the system and be noted by the patient in the throat. A blocked system will offer resistance to fluid injection or cause regurgitation from the contravertical punctum. No fluid flow in the throat indicates a complete obstruction. Fluid subsequently noted in the throat indicates that the obstruction was relieved or there had been a partial obstruction or a stenosis.

Jones 2 test: No fluid flow from the nose indicates that a complete obstruction is present. As with D & I, if regurgitation occurs from the contravertical punctum, the blockage is likely within the common canaliculus or the valve of Rosenmüller. If fluorescein is noted in the collected effluent, this indicates that the puncta, canaliculi and pump are functioning normally but there is a partial obstruction in the lower system below the lacrimal sac. The obstruction was/is likely somewhere within the nasolacrimal duct. If clear fluid exits from the system, this indicates that no dye reached the nasolacrimal sac due to blockage at the punctum or canaliculi. If regurgitation of saline occurs from the ipsivertical punctum, the blockage is likely within the canaliculus being irrigated.

6.10.6 Most common errors

1) Instilling insufficient fluorescein (Tucker & Codere 1994) or making inadequate attempts to recover fluorescein for the Jones 1 test can lead to false results.

2) Not introducing the cannula quickly enough such that the punctum closes down after dilation, making it difficult to insert the cannula.

3) Failing to respect the anatomy of the canaliculi with the dilator/cannula during dilation/irrigation, leading to patient discomfort.

4) Failing to use sufficient anaesthetic to achieve adequate anaesthesia of the punctum in susceptible individuals prior to dilation and irrigation, leading to patient discomfort.

6.11 VAN HERICK ANGLE ASSESSMENT

The van Herick angle assessment provides an estimation of the anterior chamber angle depth and is commonly used as a safety precaution against inducing acute angle glaucoma when dilating a patient's pupils.

6.11.1 Anterior chamber angle depth estimation

The most common reason for estimating the anterior angle is as a safety precaution prior to dilating a patient's pupils. The risk of inducing angle closure glaucoma with a mydriatic is minimal, providing appropriate precautions are made. An estimation of the anterior chamber angle depth may also be used in patients who are taking systemic medication known to cause pupil dilation and possible angle closure. Anterior chamber angles in older, hyperopic patients are most likely to be small and liable to closure. Hyperopic eyes, being relatively small, tend to have smaller anterior angles while the larger, myopic eye tends to have larger anterior angles. The growth of the crystalline lens throughout life means that elderly patients are much more likely to have a small anterior angle and children typically have large anterior angles. For this reason, the simple shadow test (section 6.12) can alternatively be used to assess the anterior angle in young children prior to the use of a cycloplegic drug. Exceptions include if the child is a high hyperope or there is some other indication from the case history to suggest that the anterior angle could be narrow. Although some textbooks suggest that early cataract can lead to a thicker, swollen lens and narrower anterior angle (Grosvenor 2002), the research literature indicates that early age-related cataract, particularly anterior and posterior subcapsular cataracts, typically lead to a thinner lens and a wider anterior angle (e.g. Laursen & Fledelius 1973, Wong et al. 2003).

6.11.2 Advantages and disadvantages

The van Herick anterior angle assessment is a relatively quick and simple procedure and can be part of a routine assessment of the anterior eye using the slit-lamp biomicroscope. The superior angle is the narrowest and most susceptible to closure. Although the van Herick angle assessment is unable to assess the superior angle, in most cases

the technique is sufficient to indicate whether there is a danger of angle closure (Foster et al. 2000). Only if the angle appears narrow using this assessment is gonioscopy required to determine whether dilation is safe. The van Herick assessment is a conservative one in that many patients with a narrow angle as determined by the test can be safely dilated (Pandit & Taylor 2000).

6.11.3 Procedure

1. Seat the patient at the slit-lamp biomicroscope and set up the biomicroscope with magnification at the medium setting ($\approx$16 $\times$).

2. Explain the procedure to the patient and then ask them to look straight ahead.

3. Narrow the beam to an optic section (section 6.6.4, No. 2) with the illumination system at 60° temporal to the microscope. Because you have narrowed the beam, you may need to increase its brightness.

4. Move the illumination system temporally to the very edge of the temporal limbus, keeping the cornea in focus.

5. Judge the depth of the anterior chamber by the width of the optically clear space between the cornea and the iris. Compare this width to the width of the cornea (Fig. 6.50). Record the result using a ratio or van Herick's grading system described below.

6. In a patient with a narrow angle, you may wish to repeat the measurement on the nasal anterior chamber angle. You may have to rotate both the illumination and viewing systems (keeping them 60° apart) to ensure the illumination system avoids the patient's nose.

7. Repeat for the other eye.

6.11.4 Recording

Record the result as a ratio with the cornea being unity and the anterior chamber width being a fraction of the corneal width. Alternatively, van

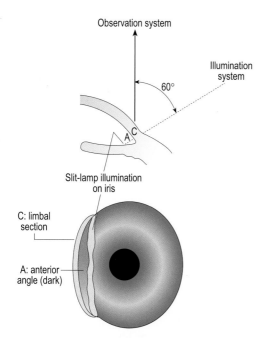

Fig. 6.50   Diagrammatic representation of van Herick's technique for anterior chamber estimation.

Table 6.2   Van Herick's anterior chamber angle grading system.

Van Herick grade	Cornea: anterior angle depth	Probability of angle closure
Grade 0	Closed	100%
Grade I	<1:1/4	Very likely
Grade II	1:1/4	Possible
Grade III	1:1/2	Unlikely
Grade IV	1:1 or greater	Impossible

Herick's grading system can be used (Table 6.2). If only one measurement is recorded, it can be assumed to be temporal. Examples:

van Herick. C/AC RE. 1:1, LE. 1:1.5.

van Herick. C/AC OD. 1: 0.5, OS. 1: 0.4.

van Herick. OD: IV, OS: III.

van Herick. RE: II T, III N. LE: III T & N.

6.11.5 Interpretation

The angle should normally be grade III or grade IV (Fig. 6.51). The prevalence of narrow angles of

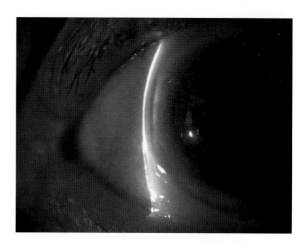

Fig. 6.51   A van Herick grade III anterior angle.

grade I and II is about 2%. If the angle is grade II or less, there is a risk of angle closure and the pupil should be dilated only if a gonioscopy examination indicates that it is safe to do so. Photographs of a range of anterior angle grades are shown on the website 🖳.

6.11.6 Most common errors

1. Failure to position the optical system as close to the limbus as possible. The measured angle will increase in size as you move away from the limbus.

2. Having the angle between the illumination system and the microscope less than 60°.

6.12 THE 'SHADOW TEST' ANGLE ESTIMATION

The shadow test provides an indication of the anterior chamber angle. A penlight positioned a few centimetres from the outer canthus and in the iris plane is shone onto the temporal iris. Narrow anterior angles have a bowed iris, so that the narrower the angle, the more the nasal iris is in shadow (Fig. 6.52).

6.12.1 Anterior chamber angle depth estimation

The most common reason for estimating the anterior angle is as a safety precaution against inducing

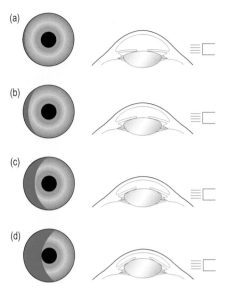

Fig. 6.52 The pen light test for anterior angle estimation. The pen light illuminates various amounts of the nasal iris depending on the size of the anterior angle. (a) Grade IV, (b) Grade III, (c) Grade II, (d) Grade I.

acute angle glaucoma when dilating a patient's pupils. The angle depth information should be considered in conjunction with the presence of any symptoms or signs of angle closure glaucoma and any family history of the disease. It is the growth of the lens throughout life that is a major cause of narrow anterior angles, so that most children have wide anterior angles. For this reason, the simple shadow test is sometimes used to assess the anterior angle in children prior to the use of a cycloplegic drug. Exceptions include where the child is a high hyperope or there is some other indication from the case history to suggest that the anterior angle could be narrow.

6.12.2 Advantages and disadvantages

This procedure is very quick and simple and is useful when a biomicroscope is not available or when a van Herick assessment may not be possible, such as with a patient in a wheelchair, or a young child. Most young children are very unlikely to have a narrow angle unless they are a high hyperope and the shadow test is ideal to use as a safety check prior to the use of a cycloplegic drug. It is unlikely to be as

Table 6.3 Anterior angle estimation by penlight grading system.

Penlight grade	% nasal iris in shadow	Probability of angle closure
Grade 0	100	100%
Grade I	75	Very likely
Grade II	50	Possible
Grade III	25	Unlikely
Grade IV	0	Impossible

accurate as van Herick's grading system with the biomicroscope.

6.12.3 Procedure

1. Dim the room lights and ask the patient to look straight ahead.

2. Hold a penlight a few cm from the outer canthus and at an angle of 100° temporally in the horizontal plane of the patient's right eye and rotate it round to 90°. The temporal side of the iris will illuminate.

3. Observe the nasal iris carefully and note how much of it is in shadow (Fig. 6.52).

4. Repeat with the left eye.

6.12.4 Recording

Grade the angle according to the percentage of the nasal iris that is in shade or use the equivalent grade (Table 6.3). For example:

Shadow test: 25% in shade RE & LE.

OD: grade IV. OS: grade III (shadow test).

6.12.5 Interpretation

See Table 6.3.

6.12.6 Most common error

Improper penlight position.

6.13 GONIOSCOPY WITH THE GOLDMANN 3-MIRROR (UNIVERSAL) LENS

Light from the anterior chamber angle is totally internally reflected by the cornea, so that the angle cannot be viewed directly. The most commonly used gonioscope lens, the Goldmann 3-mirror Universal lens (Fig. 6.53), uses a high minus contact lens to neutralise the power of the cornea and an appropriately angled mirror to allow examination of the anterior chamber angle. The Universal lens also contains two additional mirrors angled for evaluation of the peripheral and midperipheral fundus as well as a central lens for evaluation of the vitreous and posterior pole (section 6.24).

6.13.1 Gonioscopic examination of the anterior chamber angle

Gonioscopy is the standard procedure for examination of the anterior chamber angle. There is significant physiological variation between normal eyes with regard to the prominence of the various angle structures, including pigmentation. Therefore, gonioscopy should be performed frequently to be able to distinguish between normal and abnormal angle structures.

Specific indications for gonioscopy include:

- Narrow anterior chamber angles by van Herick (grade II or narrower) to assess the

relative risks for pupillary dilation. Gonioscopy is the gold standard technique against which screening tests for narrow angles are compared (e.g. Johnson & Foster 2005).

- Narrow (or closed) angle glaucoma including evaluation and documentation of peripheral anterior synechiae if present (Johnson & Foster 2005).

- Primary open angle glaucoma (POAG) and risk factors for POAG (e.g. elevated intraocular pressure) to confirm 'primary' diagnosis.

- Secondary open angle glaucoma and risk factors (e.g. pseudoexfoliation, pigment dispersion, chronic uveitis) to contribute to determination of disease severity.

- Risk of angle neovascularisation (e.g. confirmed rubeosis iridis, and ischaemic posterior segment conditions including vein or artery occlusions and diabetic retinopathy; e.g. Browning et al. 1998).

- Risk of angle recession post-blunt trauma.

- Risk of intraocular foreign body.

- Congenital or acquired structural irregularities of the iris and anomalies of the anterior chamber (e.g. iris cysts or tumours, ectopic pupil).

- Post-laser peripheral iridotomy to assess effect on angle depth.

Gonioscopy is contraindicated in patients who have experienced:

- Recent ocular trauma especially in the presence of hyphaema or microhyphaema.

- Recent intraocular surgery, including cataract surgery.

6.13.2 Advantages and disadvantages

Scleral-type lenses such as the Goldmann 3-mirror lens provide:

- Excellent optics and mirror placement allowing for the detection of subtle angle findings (e.g. early angle neovascularisation).

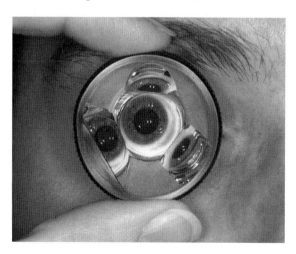

Fig. 6.53   A Goldmann 3-mirror Universal lens on the eye.

■ An undistorted view of the angle structures.

■ Excellent lens stability on the eye once inserted and good eyelid control even with a patient with blepharospasm.

■ No corneal disruption when a non-preserved coupling solution is used.

■ Better view in patients with significant loss of corneal transparency.

Disadvantages of the scleral-type lenses include:

■ Lens insertion may be more challenging to master.

■ A coupling solution is required. If a viscous preserved solution is used and not rinsed from the ocular surface, the corneal epithelium may be disrupted.

■ The thumbnail mirror must be rotated through 360° to visualise all angle quadrants (if the specific lens has only one mirror for gonioscopic assessment).

■ Compression gonioscopy cannot be undertaken with scleral-type lenses due to the area of contact with the ocular surface (see corneal-type lenses, section 6.14).

6.13.3 Procedure

A concise summary of the procedure is provided in Box 6.1.

1. Describe the specific indications for gonioscopic assessment to the patient and outline the procedure: 'I would like to use a contact lens on the front of your eye to examine the hidden part of the front of your eye. I will be putting a drop in your eyes to numb the cornea, so do not rub your eyes for at least half an hour or you could scratch your eye without feeling it.' Obtain informed consent.

2. Lens preparation: Clean and disinfect the gonioscopy lens. Fill approximately two-thirds of the concave lens surface with a viscous coupling solution, ensuring no bubbles remain to interfere with the view. These solutions provide good contact suction

Box 6.1 Summary of gonioscopy procedure

1. Disinfect the lens and fill the lens surface with viscous coupling solution.
2. Anaesthetise both eyes.
3. Align the biomicroscope illumination and observation systems. Set the magnification and the rheostat to low settings.
4. Insert the lens and (for Goldmann 3-mirror) wipe away excess solution.
5. Rotate the Goldmann 3-mirror lens through 360° to establish a good seal.
6. Place the thumbnail mirror at 12 o'clock on the cornea to view the inferior angle first.
7. Identify the *most posterior structure* observable.
8. Position the slit-beam horizontally to view the nasal and temporal sides.
9. Examine all quadrants (through 360°) in a systematic manner.
10. Remove the lens by simply releasing from contact with the cornea.

on the eye. Carboxymethylcellulose has been recommended (Nguyen et al. 1996).

3. Anaesthetise both eyes. Gonioscopy can be performed immediately following applanation tonometry so that additional anaesthetic is not necessarily required. Fluorescein does not interfere with the examination.

4. Position the patient comfortably at the biomicroscope and ensure the eye is aligned with the lateral canthal marker on the slit-lamp so that the chin rest need not be adjusted while the lens is on the eye. Consider using the lens case under your elbow or hook your little finger over the headrest bar of the biomicroscope to promote stability of the lens. This prevents unwanted force against the patient's eye.

5. Align the illumination system to be co-axial with the viewing system, set the magnification to a low power (e.g. 10×), and the rheostat to low or medium intensity. Pull the biomicroscope back toward you.

6. **Lens Insertion:** A video clip on the website illustrates the lens insertion technique .

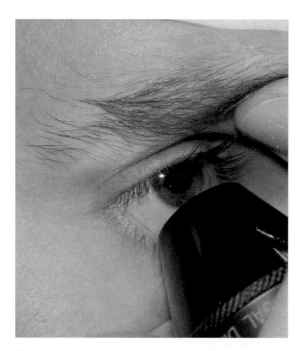

Fig. 6.54   Inserting the Goldmann 3-mirror contact lens.

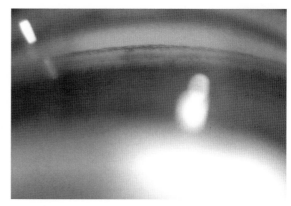

Fig. 6.55   A wide open angle of a brown iris (Asian). There is pigment on Schwalbe's line (Sampaolesi's line); iris processes overlying the ciliary body; mild pigment in the posterior trabecular meshwork and the reddish tinge is blood reflux through Schlemm's canal.

Move the microscope off to the side or reach around the microscope to insert the lens. Advise the patient that pressure and a turning feeling may be detected with the lens in place, but that there will be no discomfort. Instruct the patient to look up. Eyelid control is usually required to ensure the lens is properly inserted in one attempt. One method is to hold the eyelashes of the upper eyelids tightly against the orbital rim with the thumb, then pull the lower eyelid down and away from the globe and introduce the rim of the lens over the lower eyelid margin. Use the lens edge to pull down the lower eyelid further, while simultaneously and quickly rotating the lens upwards onto the eye (Fig. 6.54). Once the lens is on the eye, ask the patient to *slowly* look straight ahead. Keep the flat front surface perpendicular to the line of sight. If air bubbles are present, apply a little pressure and gently rock the lens to see if they can be removed. The angle can often be viewed around air bubbles, but if they remain a significant problem with the view, remove and re-insert the lens. Consider manipulating the lens through a couple of rotations with both hands to

establish the lens seal and enable smooth rotation of the lens while observing the various angle quadrants. Wipe excess solution that may have dripped onto the patient's cheek.

7. **Examination/ Observation procedure:** For examination, it is preferable to hold the lens with the left hand when examining the right eye and vice versa for the left eye. Either two hands can be used to rotate the lens to view all four quadrants, or one hand can be used with stabilisation of the lens between rotations with the middle finger.

8. Start with a vertical parallelepiped beam 1–3 mm wide. Keep the illumination moderate to reduce pupillary constriction that may decrease the perceived width of the angle and prevent patient discomfort.

9. Start with the thumbnail mirror placed in the 12 o'clock position to enable a view of the inferior angle first. The inferior quadrant is usually the widest and most pigmented, making it easier to identify the various structures.

10. In normal angles, look for the prominently discernible pigmented posterior structure, the ciliary body (CB) band, and identify the adjacent angle structures from posterior through to anterior (section 6.13.6, Fig. 6.55).

Identify the most posterior structure observable and note any abnormal findings.

11. When the ciliary body band is less visible or is not visible at all, such as with a narrow angle, with unusual pigment patterns or when peripheral anterior synechiae or neovascularisation obscure or distort the angle, use the **focal line technique** to identify Schwalbe's line (section 6.13.6), which is the last (most anterior) structure visible in a progressively narrow angle. Use a very bright optic section at a 20° angle with the mirror in the 12 o'clock position. Two separate beams representing the anterior and posterior surfaces of the cornea will be observed in the domed cornea above the angle. These two beams will collapse into one beam in the angle at Schwalbe's line. All other structures can be identified posteriorly from Schwalbe's line. This technique can also be used with the thumbnail mirror in the 6 o'clock position (superior angle examination), but it is usually not necessary if the clinician follows the structural variations through the examination of all 360° of the angle.

12. The **convex iris technique** can be used to help identify the most posterior angle structure observable before the iris inserts into the angle (section 6.13.4).

13. Use both hands and rotate the lens by 90° to observe the nasal or temporal angle. Use one hand to hold the lens to maintain contact with the eye and use the other hand to rotate the lens. The lateral angles may be more easily viewed when the slit beam is rotated horizontally.

14. Examine all quadrants (through 360°) in a systematic manner.

15. Lens removal: Instruct the patient to look toward the nose and blink forcefully (the strongest eyelid force is nasally), while simultaneously applying digital pressure through the inferior eyelid on the temporal side of the globe to introduce air beneath the lens. A popping sound may be heard as the lens releases from the eye. Repeat with more pressure temporally if the first attempt fails

to release the lens. Do not use a pulling force to remove the lens. Consider lavage of the superior and inferior cul-de-sacs with irrigating solution (or saline) if viscous, preserved coupling solution was used.

16. Always examine both eyes as relative comparison of angle structures between eyes and quadrants is important.

6.13.4 Additional examination technique: the convex iris technique

Effective gonioscopy is dynamic, requiring subtle variations in technique to observe the angles thoroughly. The convex iris technique involves changing the angle of the gonioscopy lens relative to the angle being viewed in order to visualise the otherwise obscured angle details in an eye with a shallow anterior chamber and narrow angle. This involves tilting the lens into the quadrant to be examined and/or having the patient look toward the position of the thumbnail mirror. The light from the angle can then vault over the anteriorly bowed iris to the mirror and allow the more posterior structures of the angle to be visualised. With a scleral-type lens, it is generally best to have the patient look towards the mirror (i.e. for examining the inferior angle with the mirror placed at 12 o'clock, ask the patient to look up while maintaining the seal of the lens on the eye). However, the view may still not be optimal and the lens may also need to be tilted away from the mirror being used. For *corneal*-type lenses, less movement is needed to facilitate the view into the angle as the mirrors are placed closer to the apex of the cornea. Less eye movement by the patient and more lens manipulation is generally better. However, when observing very narrow angles, it may be necessary to both tilt the lens away from the mirror and have the patient look towards the mirror.

6.13.5 Recording

The most common reason for a gonioscopic assessment is to determine the relative openness of the anterior chamber angle. There are several published grading systems but the suggested method is to use an anatomically descriptive recording system, thus eliminating the discrepancies and controversies that exist between grading systems. The anterior chamber angle is widest inferiorly and is most narrow superiorly, with the nasal and temporal quadrants in between. All quadrants should be inspected and graded independently. Recording of observations should include the following:

- Most posterior angle structure observed (e.g. posterior trabecular meshwork)

- Angular approach at the recess (approximation, in degrees)

- Iris contour (e.g. 'flat', 'steep' or 'convex' in midperipheral iris as in narrow angles; 'convex at iris root' as in plateau iris; 'convex over entire iris' as in pupillary block; or 'concave' or 'posteriorly bowed' as in pigment dispersion).

Other matters to note include:

- Amount of pigment

- Presence of iris processes, angle recession, peripheral anterior synechiae (PAS), and normal and abnormal vasculature

- Other findings: lens cortex material, naevi and surgical alterations such as sclerectomy and peripheral iridotomy (PI)

- Whether or not lens tilt (convex iris technique) was required to observe the angle properly

- To what degree the angle opens with indentation (if relevant).

Common alternative grading systems include that of Shaefer which grades the angle by the estimate of the geometrical angle between the iris and angle wall at the recess. This system most closely correlates with the van Herick angle estimation method. Grades III to IV are widely open angles of 30–40°. In both the van Herick and Shaefer systems, angles designated grade II (20°) or less are considered capable of closure. Grade 0 angles are considered closed. The Spaeth grading system uses three criteria to describe the angle. The angle is initially described in a similar way to the Shaefer system but in degrees. The peripheral iris contour is then described as being either regular (r), steep (s), or

concave (q for queer). Finally the site of iris insertion is described anatomically.

In addition to grading and describing the angle, the trabecular meshwork can be graded with respect to the degree of pigmentation. The scale is somewhat arbitrary but convention describes 0 as no pigment, 1 as trace, 2 as mild, 3 as moderate, and 4 as dense pigment deposition. The absence of pigment (grade 0) makes the angle assessment difficult as the various structures are highlighted with pigment. The focal line technique helps to delineate the faint Schwalbe's line and therefore to help determine the most posterior structure.

6.13.6 Interpretation

The website includes photographs of anterior angles with interpretation 🖱. With the mirror in the 12 o'clock position and when examining the angle in the right aspect of the mirror (i.e. 1 o'clock), the view is of the 5 o'clock position of the angle (not the 7 o'clock position). Examination of the wider inferior angle first facilitates the identification of the various structures. It is useful to approach the angle evaluation from an anterior to posterior direction as all structures are not always present:

Schwalbe's line (SL)

This is the most anterior structure of the angle and is a demarcation line marking the termination of the transparent cornea at Descemet's membrane. It is a very narrow, usually white or translucent line and is not always prominent. Sampaolesi's line is the term applied to a pigmented Schwalbe's line. It appears as pigment deposited in a wavy discontinuous fashion anterior to Schwalbe's line and is a feature of pseudoexfoliation and pigment dispersion syndromes.

Trabecular meshwork (TM)

The trabecular meshwork or trabeculum has a translucent appearance and is frequently dull grey or brown in appearance. The anterior portion of the trabecular meshwork (ATM) is usually less pigmented and is considered the non-filtering portion of the meshwork. The more posterior portion of the trabecular meshwork (PTM) overlies the Schlemm's canal and is more active in the drainage process. The posterior trabecular meshwork is pigmented and may accumulate pigment with age and in specific eye disease such as pigment dispersion and pseudoexfoliation syndromes. Trauma, uveitis and surgery are also causes of pigment deposition in the angle. It is advisable to grade the level of pigmentation in the angle, and it is usually noted that pigment deposits most heavily in the inferior quadrant. Schlemm's canal can be seen through the translucent meshwork only if blood is refluxed back into it from the venous system (Fig. 6.55). This occurs if excess pressure is applied with the gonioscope (usually a scleral-type lens) such that the pressure in the draining veins exceeds the intraocular pressure.

Scleral spur (SS)

The scleral spur is a slight protrusion of the white sclera into the anterior chamber. The trabecular meshwork attaches anteriorly and the longitudinal muscle of the ciliary body posteriorly. The scleral spur becomes more visible when the ciliary body and trabeculum are pigmented. If the scleral spur appears unusually wide, angle recession may be present.

Ciliary body (CB)

The visible band of ciliary body represents the longitudinal muscle and may appear black, brown, grey, or have a mottled appearance. If visible, the angle is widely open. In lightly pigmented eyes, blood vessels can occasionally be observed running circumferentially in the ciliary body. The presence of a very wide ciliary body band along with a history of trauma may indicate angle recession. Iris processes are strands of the iris that are seen to project anteriorly onto the ciliary body or scleral spur and occasionally even more anteriorly on to the trabecular meshwork. These are found in approximately one-third of normal eyes.

Iris root

The iris root runs from the most posterior section of the iris and inserts onto the ciliary body. It can occasionally obscure the view of the ciliary body.

Other gonioscopic findings

Peripheral anterior synechiae (PAS) are adhesions formed between the iris tissue and the trabecular

meshwork or even Schwalbe's line. Their appearance is dependent on the aetiology of the adhesion. Angle closure PAS are usually found where the angle is narrowest, whereas inflammatory PAS are often located inferiorly due to the settling of inflammatory debris. PAS may be seen adjacent to surgical incisions, such as for cataract or glaucoma surgery or in association with posteriorly located laser burns following laser trabeculoplasty.

Neovascular growth may be preceded by rubeosis iridis at the pupillary ruff; however, neovascularisation of the angle may occur without neovascularisation of the iris. Early neovascular bridging vessels across the angle can be very difficult to detect. The risk of missing neovascularisation by not performing gonioscopy in patients with central retinal vein occlusion is about 10% (Browning et al. 1998).

6.13.7 Most common errors

1. Misinterpreting angle structures. A narrow angle is the most difficult to interpret.

2. Using too little solution in the lens, causing bubbles behind the lens, limiting the view of the angle.

3. Overfilling the lens, causing the excess solution to run over the patient's eyelid and onto the cheek, which can further impede subsequent attempts at lens insertion.

4. Inappropriate lens selection. A patient with a small interpalpebral fissure may require a smaller lens size or corneal lens type.

5. Using excessive pressure on the lens. This may cause discomfort for the patient and can often be identified by blood refluxing through Schlemm's canal, seen as a pinkish band in the posterior trabecular meshwork (Fig. 6.55).

6.14 GONIOSCOPY WITH CORNEAL-TYPE LENSES

All *corneal-type* lenses (e.g. Posner, Zeiss, Sussman, Fig. 6.56) have a smaller (9 mm) and flatter area of contact on the cornea as compared to the scleral-type lenses and have four mirrors, all of which are angled to allow examination of the anterior chamber angle. These lenses are used for the general

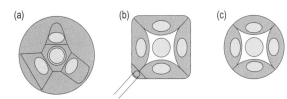

Fig. 6.56 Types of gonioscope lens (not to scale). (a) Goldmann 'Universal' 3-mirror. (b) Posner or Zeiss corneal lens with a handle. (c) Sussman corneal lens.

assessment of the anterior chamber angle and can be used quickly in the course of a regular primary care assessment.

6.14.1 Gonioscopic examination of the anterior chamber angle

Gonioscopy is the standard procedure for examination of the anterior chamber angle. There is significant physiological variation between normal eyes with regard to the prominence of the various angle structures, including pigmentation. Therefore, you should perform gonioscopy frequently to be able to distinguish between normal and abnormal angle structure. Specific indications and contraindications for gonioscopy are provided in section 6.13.1.

6.14.2 Advantages and disadvantages

Advantages include:

- Easy application of the lens onto the cornea of a cooperative patient thus facilitating a relatively quick assessment.
- Ability to perform dynamic gonioscopy.
- Essentially no lens rotation is required as all four mirrors are angled for gonioscopic assessment.
- Smaller, less concave surface enables gonioscopy without need for a viscous coupling solution.
- Corneal compressions may be undertaken to differentiate appositional from synechial angle closure (Note: *corneal*-type lenses may

also be used to therapeutically relieve appositional closure).

Disadvantages include:

- Image quality is somewhat poorer than with *scleral*-type lenses so observation of subtleties such as angle neovascularisation may be more difficult.
- The image may be more transient as the tear film seal is disrupted easily if the lens is not maintained on the central cornea (poor stabilisation due to lens sliding or eye movement).
- The clinician may identify an artificially wider angle as pressure on the cornea causes the angle to appear to widen.
- External surface-coated mirrors may be damaged if the outside of the lens is scratched.
- Corneal epithelial disruption may occur if significant lens movement occurs on the corneal surface.

6.14.3 Procedure

1. Describe the specific indications for gonioscopic assessment to the patient and outline the procedure; for example, 'I would like to use a contact lens on the front of your eye to examine the structures which drain the fluid of the eye. I will be putting a drop in your eyes to numb the cornea, so do not rub your eyes for at least half an hour or you could scratch your eye without feeling it.'

2. Lens preparation: Clean and disinfect the gonioscopy lens. No solution is absolutely required; however, a drop of solution may improve the contact and facilitate maintenance of the contact and therefore the view. A drop of saline, artificial tear or viscous solution may be used.

3. Anaesthetise both eyes. Gonioscopy can be performed immediately following applanation tonometry so that additional

anaesthetic is not necessarily required. Fluorescein does not interfere with the examination.

4. Position the patient comfortably at the biomicroscope and ensure the patient is aligned properly with the lateral canthal marker so that the chin rest need not be adjusted while the lens is on the eye. Consider using the lens case under your elbow or hook your little finger over the headrest bar of the biomicroscope to promote stability of the lens. This prevents unwanted force against the patient's eye.

5. Align the illumination system to be co-axial with the viewing system, set the magnification to a low power (e.g. 10 ×), and the rheostat to low or medium intensity. Pull the biomicroscope back toward you.

6. Lens insertion. Before applying the lens, consider the orientation of the mirrors, especially with lenses with handles (Zeiss – Unger holder, Posner – one piece). Generally, the lens is applied with the handle superior- or inferior-temporally in a 'square' pattern (Fig. 6.56b), although a 'diamond' pattern is preferred by some clinicians. Advise the patient that the lens will be felt if the lids touch it but otherwise will not be uncomfortable.

7. It is preferable to hold the lens with the left hand when examining the right eye and vice versa for the left eye. Lens stability is critical so it is important to have good arm support.

8. Instruct the patient to hold their eyes widely and to look straight ahead (a specific target to fixate on is helpful). Pull the microscope back, and bring the lens in from the patient's temporal side. Rotate the lens quickly and directly onto the central cornea so that the flat front surface is perpendicular to the line of sight. At all times, hold the lens just barely in contact with the corneal surface such that the tear prism is maintained. Do not apply excessive pressure with the lens. A wrinkled appearance through the lens indicates that folds in Descemet's membrane are occurring due to too much pressure on the lens. Maintain the flat lens

perpendicular to the cornea to maintain the tear film seal, and reposition the lens on the centre of the cornea if sliding is noted or if the patient changes fixation.

9. Position the vertical slit-beam in the mirror placed in the 12 o'clock position to enable a view of the inferior angle first. The inferior quadrant is usually the widest and most pigmented, making it easier to identify the various structures.

10. In normal angles, look for the prominently discernible pigmented posterior structure, the ciliary body (CB) band, and identify the adjacent angle structures from posterior through to anterior (section 6.13.6). Identify the most posterior structure observable and note any abnormal findings.

11. When the ciliary body band is less visible or is not visible at all, such as with a narrow angle, with unusual pigment patterns or when peripheral anterior synechiae or neovascularisation obscure or distort the angle, use the focal line technique to identify Schwalbe's line (section 6.13.6), which is the last (most anterior) structure visible in a progressively narrow angle. Use a very bright optic section at a 20° angle with the mirror in the 12 o'clock position. Two separate beams representing the anterior and posterior surfaces of the cornea will be observed in the domed cornea above the angle. These two beams will collapse into one beam in the angle at Schwalbe's line.

12. The convex iris technique can be used to identify the most posterior angle structure observable before the iris inserts into the angle (section 6.13.4) and pressure gonioscopy can be used in narrow angles to ensure there are no peripheral anterior synechiae, and to differentiate appositional and synechial angle closure.

13. Rotate the slit beam horizontally and position the beam in the appropriate mirror to observe the nasal or temporal angle.

14. Examine all quadrants (through 360°) in a systematic manner.

15. Lens removal: Remove the lens by simply releasing from contact with the cornea. No

ocular lavage is required as no viscous, preserved coupling solution is used. Examine the cornea after the procedure to ensure the epithelium is intact.

16. Always examine both eyes as relative comparison of angle structures between eyes and quadrants is important.

6.14.4 Additional examination technique: the corneal compression technique

Effective gonioscopy is dynamic, requiring subtle variations in technique to observe the angles thoroughly. The corneal compression technique is also termed compression, pressure or indentation gonioscopy. This technique can be used to differentiate if an observed angle closure is appositional (i.e. the iris is in contact with the angle structures but is not adherent) or synechial (i.e. the iris is physically and irreversibly adherent to the angle). Pressure is applied with the four-mirror gonioscopic lens directly on the centre of the cornea forcing aqueous into the peripheral chamber and forcing the iris posteriorly. Pressure on an eye with an appositionally closed angle will cause the iris to pull away from the angle to reveal some angle structures, while a synechial angle closure will remain closed. Note that only a corneal-type gonioscopy lens may be used for pressure gonioscopy; pressure on a scleral-type lens will merely retro-displace the globe.

6.14.5 Recording

See section 6.13.5.

6.14.6 Interpretation

See section 6.13.6.

6.14.7 Most common errors

1. Misinterpreting angle structures. A narrow angle is the most difficult to interpret.

2. Using excessive pressure on the lens. Unintentional pressure gonioscopy with a *corneal* type lens will indent the cornea, causing folds in Descemet's membrane as well as falsely widening the angle.

6.15 GOLDMANN APPLIANATION TONOMETRY

Applanation tonometry is based on the Imbert–Fick law, which states that the intraocular pressure is equal to the tonometer weight divided by the applanated area. Strictly, the Imbert–Fick law is only true for a spherical container with a very thin, dry and perfectly flexible and elastic membrane. However, by careful design, applanation tonometers can be made to closely approximate the Imbert–Fick law for the usual range of intraocular pressures and corneal thicknesses encountered. The Goldmann applanation tonometer measures the force needed to flatten a 3.06 mm diameter circular area of the cornea to provide a measure of the pressure in the eye. An area of diameter between 3–4 mm was chosen as it was found that at such a diameter the surface tension attraction of the Goldmann probe was equal and opposite to the force required to counteract corneal rigidity for an average thickness cornea. The calibration of the instrument should be checked on a regular basis.

6.15.1 Intraocular pressure measurement

Although tonometry is now known to be a poor screening test for glaucoma compared to optic nerve head and visual field assessment, high intra-ocular pressure remains an important risk factor and tonometry provides useful additional information when used in conjunction with the other assessments (e.g. Harper & Reeves 1999). Routine tonometry helps to identify ocular hypertensive patients who should subsequently be monitored more closely. Tonometry must be performed in any patient with glaucoma or 'at risk' of glaucoma, e.g. suspicious discs, family history of glaucoma, central visual field defect, narrow anterior angles, etc.

6.15.2 Advantages and disadvantages

Goldmann has long been the gold standard for intraocular pressure (IOP) measurements and its accuracy is such that it is used to determine the validity of other tonometers. It does, however, have the disadvantage that it only provides valid measurements for corneas with near average thickness. For a very thick cornea, GAT tends to overestimate IOP, and for very thin corneas it underestimates IOP. For example, Johnson et al. (1978) reported details of a 17-year-old patient with GAT readings between 30 and 40 mmHg due to extremely thick corneas of 0.90 mm (compared to a normal average of 0.54 mm; Doughty & Zaman 2000) whose 'real' IOP was 11 mmHg. This inaccuracy of GAT has been known for some time (Ehlers et al. 1975), but has come to the fore since the findings of significant IOP reductions due to the corneal thinning induced for refractive surgery (Doughty & Zaman 2000). The influence of central corneal thickness on applanation IOP may lead to the classification of some normal subjects with thick corneas as ocular hypertensives (Brandt et al. 2001) and several reports have suggested that central corneal thickness should be measured in ocular hypertensives (Doughty & Zaman 2000, Johnson et al. 1978). Some reports have suggested that non-contact tonometry provides even higher IOP values than Goldmann tonometry in patients with thick corneas (Matsumoto et al. 2000, Tonnu et al. 2005). In addition, this effect could also mean that some patients diagnosed as having normal tension glaucoma using GAT may actually be patients with high IOP but a thin cornea (Emara et al. 1999). In this regard, a recent clinical note reports two cases of post-LASIK patients with steroid response progressing to end-stage glaucoma, and that the late detection may have been partly caused by unreliably low IOP after surgery (Shaikh et al. 2002). Attempts have been made to determine the relationship between corneal thickness and GAT to provide a validated correction factor, but there is wide disagreement among investigators (Herndon 2006). Another approach has been to discover alternative tonometers that are independent of corneal thickness. At present, the dynamic contour tonometer (Pascal tonometer) appears to be the most useful in this regard, in that it is independent of corneal thickness and has low intra- and interobserver variability (Herndon 2006, Kaufman et al. 2004).

6.15.3 Procedure

1. Make certain that the tonometer probe tip has been appropriately disinfected. Check the integrity of the cornea for any contraindications to performing the technique.

2. Explain the test to the patient and obtain informed consent. Ask about any sensitivity to the anaesthetic. For example: 'I am now going to measure the pressure in your eye, which is one of the tests for glaucoma. This involves putting a drop in your eye. Have you ever reacted badly to drops or an anaesthetic before at an optometrist's or dentist's office?'

3. Inform the patient that the drops will sting at first but that the stinging will disappear very quickly. Instil one drop of anaesthetic or anaesthetic/fluorescein solution in each of the patient's eyes (section 6.17). You may suggest that the patient closes their eyes as this can be more comfortable. Keep a tissue handy to dab the patient's tears subsequently. Allow approximately 30 seconds for the anaesthetic to work.

4. Position the patient comfortably at the slit-lamp, with their lateral canthus aligned with the marker on the headrest and with the patient's chin in the chin rest and forehead against the headrest.

5. If required, add a small amount of fluorescein to both conjunctivae. Fluorets can be wet with preserved saline or drop of the anaesthetic, although the pH of the anaesthetic will reduce the fluorescence of fluorescein. Insufficient fluorescein will result in poorly visible mires.

6. With the fluorescein in place, check for corneal staining prior to performing tonometry. Ensure there are no conditions that would contraindicate applanation tonometry, such as a serious corneal injury (this is likely to have been identified in the case history).

7. Insert the tonometer probe into the Goldmann tonometer and align the white line on the carrier with the 0°/180° line on the probe. Astigmatic corneas produce an error of 1 mmHg for every 4 D of corneal cylinder. To reduce this error, adjust the tonometer head to 43° from the flattest corneal meridian if the corneal cylinder is greater than 3 D. If astigmatism is with-the-rule or against-the-rule, the probe can be aligned with the red line on the probe carrier (at 43°).

8. Goldmann tonometry is a monocular technique. Position the Goldmann probe in front of the slit-lamp eyepiece that corresponds to your dominant eye. For example, if you are right eye dominant, insert the tonometer body into the right-hand hole on the slit-lamp tonometer plate, so that you will view the probe image through the right eyepiece.

9. Set the tonometer scale to an average setting of about 16 mmHg (1.6 g on the GAT scale), so that minimal movement of the tonometer scale is subsequently required. Use low (≈10 ×) to moderate (≈16 ×) magnification, turn the illumination system to 45°–60° to the temporal side of patient, and adjust the system to the widest beam and the cobalt blue filter. You may need to increase the slit-lamp illumination.

10. Adjust the biomicroscope to align the probe with the centre of the patient's cornea.

11. Encourage the patient to blink a few times, then to stare straight ahead.

12. Bring the probe toward the cornea. Corneal contact is signalled by either a green glow on the peripheral cornea when you are looking outside the instrument or by the appearance of two green arcs when you are looking into the eyepiece.

13. At first contact, two green hemispherical pools of fluorescein may be seen. These are caused by the tears filling in the gap between the cornea and the tonometer probe. If these are seen, move the probe very slightly further forward to applanate the

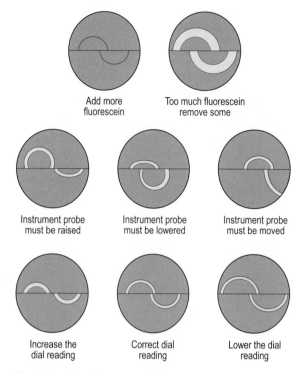

Add more fluorescein

Too much fluorescein remove some

Instrument probe must be raised

Instrument probe must be lowered

Instrument probe must be moved

Increase the dial reading

Correct dial reading

Lower the dial reading

Fig. 6.57   Possible appearances of the Goldmann applanation tonometry pattern.

cornea. The probe and its arm will then be seen to move backwards.

14. Determine whether you have the correct amount of fluorescein by assessing the diameter of the green arcs. Their thickness should be about 1/10 the size of the diameter of the arcs (Fig. 6.57). If the arcs are too thin, there is insufficient fluorescein and more should be instilled. If the arcs are too thick, a tear meniscus has formed around the outside of the probe and you should attempt to remove excess tears from the eye and probe using a tissue. This is a common problem in patients with a large tear volume and/or ectropion.

15. If the arcs can both be seen, but are not correctly positioned (Fig. 6.57), move the probe while it is still in contact with the cornea until the two green arcs are of equal size above and below the horizontal line of the probe beam splitter and are centred in your view (Fig. 6.57). Always move the probe towards the larger ring. If only one (or

neither) arc can be seen, remove the tonometer tip from corneal contact to make small adjustments to the position of the tonometer probe until both arcs can be seen.

16. It may be necessary to hold the superior eyelid if the patient is apprehensive and cannot hold their eyes open without blinking. Direct the patient to look downwards and then use your thumb to pin the upper eyelid against the supraorbital ridge. Alternatively, use the ring finger to immobilize the superior eyelid and the thumb to draw the lower eyelid downwards. Do not put pressure on the patient's globe as this will affect the intraocular pressure.

17. Adjust the tonometer scale until the inner edges of the green arcs are just touching, then remove the probe from the patient's eye. If a pulsation is perceived, adjust the scale such that the pulse centres on the correct alignment pattern.

18. Take the tonometry reading. The dial is calibrated in grams, with each gram being equivalent to 10 mmHg. A reading of 1.6 g therefore indicates an IOP of 16 mmHg.

19. Examine the cornea for unintentional damage. Examine the depth of any abrasion using an optical section technique (section 6.6.4 No. 2). Deep and/or extensive abrasions made by novices may need analgesic treatment and should be monitored.

20. Inform the patient not to rub their eyes and avoid dusty or windy environments for at least half an hour because of the anaesthetised cornea. Contact lens wearers must be warned to not wear their contact lenses for at least the same time period.

21. Disinfect the probe.

6.15.4 Alternative procedure: Perkins tonometry

1. The Perkins tonometer uses the same principle as the GAT, but is a hand-held

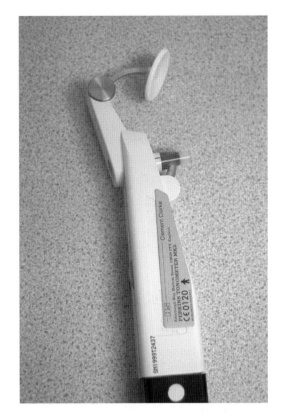

Fig. 6.58 A Perkins tonometer.

tonometer and does not require a slit-lamp biomicroscope (Fig. 6.58).

2. Its advantages are that it is portable, can be used on domiciliary (home) visits and being hand-held may be used with the patient either sitting up or lying down (note that the IOP will be higher when the patient is lying down). In addition, some patients are less apprehensive with this technique.

3. Its disadvantages include that it is less stable than the biomicroscope-mounted instrument, has a fixed low magnification for viewing the mires, does not allow for efficiently examining the cornea before and after the test as the patient is not already at the biomicroscope and it is easier to be off-axis and on the thicker peripheral cornea.

4. The procedure is the same as that with GAT, except for the setting up of the instrument.

5. Adjust the chair so that the patient is slightly below your eye level.

6. Instruct the patient to look at the duochrome or other target that fixes the eyes in a slightly elevated position looking towards the instrument.

7. Rest the instrument on the patient's forehead and pivot the instrument so that the probe can make contact with the centre of the cornea.

8. Hold the patient's eyelids apart if needed.

9. The remainder of the procedure is the same as for Goldmann tonometry. Contact time must be kept to a minimum as there is a greater possibility of abrasion with Perkins compared to GAT.

6.15.5 Recording

Record the tonometer readings for the right and left eyes on the right and left side respectively of a capital letter 'T'. Also indicate that you used a Goldmann or Perkins tonometer and the time of day (as intraocular pressure varies diurnally). For example:

$_{15}T_{16}$ – Goldmann – 11.30 a.m.;
$_{18}T_{16}$ – Perkins – 2.30 p.m.

6.15.6 Interpretation

The range of normal Goldmann IOPs is from 7 to 20 mmHg (mean of about 13 mmHg). However, note that Goldmann readings are influenced by central corneal thickness (Doughty & Zaman 2000) and provide a significant underestimation with corneal epithelial oedema (Whitacre & Stein 1993). Various systemic drugs can alter IOP, including systemic and topical steroid use that can significantly raise IOP in steroid 'responders' and beta-adrenergic blockers that can lower IOP. IOPs below 7 mmHg may suggest conditions such as retinal detachment, uveitis or wound leak. IOPs above 20 mmHg indicate ocular hypertension and may suggest glaucoma. However, note that patients can have primary open-angle glaucoma and have a normal IOP below 21 mmHg. The difference in IOP

between the two eyes should not exceed 4 mmHg. IOPs vary diurnally, with the highest IOP generally measured in the mornings. If a suspected glaucoma patient has a normal IOP in the afternoon, ask the patient to return on another day in the early morning, so that IOPs can be remeasured at that time.

6.15.7 Most common errors

1. Obtaining high IOPs because of patient apprehension. Describing the procedure to the patient in non-threatening terms can help.

2. Pressing on the globe while holding the eyelids open.

3. Taking a reading when a tear meniscus has formed around the probe leading to two thick tonometer arcs and an invalid, low pressure measurement.

4. Taking measurements with the patient having too tight a shirt collar.

5. Taking measurements with the patient holding their breath.

6. Repeating the applanation, which reduces IOP due to the tonographic effect.

6.16 NON-CONTACT TONOMETRY (NCT)

Non-contact tonometry also measures the force needed to flatten a small area of the cornea to provide a measure of the pressure in the eye. However, the cornea is flattened by a puff of air, so that there is no probe contact with the eye. The pressure of the air increases linearly over time and the instrument determines the time at which the corneal area is flattened and provides an IOP reading.

6.16.1 Intraocular pressure measurement

Although tonometry is now known to be a poor screening test for glaucoma compared to optic nerve head and visual field assessment, high intra-ocular pressure remains an important risk factor and tonometry provides useful additional information when used in conjunction with the other assessments (e.g. Harper & Reeves 1999). Routine tonometry helps to identify ocular hypertensive patients who should subsequently be monitored more closely. Tonometry must be performed in any patient with glaucoma or 'at risk' of glaucoma, e.g. suspicious discs, family history of glaucoma, central visual field defect, narrow anterior angles, etc.

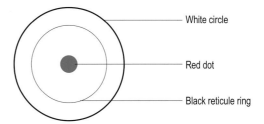

Fig. 6.59   The correct pattern observed through the eyepiece when the non-contact tonometer is in correct alignment and focus.

6.16.2 Advantages and disadvantages

Non-contact tonometry is easier to perform than Goldmann or Perkins tonometry, does not require corneal anaesthesia, and can be performed by trained clinical assistants. However, results are typically less reliable than GAT. A useful protocol may be to screen all patients who do not show any risk factors for glaucoma using NCT measurements taken by a clinical assistant and to repeat any measurements which are high, unequal or increased from previous visits using GAT. Any patient with glaucoma or any risk factors for glaucoma should have pressures measured by contact tonometry.

6.16.3 Procedure (for Reichart NCT)

1. Explain what you are going to do and why.

2. Seat the patient comfortably behind the machine and ask them to remove any spectacles.

3. Turn the instrument on and focus the eyepiece using the black graticule.

4. Turn the power switch to the demonstration position. Ask the patient to place a finger or hand in front of the instrument nozzle. Explain that you are going to demonstrate the air puff on their hand/finger, and then trigger the instrument. The demonstration also clears the air passage of dust, and allows you to check the machine's calibration reading. It should be 49 ± 1 (this will vary slightly depending on the instrument that is used). If it is not correctly calibrated, the machine should not be used.

5. Ask the patient to move forward and place their chin and forehead against the rests. If

proper head position has been obtained, a click should be heard. Align the patient's left canthus with the mark on the left upright support.

6. Ask the patient to close their eyes. With the safety lock raised, move the tonometer forward until the nozzle is about 1 cm from the eye. Lower the safety lock, making sure it clicks into place, and check that the tonometer stops at the correct location. Ask the patient to open their eyes.

7. Adjust the height and lateral position of the instrument so that the bright red spot from the instrument is positioned in the centre of the pupil and the patient should be able to see the red fixation light. If the patient has high ametropia and has difficulty viewing the target, a correction adjustment knob is available on the side of the instrument. If the patient has poor vision in the tested eye, use the fixation light in front of the fellow eye.

8. Move the focus in and out with the joystick, until the red dot in the white circle is in focus and inside the black reticule ring (Fig. 6.59). Press the button for a reading when the focus and alignment are correct. If the patient is not correctly aligned the instrument will not fire. If you are too far away from the patient's eye, the red dot may be seen in front of an undefined white area and may appear aligned to the novice. However, when the instrument is moved towards the patients eye, a donut shaped white ring and subsequently the alignment white circle will come into view.

9. If a reading of 99 is displayed, the patient blinked during the test. The override switch can be used if the patient is uncooperative and exact alignment is not possible. This should not be used unless it is necessary.

10. Repeat the reading at least three times for each eye.

6.16.4 Alternative procedure: Pulsair

The Pulsair is a portable (particularly recent versions), hand-held non-contact tonometer and may be used with the patient either sitting up or lying down (note that the IOP will be higher when the patient is lying down). It may be liable to a long-term drift in accuracy with use and regular re-calibration is recommended (Atkinson et al. 1992). In addition, some Pulsairs, perhaps needing adjustment, are extremely sensitive to the correct positioning and do not take a reading for long periods, leaving the optometrist or clinical assistant feeling frustrated.

The procedure is similar to the Reichart NCT except:

1. Have the patient seated comfortably in the examination chair.

2. Raise the chair so that the patient is slightly below your eye level.

3. Instruct the patient to look at a suitable target so that the patient's eyes are slightly elevated and looking towards the instrument.

4. Steady the tonometer by placing one hand on both the instrument and the patient's forehead and align the red corneal reflex with the centre of the eyepiece by direct observation.

5. Move the tonometer head to about 20 mm from the patient's cornea and directly along the visual axis. Instruct the patient to look at the red target light.

6. Look through the eyepiece and make appropriate adjustments based on the reflex seen (Fig. 6.60). The tonometer will take measurements automatically once the tonometer is correctly aligned.

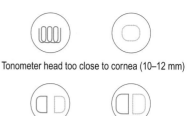

Tonometer head too close to cornea (10–12 mm)

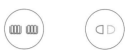

Tonometer head at correct distance from cornea (13–16 mm)

Tonometer head too far away from cornea (17–20 mm)

Fig. 6.60 Appearance of the reflex with the Pulsair tonometer.

7. Press the reset switch and take three readings (McCaghrey & Matthews 2001) and calculate an average (this is done automatically on the latest versions of the Pulsair).

8. If the IOP exceeds 30 mmHg, switch to the 30+ position and repeat the measurement.

6.16.5 Recording

Record the three tonometer readings for the right and left eyes on the right and left side respectively of a capital letter 'T'. Also indicate that you used a NCT or Pulsair tonometer and the time of day (as intraocular pressure varies diurnally). For example:

$$_{15,16,17}T_{16,14,17} - \text{NCT} - 11.30 \text{ a.m.;}$$
$$_{12,10,14}T_{16,10,12} - \text{Pulsair} - 2.30 \text{ p.m.}$$

6.16.6 Interpretation

The range of normal NCT IOPs is from 7 to 20 mmHg (mean of about 13 mmHg). There are several studies that have compared relative readings from the GAT with the other tonometers and these report slight differences that are model dependent. You should check the literature for information regarding the model type you have. It is important to regularly re-calibrate non-contact tonometers (Atkinson et al. 1992). Three readings are required to average the effects of the arterial pulse, which varies IOP by over 4 mmHg. Occasionally, successive readings can become lower due to the tonographic effect. If high, unequal or increased results are found, the pressure should be rechecked with GAT (section 6.15).

6.16.7 Most common errors

1. Obtaining high IOPs because of patient apprehension. Describing the procedure to the patient in non-threatening terms can help.

2. Not explaining the procedure and demonstrating it to the patient, so that he or she is unnecessarily startled.

3. Taking fewer than three readings on each eye.

4. Using the override switch on the NCT without taking the time to position and align the patient adequately.

5. Not checking the calibration of the NCT/Pulsair.

6.17 INSTILLATION OF DIAGNOSTIC DRUGS

6.17.1 What are the risks with diagnostic drugs?

Diagnostic drugs are available to the majority of optometrists and other primary eye care practitioners throughout the world. The three major types of diagnostic drugs available are anaesthetics, cycloplegics and mydriatics. Staining agents are discussed in the dry eye related sections 6.7 and 6.8. The advantages to be gained by using these drugs far outweigh the possible adverse ocular and systemic effects that rarely occur. For example, in a systematic review of published research between 1933 and 1999, Pandit & Taylor (2000) concluded that the risk of inducing acute glaucoma following mydriasis with tropicamide alone is close to zero, and the risk with long-acting or combined agents is between 1 in 3380 and 1 in 20 000. Mydriasis with tropicamide alone is safe even in patients with primary open-angle glaucoma. To compound this point, it should be noted that the most common cause of malpractice claims in the US is misdiagnosis of intraocular

disease, principally retinal detachment, open-angle glaucoma, and tumours. The great majority of claims alleging misdiagnosis involve optometrists who have failed to use diagnostic drugs for dilation of the pupil, with very few claims being due to adverse responses to ophthalmic drugs (Classé 1989). Of course, precautions must always be taken when using any of these drugs to ensure that the patient is at minimal risk.

6.17.2 Obtaining informed consent

1. Using lay terms, inform the patient about the technique you wish to use and the rationale for doing so.

2. Inform the patient whether the drops will sting, how long any side effects (e.g. near blur and photosensitivity with mydriatics) will last and the chances of an adverse reaction.

3. If you wish to use a mydriatic or cycloplegic, ask the patient whether they are going to operate heavy machinery or drive or perform a similar activity requiring good vision following the eye examination. Ideally, patients should be informed not to drive after the examination if possible and, if pupillary dilation is likely, it is good practice to advise patients to bring a driver with them or use alternative transport to get to the practice. Indeed, if pupillary dilation is routine, this advice can be provided to patients when they make the appointment and printed on their appointment card. If driving is their only option for transport home, allow sufficient time for them to adapt to a dilated pupillary state and recommend that they drive only on familiar roads. Commercially available paper sunglasses or attachments could be provided if it is sunny. If the patient has to operate heavy machinery or perform a similar possibly dangerous task, make another appointment for them when they can have their pupils dilated.

6.17.3 Safety checks

1. Case history/case history notes. If the following information is not included in your

initial case history notes, make sure you ask about them prior to instillation of the drops.

a) Does the patient report symptoms suggestive of angle closure?

b) Does the patient have any systemic or ocular disease that could be aggravated by the use of a diagnostic drug? For example, patients with angle closure glaucoma, with or without surgical or laser treatment, should be dilated with caution.

c) Does the patient have a systemic condition that could be aggravated by the instillation of a diagnostic drug? For example, one case highlighted the need to avoid hyperextending the neck of a child with Down's syndrome when instilling drops to prevent spinal cord injury (Nucci et al. 1996).

d) Has the patient been given similar drops before and did they have a reaction to them?

2. Visual acuity. Make sure that you record distance visual acuity before any procedure is carried out on the patient. If you have not already measured visual acuity, make sure that it is measured prior to instillation of the drops.

3. Anterior angle assessment. You should estimate the size of the anterior chamber angle before using any drug that has mydriatic effects. A van Herick assessment (section 6.11) may not be possible with some patients such as young children and a penlight shadow assessment of the angle (section 6.12) could be used. A grade II van Herick angle or less indicates an eye at risk of angle closure and gonioscopy (sections 6.13 and 6.14) should be performed to ensure that dilation is safe. If, during gonioscopy, half or less of the trabeculum is visible in all quadrants, there is a risk of angle closure. Do not use miotics after mydriasis as it is generally unnecessary and pilocarpine can even cause angle closure by producing a mid-dilated pupil (Mapstone 1977, Pandit & Taylor 2000). As indicated previously, the risk of inducing acute angle glaucoma using a mydriatic is very low. Indeed, some clinicians take the view that it is better for patients to have a mydriatic-induced angle closure in

their office/practice, where appropriate treatment can be provided, than in the patient's home. In situations where you dilate a pupil of a patient 'at risk' of angle closure, make sure that you obtain informed consent (Classé 1992), and be prepared to manage any subsequent angle closure. Angle closure is even less likely to occur with mydriasis due to a cycloplegic, as cycloplegia is generally used on a much younger population than mydriatics. The anterior angle is wider in children and young adults and gets smaller throughout adulthood due to the increase in size of the lens.

4. Slit-lamp examination. Prior to mydriatic instillation, check for the following: iris supported intraocular lens implant, synechiae, subluxated crystalline lens, dislocated intraocular lens implant, exfoliation or pigmentary glaucoma (dilation can significantly liberate pigment into the anterior chamber). If any of these conditions are found, avoid mydriasis if possible or proceed with great caution.

5. Assessment of the cornea. Determine the integrity of the cornea before any drops are instilled and after any procedure involving the cornea, such as contact tonometry or gonioscopy.

6.17.4 Choosing the appropriate drug and dosage

1. Case history/case history notes. If the following information is not included in your initial case history notes, make sure you ask about them to help you choose the appropriate drug and dosage.

a) Does the patient have any systemic or ocular disease that could be aggravated by the use of a diagnostic drug? For example, phenylephrine 10% should not be given to patients with severe cardiac disease, systemic hypertension and hypotension, insulin-dependent diabetes, aneurysms or advanced arteriosclerosis. Phenylephrine 2.5% should only be used with great caution in these patients. There have also been reports of similar problems after the use of hydroxyamphetamine hydrochloride 0.25% used in combination with tropicamide 0.25% (Gaynes 1998).

b) Does the patient have any systemic or ocular disease that could have an influence on the choice of a diagnostic drug? For example, it is often difficult to obtain satisfactory mydriasis in diabetic patients and they may require additional mydriatic drops and/or a combination of mydriatics drops (tropicamide 0.5% or 1% plus phenylephrine 2.5%). Patients with kidney disease can have unusually slow detoxification and elimination of ocular diagnostic drugs systemically absorbed and care should be given to use the lowest necessary dosage of the drug. Conversely, note that patients with a compromised corneal epithelium can have enhanced penetration of a diagnostic drug.

c) Is the patient taking systemic medication that could interact with a diagnostic drug? For example, phenylephrine should not be given (or given with great caution) if the patient is under medication with monoamine oxidase inhibitors or trycyclic antidepressants.

d) Has the patient had an allergic reaction to eye drops previously?

2. Iris colour. In general, patients with lighter irides will respond quicker and to a greater degree than those patients with dark irides. Therefore, give a higher drug dosage to a patient with dark irides and/or use a combination drug approach.

3. The drug(s) and dosage (concentration and number of drops) will depend on the procedure you are going to perform. You may even choose to use a combination drug procedure to provide the desired effect. For example, when greater dilation is required, such as when using head-band binocular indirect ophthalmoscopy, one drop of phenylephrine 2.5% and one drop of tropicamide 0.5% (or 1%) could be used.

4. Instilling a topical ocular anaesthetic prior to the use of a mydriatic or cycloplegic agent (one may have been used for contact tonometry)

results in an enhanced mydriatic/cycloplegic effect. The anaesthetic, as well as reducing possible discomfort, can reduce lacrimation and thus reduce drug washout for subsequently instilled drugs. It has also been suggested that the mildly toxic effects of a topical anaesthetic on the cornea opens up the intracellular spaces and aids penetration of other drugs.

5. In all cases, choose the drug with the least possible adverse effects and the lowest concentration that will allow you to efficiently attain the cycloplegia or mydriasis that you require. For example, research has suggested that cyclopentolate 1% is sufficient to produce good cycloplegia, with an effect similar to atropine 1%, in patients with accommodative esotropia (Celebi & Aykan 1999) and that tropicamide 1% is as effective as cyclopentolate 1% for the measurement of refractive error in most healthy, non-strabismic infants (Twelker & Mutti 2001).

6.17.5 Checks prior to instillation

1. Ensure that you have performed all the procedures prior to instillation of the diagnostic drug that would not be possible after it has been instilled. For example, make sure that you assess pupil reflexes, near muscle balance and accommodation prior to using a cycloplegic and tonometry prior to a mydriatic.

2. Carefully identify any drops before instillation by checking the brand name, ingredients, and expiration date and checking for discoloration and precipitates. If the expiration date has passed, or if there are precipitates, discoloration or other signs of contamination, the suspect container should be discarded and a new one obtained.

3. Before the instillation, record the drug type (preferably by its brand name) and dosage (concentration and number of drops used in each eye). The use of the brand name is useful since it uniquely identifies the particular preparation that has been used. Different

brands may well have different preservatives or other non-active ingredients.

4. Recheck the container of the diagnostic drug for its identity and remove the cap in preparation for drug instillation. If a dropper bottle is being used, do not place the dropper cap on any surface in such a way as to risk contaminating the inside of the bottle cap. It is best if you hold it in your hand.

6.17.6 Drug instillation procedure

1. The patient should be seated in a fixed chair with a proper back support and arm rests. There is a chance that upon instillation, the patient (especially a child) will move violently. Therefore do not use a stool or a chair on casters.

2. Ask the patient to tilt their head backwards with the chin raised slightly.

3. Gently pull down the lower eyelid or pull it forward slightly to form a pouch.

4. Instil a drop or drops into the temporal side of the pouch. Avoid touching the eyelashes, eyelids or conjunctiva with the dropper tip. Gently release the lower eyelid.

5. In the case of ointment, gently squeeze a 1.5 cm ribbon of ointment inside the lower fornix.

6. Ask the patient to look downward and gently release the upper eyelid over the eye.

7. Press firmly over the lacrimal sac (just medial to the inner canthus) for at least 10 seconds. Nasolacrimal occlusion prevents any excess drug entering the nasolacrimal duct, keeping systemic absorption to a minimum. Nasolacrimal occlusion is not required when an ointment is used. Make sure that you wipe any excess drops/ointment away from the eye with a tissue.

8. If two drops are to be used, wait at least 3 minutes between drops. Instilling two drops consecutively without this wait overfills the lacrimal lake and negates the theoretical effect of applying more drug.

6.17.7 Post-drug installation procedure

1. Return the cap to the bottle (and screw on securely) or dispose of single dose products such as Minims.

2. Anaesthetics: Inform the patient not to rub their eyes and avoid dusty or windy environments for at least half an hour after use of an anaesthetic. Contact lens wearers must be warned to not wear their contact lenses for at least the same time period.

3. Mydriasis: Measure intraocular pressure post-mydriasis for patients at risk of angle closure. A rise of more than 5 mmHg should be monitored until it returns to normal levels.

4. Provide commercially available paper sunglasses or attachments after mydriasis when necessary to avoid photophobia.

5. Use appropriate follow-up procedures and/or emergency care should any untoward reactions or sequelae occur. All these drugs (with the exception of tropicamide, for which no serious adverse effects have been recorded) can give rise to systemic effects such as altered mental states and increased heart rates. Patients may also faint. Note that an unwanted reaction such as a rise in IOP due to pupil block post-mydriasis can develop some hours later, and 'at risk' patients should be told whom to contact in case of an emergency.

6.17.8 Recording

Record the time, the number of drops instilled into each eye and the drug and its concentration. For example:
9.30 a.m.: 2 drops 0.5% tropicamide.

6.17.9 Most common errors

1. Instilling two drops consecutively without waiting for 3 minutes after the first drop.

2. Not checking drops carefully enough before instillation by forgetting to check the brand

name, ingredients, and/or expiration date and/or not checking for discoloration and precipitates.

3. Not using mydriatics because of a worry of inducing closed-angle glaucoma.

6.18 PUPIL LIGHT REFLEXES AND SWINGING FLASHLIGHT TEST

Observing the pupil reflexes as a light is shone into an eye (the direct reflex) and the fellow eye (consensual reflex) can indicate abnormalities affecting the afferent or efferent neurological pathways responsible for pupillary function. The swinging flashlight test (Levatin 1959) accentuates small defects in a unilateral direct pupil reflex that could otherwise easily be missed.

6.18.1 Pupillary function

Evaluation of pupillary function provides valuable information about the integrity and function of the iris, optic nerve, posterior visual pathways and the third and sympathetic nerves to the eye, and some of the conditions that cause pupil reflex abnormalities are life threatening. Afferent pupillary defects are caused by lesions in the 'front end' of the pupillary light reflex pathway and most commonly by lesions in the retina and optic nerve. The afferent pupillary pathways leave the visual pathways in the last third of the optic tracts to reach the pretectal nuclei (Fig. 6.61). Afferent pupillary defects do not cause anisocoria (different pupil sizes), but may produce abnormal pupillary light reflexes. Efferent pupillary defects produce anisocoria and are caused by lesions to the motor neurone system, which carries signals from the central nervous system to the iris via the third cranial nerve.

6.18.2 Advantages and disadvantages

These tests are quick and simple and can be performed without the need for any additional equipment. Pupil size should be assessed in both bright and dim illumination to investigate any anisocoria.

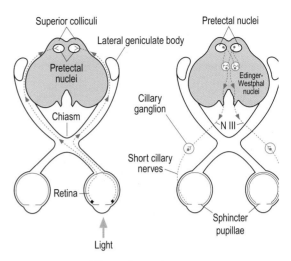

Fig. 6.61   The pupillary reflex pathway.

The swinging flashlight test (Levatin 1959) provides a sensitive assessment of any unilateral or asymmetric afferent defects, and has been shown to be superior to the Marcus Gunn test (redilation under sustained illumination) for detecting relative afferent pupillary defects (Enyedi et al. 1998). There is no condition in which the near reflex is defective or lost when the light reflex is normal. Therefore the near reflex need only be checked if the light reflex is abnormal. Patients can show an abnormal light and near pupil reflex or an abnormal light reflex with a normal near reflex (light–near dissociation).

6.18.3 Procedure

1. Ask the patient to take off their glasses, and look at a letter on the distance visual acuity chart that both eyes can see easily. If the worst monocular visual acuity is less than about 6/18 (20/60), ask the patient to look at a spot of light on the distance chart.

2. Sit in front and to the side of the patient, so that you can easily observe the patient's pupils, but you are not obscuring fixation of the target.

3. Keep the room lights on and check the size, shape and location of both pupils. Compare the

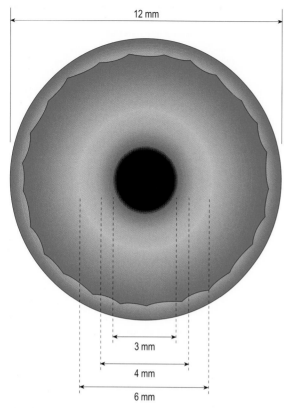

12 mm

3 mm

4 mm

6 mm

Fig. 6.62   The size of the pupil can be estimated using the iris as a 12 mm reference scale.

size of both pupils carefully. You can estimate the size of the pupil using the iris as an approximate 12 mm reference scale (Fig. 6.62).

4. If the pupil sizes are unequal in bright light conditions, measure the pupil sizes with a millimetre ruler or a hemisphere scale. In addition, dim the room lights but keep the light levels high enough so that you can clearly see the patient's pupils, and measure the size of the patient's pupils again. An ultraviolet lamp, such as a Burton lamp used for contact lens fitting, can be used with patients with dark irides as the lens fluoresces to allow pupil sizes to be measured.

5. Direct and consensual light reflexes:
    a) Ask the patient to keep fixating a letter or spotlight on the distance chart.
    b) Shine a penlight or direct ophthalmoscope into the right pupil from the inferior

temporal side from a distance of 5 to 10 cm. Observe the extent and speed of constriction of the right pupil (direct light reflex) and left pupil (consensual reflex). Remove the light and observe the direct and consensual dilation. Check this several times as dramatic fatigue can occur in an abnormal eye that at first shows a normal response.
    c) Shine the light into the left pupil from the inferior temporal side from a distance of 5 to 10 cm. Observe the extent and speed of constriction of the left pupil (direct light reflex) and right pupil (consensual reflex). Remove the light and observe the direct and consensual dilation. Check this several times.

6. Swinging flashlight test:
    a) Ask the patient to keep fixating a letter or spotlight on the distance chart.
    b) Shine a penlight or direct ophthalmoscope into the right eye from below the patient's eyes from a distance of 5 to 10 cm. Pause for 2–3 seconds and then quickly switch the light to shine into the left eye.
    c) Repeatedly alternate between the two eyes, pausing for 2–3 seconds on each eye, and look for any change in pupil size as the light is alternated.
    d) A normal response is that both pupils will constrict as the penlight is shone in one eye. As the light is moved off the eye on its way to the fellow eye, both pupils will dilate. As the light reaches the fellow eye, both pupils constrict. After the light has been shone on a pupil for 1–2 seconds, the pupils may redilate slightly, so it is important to observe the pupils at the instant the light first falls on them.
    e) An eye with a relative afferent pupillary defect (RAPD) will dilate as the eye is first turned upon it, as the consensual dilation response due to the light moving off the good eye overpowers the poor constriction response from the affected eye.
    f) The RAPD can be quantified by adding successively increasing neutral density filters to the 'good' eye, until a normal swinging flashlight response is seen.

7. Near reflex: This need only be measured if the light responses are abnormal or sluggish.
   a) Ask the patient to keep fixating a letter or spotlight on the distance chart.
   b) Ask the patient to then look at a target such as the patient's own thumb about 15 cm from his or her eyes.
   c) Observe the extent and speed of pupillary constriction as the patient changes fixation from distance to near.
   d) Ask the patient to look back at the distance target and observe the dilation as this occurs.

6.18.4 Recording

Pupil shape and size: record any irregularity in pupil shape and any anisocoria.

Pupil reflexes: a 0 to 4+ grading system can be used for direct (D) and consensual (C) reflexes, where 0 indicates no pupil response, 1+ (or +) indicates a very small, just visible response, 2+ (++) indicates a small, slow response, 3+ (+++) indicates a moderate response and 4+ (++++) indicates a brisk, large response typical of a healthy young patient. An alternative is to use the acronym PERRL (Pupils Equal Round and Respond to Light), but this does not differentiate between a just visible response and a large, brisk one. If the light reflex is abnormal, the near reflex must be checked. Some disorders produce an absent light reflex with a normal near reflex (light–near dissociation).

Also record the result of the swinging flashlight test as +ve RAPD (if an RAPD is indicated) or −ve RAPD (this indicates that there is no problem). If +ve RAPD is found, record which side was defective. If the defect is quantified using a neutral density filter, indicate the filter density in log units. Examples:

RE 6, LE 6. D & C 4+ R & L, −ve RAPD.

OD 4, OS 4. D & C 3+ R & L, +ve RAPD OD.

RE 6, LE 4 bright, 7/6 dim. RE D & C 1+, LE D & C 3+.

OD 5, OS 5. PERRL, −ve RAPD.

RE 5, LE 4 bright, 6/5 dim. PRRL, −ve RAPD.

OD 4, OS 4. PERRL, +ve RAPD LE, 0.3 ND filter.

6.18.5 Interpretation

Pupils are normally equal in size and typically vary from 3 to 6 mm in diameter in bright light to about 4 to 8 mm in dim light and show slight physiological fluctuations in size or hippus. The pupil gets smaller with age. Physiological anisocoria is seen in about 20% of normal patients and is generally the same in dim and bright illumination, usually small (<1 mm), shows normal pupil reflexes and has been present for years. If the diagnosis is in any doubt, this can be checked by asking the patient to bring in some old close-up photographs of themselves looking straight ahead. Pathological anisocoria is due to an abnormality in the efferent or motor pupil pathway. Anisocoria that is greatest in bright light will generally show an abnormal direct and consensual light reflex. This indicates a problem in the motor leg of the light reflex pathway, such as in the third nerve, ciliary ganglion (including Adie's tonic pupil) or iris, or could be drug induced.

An abnormal direct light response in a pupil capable of a normal consensual response indicates an afferent (visual pathway) defect. There is generally no anisocoria. The swinging flashlight provides a more sensitive assessment of any unilateral or asymmetric afferent defects. It compares each eye's direct response (reflecting the normality of its visual pathway) with its consensual response (reflecting the normality of the other eye's visual pathway). Symmetrical afferent defects do not show a positive RAPD. Some normal subjects may show a persistent but small RAPD in the absence of detectable pathologic disease. Therefore, an isolated RAPD in the range of 0.3 log unit that is not associated with any other significant historical or clinical finding should probably be considered benign (Kawasaki et al. 1996). Similarly, patients with unilateral cataract may show a RAPD in the non-cataractous eye that is not reflective of visual pathway disease (Lam & Thompson 1990).

6.18.6 Most common errors

1. Using too slow a swing in the swinging flashlight test.

2. Using too low a light level to observe the contralateral eye, especially with a darkly pigmented iris.

3. Forgetting to check pupil reflexes prior to instilling a mydriatic or cycloplegic.

4. Blocking the patient's view of the visual acuity chart and stimulating accommodation and subsequent pupil constriction.

6.19 INDIRECT FUNDUS BIOMICROSCOPY

Various direct and indirect techniques are available for the assessment of the posterior pole and the rest of the vitreous and fundus. Stereoscopic techniques are the clinical standard for fundus examination, and fundus biomicroscopy with a high plus lens is the standard for assessment of the posterior pole, including the disc, macula and vasculature. This indirect technique may also be used for peripheral assessment, and is often employed to enable a more magnified, stereoscopic view of small, peripheral lesions noted on general assessment with the head-band binocular indirect ophthalmoscope (section 6.22). Some clinicians use this modified technique for examination of the entire fundus, including the periphery.

6.19.1 Stereoscopic examination of the posterior pole

The traditional assessment of the fundus by direct ophthalmoscopy is inadequate not only because of the limited field of view but also because the view is strictly two-dimensional. For example, the neuroretinal rim tissue and the cup-to-disc ratio cannot be evaluated properly without stereoscopic observation of the depression of the cup in relation to the disc structure. Often the depression of the cup extends beyond the area of pallor and this is very difficult to detect without observing the disc stereoscopically (Varma et al. 1992). Therefore, the assessment of the cup-to-disc ratio with the direct ophthalmoscope, using monocular cues to attempt to determine depth and contour, can be considered an estimate only. 2-D digital fundus images also provide slightly smaller assessments of cup-to-disc ratio than fundus biomicroscopy (Hrynchak et al. 2003). In addition, non-stereoscopic assessment cannot consistently or accurately determine the presence

of more subtle elevations such as oedema of the retina or macula (Grey & Hart 1996).

6.19.2 Advantages and disadvantages

Advantages of fundus biomicroscopy for general assessment of the posterior pole of the fundus include (Table 6.4):

- Stereoscopic viewing is possible through dilated and undilated pupils. In addition to a more accurate assessment of the disc and macula region, this allows immediate assessment of any lesion/feature that requires stereoscopic examination.

- A larger field of view is available compared to direct ophthalmoscopy, even through an undilated pupil (Raasch 1982).

- The technique is dynamic and all parts of the fundus can be viewed with only minor cooperation from the patient.

- A superior view is obtained through media opacities as compared to direct ophthalmoscopy and this is particularly useful to assess the fundi behind cataract.

- Varied lens diameters and powers are available. The +90D or SuperPupil™ and other smaller, higher-powered lenses can facilitate examination when the pupil is undilated or otherwise small or provide a better field of view for examination of the peripheral retina. The Super66™ or +78D and other lower-powered lenses allow more magnification and better stereopsis for viewing details of the optic nerve, macula, and specific lesions.

- Variable magnification settings on the slit-lamp allow for varied viewing conditions with the same lens, and a very wide range of magnification options when various lenses are employed.

- The view is relatively independent of ametropia. This is particularly useful in moderate to high myopia, where the high magnification when using direct ophthalmoscopy can limit the field of view substantially. A better estimate of optic disc size can also be obtained. The slit-lamp beam

Table 6.4 Optical and observational characteristics of various fundus examination techniques.

Method	Image	Stereopsis?	Diameter (approx.) (mm)	Image mag.*	Mag. in slitlamp (16 ×)	Static field of view*	Extent of fundus visible†
Direct ophthalmoscope	Erect	No	N/A	15× ‡		~5°‡	To equator
Monocular indirect	Erect	No	N/A	5×		~12°	Beyond equator
SuperPupil™	Reversed and inverted	Yes. Detail in stereopsis improves with lower power (higher magnification); best with 'Super' series	15	0.45×	7×	Variable (generally higher with higher powered lenses)	Beyond equator (generally facilitated with higher powered lenses)
Super ViteroFundus™			25	0.57×	9×		
SuperField™			30.2	0.76×	12×		
Super66 Stereo Fundus Lens™			35	1.0×	15×		
+90 D			19	0.76×	12×		
+78 D			29	0.93×	14×		
+60 D			30	1.15×	18×		
BIO, +20 D	Reversed and inverted	Yes	48	3×	–	~45°	Entire retinal surface
Fundus contact lens	Reversed	Yes	–	Variable	Variable	–	Entire retinal surface

* Various manufacturers' claims.

† Through a dilated pupil, with direction of patient fixation to regions to be viewed and with manipulation of the slit-lamp.

‡ Varies with refractive error.

height can be used to increase the accuracy of disc size estimates when used with appropriate magnification factors (Garway-Heath et al. 1998).

■ A red-free filter and various magnification settings facilitate the assessment of the retinal nerve fibre layer.

■ A yellow filter attachment facilitates examination of individuals who are photosensitive. Clinicians have varied opinions on whether or not to use a yellow filter as some find the colour rendering properties of the filtered lenses unacceptable and question the necessity in a routine, quick assessment. Students first learning the technique, however, should use a yellow filter to reduce the discomfort and exposure of their subjects (Bradnam et al. 1995).

These advantages outweigh the mild inconvenience of the aerial inverted and reversed image, the interpretation of which is soon learned.

6.19.3 Procedure

A concise summary of the procedure is provided in Box 6.2 and a video clip of the technique is available on the webside .

1. Note that the procedure for fundus biomicroscopy is the same in undilated or dilated pupils. Maintaining a stable, binocular image is easier when the pupil stop is larger; however, with practice, the ability to maintain excellent views through a small pupil improves.

2. Explain the test to the patient: 'I am going to examine the health of the inside of your eyes with a microscope and a lens held close to your eye. The light will be bright, so please let me know if you would like a break.' If dilation of the patient's pupils is required, follow the informed consent procedure for the instillation of a mydriatic drug (section 6.17).

Box 6.2   Summary of fundus biomicroscopy procedure

1. Dilate the patient's pupils (if required and unless contraindicated).

2. Prepare the slit-lamp biomicroscope and clean your lens.

3. Place the illumination system in line with the eyepieces, use a parallelepiped and set the magnification low (≈10×). Direct patient fixation.

4. Introduce the lens, ensuring that the light enters the pupil through the lens.

5. Look through the biomicroscope and pull the joystick straight back, first noticing the lens itself in focus, then the red reflex of the retina also coming into focus.

6. Increase the magnification and broaden the illumination as required.

7. Evaluate the optic nerve head and its immediate surroundings.

8. Systematically examine the rest of the posterior pole while maintaining lens stability.

9. Examine the light-sensitive macula last.

10. Examine the posterior vitreous by pulling even further back on the joystick.

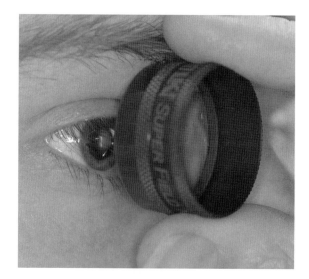

Fig. 6.63   Holding the condensing lens for fundus biomicroscopy.

3. Set the slit-lamp biomicroscope up for yourself and your patient if this has not already been done, and ask them to remove any spectacles. Choose an appropriately powered lens for the type of examination required and make sure that it is clean.

4. Place the illumination system in line with the eyepieces of the biomicroscope (zero degrees displacement). Use a parallelepiped of moderate width, moderate height, and low to medium intensity. Set the magnification to low (≈ 10×), and dim or turn off the room lights. If you are examining the patient's right eye, ask the patient to look at your right ear with their left eye. If you are examining the patient's left eye they should look at your left ear. If the patient is monocular or low-visioned, advise the patient to look in a general straight ahead direction. Most patients can maintain a stable eye position fairly well.

5. Look through the biomicroscope and reduce the height of the slit to the size of the pupil.

6. Either rest your elbow on the biomicroscope table (or on the lens holder placed on the table) or hook your little finger over the forehead rest of the biomicroscope to take the strain off your arm. Holding the lens manually offers more flexibility in manipulation of the lens and therefore the view, than using one of the available lens mounts.

7. Hold the lens with your thumb and first finger. Generally, use your left hand for examination of the patient's right eye and vice versa. The lens should be oriented with the back of the lens facing the patient (i.e. the V of 'Volk' points towards the patient).

8. Introduce the lens into the light path, within 5 mm of the patient's cornea. The optimum lens-to-cornea distance is greater for lower plus lenses (range 5–11 mm); however, being closer and pulling away slightly is preferred to being too far from the eye where the pupil stop prevents a stereoscopic view and reduces the field of view. Make sure that the light enters the pupil through the lens. Rest your other fingers on the patient's cheek and/or bridge of the nose and brow to help stabilise the lens (Fig. 6.63).

9. Once you see the light enter the pupil and the lens is stable, look again through the biomicroscope. The real image is created by the lens between you and the patient so the biomicroscope joystick must be pulled straight back until the biomicroscope is focused on this aerial fundus image. As the slit-lamp is being pulled back, the surface of the lens itself will first come into focus, then the blurred red reflex of the retina should be seen. While maintaining lens stability, continue to pull back until the fundus structures come into focus. The extent of this movement varies with the power of the condensing lens. The lower dioptric powered lenses will create an image farther from the patient's face so the biomicroscope must be pulled back more than with higher-powered lenses. Novices must learn *not* to move the lens back at the same time as the slit-lamp is pulled back.

10. Increase the magnification and broaden the illumination as required. Reflections can be reduced by tilting the lens and/or tilting the illumination system.

11. Encourage the patient to blink normally throughout the procedure but to hold their eyes open wide between blinks. Make sure the patient keeps both eyes open and that the eye not being examined has a clearly visible fixation target as this assists the patient in holding the eyes open. If the patient's eyelids are blepharospastic or ptotic, hold the upper eyelid with the fourth finger of the hand that is holding the lens. You can facilitate examination of the photophobic patient by reducing the illumination intensity, beam width and beam height, and by using a yellow filter.

12. Evaluate the optic nerve head and its immediate surroundings (Fig. 6.64). Note whether the disc is particularly large or small and note its shape and colour and the clarity of the disc margins. Make sure you are viewing the cup stereoscopically and estimate the cup- to-disc ratio along the horizontal and vertical meridians and note the location, slope and depth of the cup. Assess the neuroretinal rim, noting the

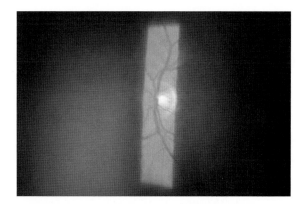

Fig. 6.64   A right optic disc seen with fundus biomicroscopy.

relative width of the superior, inferior, nasal and temporal rims if possible. Note the presence of any anomalies/abnormalities of the disc or its immediate surroundings.

13. Systematically examine the rest of the posterior pole. Follow the arcades (either inferiorly or superiorly) around the macula, to the opposite arcades and back to the nerve head. As the illumination system of the biomicroscope is moved down with the joystick of the slit-lamp through the high plus lens, the light will go up behind the high plus lens to illuminate the superior retina. To maintain the image stability, as you move the light with the biomicroscope, move or tilt the lens slightly in the same direction as the light source in order that the cone of light from the lens continues to go straight through the pupil. Because the image is inverted and laterally reversed, what appears to be the inferior fundus in the view is actually the superior fundus and vice versa.

14. Note the colour and tortuosity, and any general or focal narrowing or dilation of the blood vessels. Also carefully examine the arteriovenous crossings and look for abnormalities such as venous nipping or right angle crossings (venule deviations due to an overlying hardened arteriole). Estimate the relative width of the arteries and veins between one and three disc diameters from the disc (the AV ratio) as a percentage (Wolffsohn et al. 2001) rather

than using the traditional two-thirds or three-quarters. If the AV ratio is 50% or less, determine whether this is due to narrowed arterioles (usually representative of hypertensive changes) or distended venules (usually representative of venous stasis). At the same time, examine the surrounding fundus and look for any abnormalities.

15. Some practitioners recommend that the light-sensitive macula should be examined last. Note that the after-image produced can make patient fixation of the second eye examined difficult.

16. Examine the posterior vitreous by pulling even further back on the joystick with the patient's gaze in primary position. The most common and prominent finding is the Weiss ring representing the posterior vitreous that has pulled away from the optic disc. Other abnormalities include opacities, blood cells from haemorrhage and retinal pigment epithelial cells from retinal breaks.

17. If a binocular or adequate view of any part of the fundus and particularly the optic nerve and macula is not obtained, or any lesions are noted or a condition such as glaucoma is suspected, the patient's pupils should be dilated. If a patient refuses mydriasis, counselling on the relative risks should be undertaken and carefully documented.

6.19.4 Additional examination techniques

Midperipheral and peripheral fundus assessment can be mastered with the high plus lenses at the slit-lamp. With good technique and lens stability, midperipheral views through undilated pupils are relatively easy to obtain. Far peripheral views may be improved with pupillary dilation. As with head-band binocular indirect ophthalmoscopy with a +20 D lens, the patient's gaze is directed toward the sector that the examiner wishes to view. All eight sectors of the fundus are examined in a systematic order (for example: view the superior fundus first, then the superior-nasal, nasal, inferior-nasal, inferior, inferior-temporal, temporal and finally the superior-temporal fundus). To view the superior

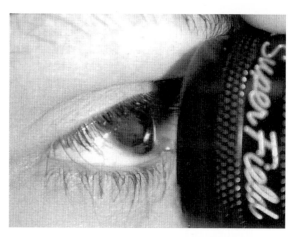

Fig. 6.65 Examining the superior fundus using fundus biomicroscopy with a SuperField lens. Note that the patient is looking upwards, and the lens is tilted slightly to maintain coaxial illumination while evaluating the superior fundus.

periphery, ask the patient to look up, centre the lens and light to enter the patient's pupil and pull the slit-lamp back, as per instructions for the posterior pole assessment. To view further into the periphery, move the biomicroscope down (the light will be directed up behind the lens) and tilt the lens slightly to maintain coaxial illumination (Figs 6.65 and 6.66). Although the view of the superior retina will be inverted and reversed, it is helpful to remember that, if you are directing the light towards the superior retina with the patient looking upwards, you will be looking at the superior retina (Figs 6.65 and 6.66).

Examination of the retinal nerve fibre layer (NFL) with the red-free filter is useful, and is especially important in patients in whom you suspect optic neuropathies including glaucoma. As the filter decreases the brightness of the image, the slit-lamp illumination should be increased. A 'bright–dark–bright' pattern is noted in normal individuals, as noted by the light band of white striated nerve fibres inserting into the superior-temporal and inferior-temporal poles of the disc, and a darker pattern through the macular area. 'Slit' defects appear as slightly darker bands in the striated nerve fibre layer band and are approximately one blood vessel width across. These defects can be normal in some individuals. 'Wedge' defects appear as a darker band that widens as it extends away from the optic disc into the nerve fibre layer. These

(a)
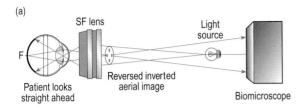

Patient looks straight ahead

(b)
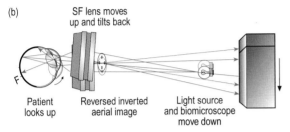

Fig. 6.66 (a) Optics of fundus biomicroscopy with a high-plus lens. The real image is reversed and inverted and lies between the hand-held lens and the observer at the slit-lamp. The image is therefore in focus when the slit-lamp biomicroscope is pulled back towards the observer. (b) Observation of the superior fundus is facilitated by having the patient look up.

can be accompanied by a focal loss in the neuroretinal rim tissue. Diffuse loss of the striations of the NFL can also be noted. Note that the fine tertiary retinal vessels can be seen more prominently in regions of NFL loss and are less visible within the healthy NFL. Nerve fibre loss with age decreases the robustness of the 'bright–dark–bright' pattern, as does media opacity and observation with a lens with a yellow filter (Jonas et al. 1999).

6.19.5 Recording

Keep in mind that the image is real, inverted and aerial, so vertical and lateral directions must be reversed for recording. Two methods may be employed for documentation of the findings with indirect fundus biomicroscopy with a high plus lens. The first involves mentally reversing and inverting the image before drawing the findings. This requires a significant amount of practice and is prone to errors in interpretation. The second and often more accurate method is to place the examination form upside down to compensate for the reversed inverted image, and draw exactly what is seen in the lens (this technique is demonstrated for

headband BIO in section 6.22.4). If digital imaging is available, abnormalities/anomalies should be photographed when possible and the image stored for future comparisons.

Optic nerve head

Record the following:

1. Distinctness of the optic disc margins.

2. Optic nerve head size and shape. Indicate whether the optic disc size is small, average or large (compare Figs 6.6, 6.7 and 6.8).

3. The size, configuration and location of any peripapillary chorioretinal atrophy, both zone alpha and zone beta.

4. The health of the neuroretinal rim (NRR) tissue by its colour, thickness and uniformity. Whether or not the 'ISNT' rule is followed should be documented (section 6.19.6).

5. The optic cup size. Draw the shape, size and location of the physiological cupping on a diagram of the disc. Include a horizontal cross-section of the cupping showing the depth and shape, and a vertical one if necessary. Record the size of the optic cup as a decimal fraction of the optic nerve in both the horizontal and vertical dimensions. The disc is considered one unit and the cup is a fraction of that unit and should be recorded in 0.05 steps, e.g. 0.60 horizontally and 0.65 vertically. In general, when the cup is smaller than one-third of the overall optic nerve head, the cup can be visually superimposed on the rims to determine the ratio, and certain mathematical relationships hold. For a 0.20 cup, four more of the same sized cups should be able to fit into the available rim tissue (Figs 6.67 and 6.68), although not necessarily symmetrically. For a 0.25 cup, three more should be able to be superimposed on the rims. For a 0.33 cup, the cup would be the same size as equally sized rims (Fig. 6.67). A 0.30 cup is slightly smaller than one-third of the optic disc, whereas a 0.35 cup is slightly larger than one-third. The assessment of larger cups is often considered more challenging. In larger cups where the rims are smaller than the width of the cup, the rims can be superimposed on the cup to help to determine the ratio. With a 0.50 cup, both of

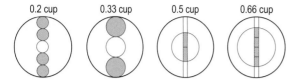

0.2 cup   0.33 cup   0.5 cup   0.66 cup

Fig. 6.67   Mathematical relationships that can help to determine the cup-to-disc ratio.

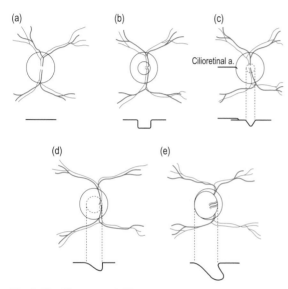

(a)   (b)   (c)

Cilioretinal a.

(d)   (e)

Fig. 6.68   Diagrams of different sizes and types of optic nerve cupping. (a) No cup. (b) 0.4 cup-to-disc ratio (CD) in both the horizontal and vertical meridians. Deep, with clearly demarcated edges. (c) Shallow cup with gently sloping edges and a CD of 0.30 H and 0.25 V. (d) CD of 0.60 H and 0.50 V, with nasal displacement of the vessels and a gentle slope temporally. (e) Advanced glaucomatous cupping with a CD of 0.90 and a deep 'bean-pot' shape. There is no healthy rim of tissue temporally.

the rims can be superimposed onto the cup and add up perfectly to the cup size. For a 0.65 cup, both rims superimposed within the cup add up to half of the total cup (Figs 6.67 and 6.68). Photographs of optic nerve heads with a range of CD ratios are available on the website 🖱.

6. In the same diagram, include all anomalies/abnormalities of the disc such as coloboma, crescents (Figs 6.9 and 6.10), drusen, disc swelling, haemorrhages,

myelinated nerve fibres (Fig. 6.12), narrowing of blood vessels as they cross the disc, pallor, pits and disc tilting (Figs 6.10 and 6.11). Digital imaging should be used when available. The differential diagnosis of drusen in the disc can be helped by using cobalt blue light and a yellow filter as they autofluoresce. Note the presence of the lamina cribrosa (Figs 6.9 and 6.13) and spontaneous venous pulsation.

Example: The recording of a normal optic nerve head would include text such as:
    Margins – distinct, NRR – healthy (follows ISNT rule), CD 0.35 H, 0.40 V and could include a plan and cross-sectional diagram of the disc.

Nerve fibre layer

Record the relative brightness and width of the pattern in the superior-temporal and inferior-temporal nerve fibre layer. Note any diffuse loss, as well as any slit- or wedge-type defects. Note that the visibility of the tertiary vessels in this area is helpful in determining the relative loss of tissue. Patients with a more darkly pigmented retinal pigment epithelial layer often have a more prominent appearance of the nerve fibre layer than those with less pigment (Figs 6.9 and 6.10).

Blood vessels

Record the relative size of the arteries and veins between one and three disc diameters from the disc (AV ratio) as a percentage (Wolffsohn et al. 2001). Record or photograph any abnormality of the blood vessels such as attenuation (local or generalised) or dilation (specific vessels or all venules, presence of segmentation or beading), emboli (cholesterol, fibrin-platelet, calcific), broadened reflex or copper/silver wiring, or vascular sheathing. Note or photograph any abnormalities of the artery–vein crossings such as venule deflections (90° crossings, Figs 6.31–6.33) and nipping (venule pinching by hardened arteriole, Figs 6.31 and 6.33). Note or photograph any tortuosity of the arterioles (often congenital) and venules (often acquired). Indicate the location of all findings in a diagram. If no abnormalities are detected, record 'No abnormalities detected' (NAD) or 'Negative', or equivalent.

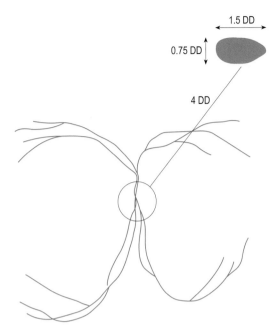

1.5 DD

0.75 DD

4 DD

Fig. 6.69 Diagrammatic representation of a choroidal naevus located 4 disc diameters (DD) at 1 o'clock from the disc. Its size is 1.5 DD by 0.75 DD.

Fundus (posterior pole, equator and periphery)

Unless digital imaging is available, draw the abnormality on a fundus diagram. Note the size, shape, location, colour, elevation and depth of any abnormality. The size of a lesion and its location with respect to the disc is usually specified in disc diameters (DD). For example, the lesion may be 2 DD × 1 DD wide. It may be located 4 DD at 4 o'clock from the disc. Record this on the diagram (Fig. 6.69). Describe the general appearance of the fundus, including whether it is tessellated and lightly or darkly pigmented. If no abnormalities are detected, record 'No abnormalities detected' (NAD) or 'Negative', or equivalent. Record this separately for the posterior pole and the periphery/ midperiphery. Determining the appropriate anterior-to-posterior location in the peripheral fundus can be facilitated by certain normal landmarks (Fig. 6.69).

Macula

Record any findings or abnormalities noted at the macula such as drusen (Figs 6.31–6.33), pigmentation changes (Fig. 6.31), haemorrhages, exudates, cotton wool spots, subfoveal neovascular membranes and thickening (oedema). If no abnormalities are detected, record 'No abnormalities detected' (NAD) or 'Negative', or equivalent. Pertinent negative findings should be recorded in certain situations, e.g. 'No clinically significant macular edema' in those patients who are diabetic.

Vitreous

Record any findings or abnormalities noted in the posterior vitreous such as posterior vitreous detachment (Fig. 6.30), floaters or cells. If no abnormalities are detected, record 'clear' or 'No abnormalities detected' (NAD). Note that the anterior vitreous is examined with the slit-lamp without an auxiliary lens.

6.19.6 Interpretation

See sections 6.4 and 6.5.

ISNT rule: The optic nerve head should have a pink rim of tissue surrounding the physiological cupping. The neural retinal rim (NRR) tissue should be approximately 1.5–2.0 times wider superiorly and inferiorly than temporally. The mnemonic 'ISNT' is often used and indicates that in most normal discs the thickest part of the rim is the *Inferior-temporal*, followed by the *Superior-temporal*, then *Nasal* and the thinnest is the *Temporal*. The thickness of the temporal NRR is variable and of limited clinical use. In glaucoma, the NRR often becomes thinner at the superior and inferior (temporal) poles first and a 'notch' indicates the localised loss of the NRR. If this occurs, the NRR will not obey the ISNT rule. This preferential damage to the superior and inferior (temporal) poles of the NRR in glaucoma causes the vertical CD ratio to increase (Jonas et al. 1999), which means that the vertical CD ratio is more important clinically.

6.19.7 Most common errors

1. Misaligning the indirect optical system causing a poor view and a view with only one eye (no stereopsis). Stability of the lens is critical and is facilitated by resting

your fingers on the patient's cheek and/or bridge of the nose and brow to help stabilise the lens.

2. Holding the lens too far from the cornea, causing the pupil stop to limit the view and/or a view with only one eye (no stereopsis). You need to learn *not* to move the lens back from the eye when the slit-lamp is pulled back from the eye.

3. Exaggerating the extent or misrepresenting the location of the abnormality (more common with high magnification).

4. Inaccurately documenting the lesion because of the inverted and reversed image. Drawing the lesion as it is seen through the lens with the exam form upside down (allowing for superior, inferior, temporal or nasal fixation) eliminates errors incurred by attempting to mentally reverse and invert the image before documenting.

5. Holding the lens too close such that the patient's lashes touch the lens. Patients may be concerned about the lens touching their eye so may either blink frequently or may pull back from the headrest. You may also get condensation on the lens surface, which will obscure your view.

6. Having insufficient range of the slit-lamp such that it cannot be pulled back far enough to focus the image. Choosing a higher-powered lens will usually solve this problem.

6.20 DIRECT OPHTHALMO-SCOPY

The direct ophthalmoscope was first proposed by Jan Evangelista Purkinje in 1827, invented by Charles Babbage in 1847 and first used in a clinical way by Herman Helmholtz in 1851. This invention revolutionised eye examinations by allowing observation of the fundus and replacing the diagnosis of 'amaurosis' (an outwardly healthy eye with poor vision) with a multitude of others for which an aetiology and treatment could be sought.

6.20.1 Lens, vitreous and general fundus examination

An assessment of ocular health is a legal requirement of the primary eye care examination and allows the early detection of ocular disease. In addition, the ocular effects of certain systemic diseases can be observed. Over many years, various techniques for fundus examination have been introduced and modified with a view to maximising the view and minimising the time required to examine the eye efficiently. Features of these techniques to consider include stereopsis, field of view, magnification, effect of media opacities on the view and ease of use. The advantages and disadvantages of the various techniques are discussed in sections 6.19.2, 6.20.2, 6.21.2, 6.22.2 and 6.23.2.

6.20.2 Advantages and disadvantages

Direct ophthalmoscopy has the advantage of being a simple technique to perform, providing an erect view of the fundus with moderate to high magnification (15× with an emmetrope), not requiring a dilated pupil and can easily be performed with the patient sitting upright. It uses a hand-held instrument that is easily portable. It can also be used in combination with fundus biomicroscopy. It provides a better retro-illumination picture of cortical and posterior subcapsular cataract and vitreous floaters in an undilated pupil than slit-lamp biomicroscopy and can provide a useful estimate of a patient's visual dysfunction due to cataract. It can also provide a useful assessment of small lesions such as microaneurysms and neovascularisation when the pupil is not dilated. It can be used to observe spontaneous venous pulsation at the disc, which is not as easily seen with fundus biomicroscopy. This can help in the differential diagnosis of true papilloedema from pseudopapilloedema, since the spontaneous venous pulse is absent in true papilloedema. Also, the loss of spontaneous venous pulsation can suggest an impending closure of the central retinal vein.

The direct ophthalmoscope should not be used as the only assessment of the anterior segment as it provides a 2-D, fixed, low magnification view with limited control of illumination. The magnification for corneal assessment is only about 2.5× and is created by the working distance lens used. The magnification is higher for lens assessment due to the additional magnification provided by the cornea and is about 15× for the emmetropic fundus examination due to the magnification from the cornea and the lens.

For fundus assessment, the extent of the fundus that is visible is limited so that significant fundus lesions can be missed because of the difficulties in scanning the retinal surface with the small field of view provided (Parisi et al. 1996, Siegel et al. 1990). The assessment available does not compare to modern digital fundus cameras that can produce a 2-D photograph of the posterior pole of the fundus through an undilated pupil (view the photographs in sections 6.4 and 6.5, virtually all taken through non-dilated pupils). This is particularly the case with myopes, where the increased magnification with direct ophthalmoscopy comes with an additionally reduced field of view. Digital fundus camera systems also have the facility to store images for subsequent analysis and comparison, allow a presentation of the photograph with an explanation to the patient, allow images to be transferred between healthcare professionals, and facilitate quality control and auditing. As a monocular technique, direct ophthalmoscopy provides a non-stereo view of the fundus and therefore is not as valid as stereo techniques at assessing important fundus features such as cup-to-disc ratio (Watkins et al. 2003), macular oedema and depth or elevation of lesions. In addition, direct ophthalmoscopy provides a much poorer image through media opacities than indirect ophthalmoscopy. It also requires a very close working distance, which some patients find unsettling (students need to learn to overcome the natural avoidance of invading a patient's 'personal space') and if the examiner or patient is ill it may be necessary for the examiner to wear a surgical mask to prevent the spread of infection. Finally, the bending required can lead to strain injury to the back of the examiner over the long term.

6.20.3 Procedure

1. Familiarise yourself with the controls of the direct ophthalmoscope. Learn how to vary the intensity of the light beam, its size, shape and colour. A green ('red-free') filter increases the contrast of blood vessels and vascular lesions (they appear dark against the light background of the fundus) and therefore can be useful when assessing patients with diabetes or other vascular disease. Some instruments also have settings that will project a target with the light beam such as an eccentric fixation target. A slit aperture is sometimes provided to determine the elevation or depression of a lesion using the monocular cue of the beam bending. A polarising filter and a half circle aperture are often available to help decrease annoying reflections from the corneal surface, although the image with the polarising filter is limited in that the luminance across the image becomes variable (in a 'maltese cross' pattern due to corneal birefringence) and significantly reduced. Direct ophthalmoscopes include focusing lenses with ranges that differ depending on the instrument used, but are typically from about +30 to −30 D. The power of the lens being used is displayed, with the red numbers indicating minus lenses and the black numbers indicating plus lenses. Some instruments have a second wheel of lenses or a setting for additional lenses that, when used in combination with the first wheel of lenses, allows for a higher total dioptric range.

2. Raise the chair to such a position that you can comfortably look into the patient's eye (from the patient's temporal side) by bending over only slightly. This is important to avoid a long-term strain injury to your back.

3. Inform the patient that you are going to examine the health of their eyes.

4. Use the largest aperture beam for patients with large pupils as it provides the largest field of view. For patients with smaller pupils, typically the elderly, the intermediate size aperture is preferred as the field of view is limited by the pupil and the larger aperture creates a larger corneal reflex.

5. Set the lens wheel to about +10 D (if you remove your spectacles for this technique, you must take this into account, i.e. a −6 D myopic examiner should start with a +4 D lens). Make sure that any auxiliary lenses are set at zero.

6. Ask the patient to remove their spectacles and remove your own. If a patient wears contact lenses, it may be easier to perform direct ophthalmoscopy with the patient wearing the lenses, particularly with highly myopic patients. If you have an unusually large astigmatic or myopic correction it may be necessary to wear spectacles or contact lenses while using the direct ophthalmoscope.

7. Dim the room lights. Hold the ophthalmoscope in your right hand and use your right eye to examine the patient's right eye. Your left hand and left eye should be used to examine the patient's left eye. It may take some practice to become comfortable with this, especially with your non-dominant eye and hand. If you have reduced visual acuity in one eye it will be necessary to use your better seeing eye to evaluate both the patient's eyes. This will take some practice to avoid bumping the patient's nose and to obtain an adequate view of the fundus on your affected side.

8. Instruct the patient to look up and temporally (usually at the corner of the room). Some practitioners find this places less strain on the examiner's back than if the patient looks straight ahead at a target such as the duochrome.

9. Place the top of the ophthalmoscope against your brow. You should now be able to view through the aperture. Rotate the ophthalmoscope handle approximately 10° to 20° from the vertical to avoid the patient's nose. Position the ophthalmoscope about 15° temporal to the patient's line of sight. Both of your eyes should be kept open to relax your accommodation. It will take some practice to suppress the other image, especially when you are using your non-dominant eye.

10. Place the hand not holding the ophthalmoscope on the back of the examination chair for stability. With the total dioptric power set at about +10 D (step 2) move closer to the patient until the anterior segment of the eye is in focus (at approximately 10 cm). Now observe the clarity of the media. Opacities will appear as dark areas against a bright red background (the red reflex; Figs 6.25 and 6.27). You can estimate the location of the opacity by using the principle of parallax motion. Choose a point of focus, e.g. the iris. If the opacity is **A**nterior to the iris, '**A**gainst' motion will be observed when you move the beam. If the opacity is posterior to the iris, 'with' motion will be observed when you move the beam. If you note that the opacity is anterior (e.g. on the cornea) ask the patient to blink. If the opacity moves, it is floating in the tears (e.g. mucus or debris). If it does not move it is a true corneal opacity. Instruct the patient to look up, then left, then down and then right while directing your view in the same direction to view opacities in the lens behind the iris. Cortical lenticular opacities are most commonly found in the inferior nasal aspect of the crystalline lens so care should be taken to inspect this quadrant. Anterior segment abnormalities should be assessed in more detail using slit-lamp biomicroscopy.

11. Move in closer to the patient on a line 15° temporal to the patient's visual axis and decrease the dioptric power of the focusing lens as you move closer. By doing this, opacities in the vitreous may be observed, such as floaters, haemorrhage and asteroid bodies. To look more carefully for floaters, ask the patient to look up and down, and watch for any floaters moving in your view.

12. You should now be as close as possible to the patient without touching the patient's eye. This may feel uncomfortably close for both you and the patient but it is important as the further away you are from the patient, the smaller the field of view you will obtain. Also, if you are closer to the patient the corneal reflex will move further from the viewing axis, making the view less obstructed. If you are viewing 15° temporally from the patient's line of sight, the disc or retinal vessels should now be in view.

13. If both you and the patient are emmetropic and your accommodation is relaxed, the dioptric value of the lens wheel should be close to zero. If you and/or the patient are uncorrected and ametropic, the lens power necessary to focus on the fundus (i.e. the power in the lens wheel) will be the sum of the refractive errors and your accommodative state. Some practitioners use this as an approximate estimation of the patient's spherical refractive state.

14. If you do not see the disc straight away but can focus on the vessels, follow the vessels backward towards the disc. The bifurcation of the vessels forms a 'V' and this will point in the direction you should move to get to the disc.

15. Once you see the disc, focus it clearly using the lens wheel. Bracketing several lens positions may be required before deciding on the optimal focus. Note the size of the disc by comparing it to the illuminated area provided by the intermediate aperture on your ophthalmoscope (Gross & Drance 1995). If it is a small disc it will be significantly smaller than the illuminated area. Note that this technique is only valid for low powers of ametropia (<5.00 DS). For higher powers, the magnification induced by ametropia with the direct ophthalmoscope invalidates this assessment.

16. Determine whether the neuroretinal rim (NRR) follows the ISNT rule (section 6.19.6) and estimate the vertical and horizontal CD ratios (Figs 6.67 and 6.68). The cup margins should be determined by kinking of the vessels as they pass over the margin. Do not assess the cup as the area of pallor, as the cup can extend beyond this area. This is difficult as you are trying to make judgements about a 3-D structure with a 2-D image. In deep cupping, the bottom of the cup will focus with less plus than the neuroretinal rim tissue and it can appear grey with central mottling (the lamina cribrosa, Figs 6.9 and 6.13). Slight parallax movements may help in determining the cup. Note the relative position of the vessels to the cup. The website includes a series of photographs of optic nerve heads with a range of CD ratios .

17. Evaluate the optic nerve head and its immediate surroundings (Figs 6.6–6.14). Note its shape and colour and the clarity of the disc margins. Observe the veins as they leave the optic cup and look for venous pulsation. Note the presence of any anomalies/abnormalities of the disc or its immediate surroundings.

18. Systematically examine the vascular arcades and rest of the posterior pole. Follow the arcades (either inferiorly or superiorly) around the macula, to the opposite arcades and back to the nerve head. Carefully note any tortuosity and/or focal narrowing of the arterioles as they appear to be relatively sensitive indicators of vascular damage caused by high blood pressure (Wolffsohn et al. 2001). Also examine the arteriovenous crossings and look for abnormalities such as venous nipping or right angle crossings (Figs 6.31–6.33). Estimate the relative width of the arteries and veins between one and three disc diameters from the disc (the AV ratio) as a percentage (Wolffsohn et al. 2001) rather than using the traditional two-thirds or three-quarters. If the AV ratio is 50% or less, determine whether this is due to narrowed arterioles or distended venules. At the same time, examine the surrounding fundus and look for any abnormalities.

19. Examine the retina more peripherally. Ask the patient to look into various positions of gaze (up, up and right, right, down and right, down, down and left, left and up and left) and systematically examine the retina with a moderately wide beam of light. You must look in the same direction as the patient. For example, when the patient looks up, you must position the ophthalmoscope slightly below the pupil and aim the ophthalmoscope beam upwards, towards the superior retina (Fig. 6.70). It is important to be careful, as moderately large abnormalities can be missed easily due to the direct ophthalmoscope's high magnification and narrow field of view.

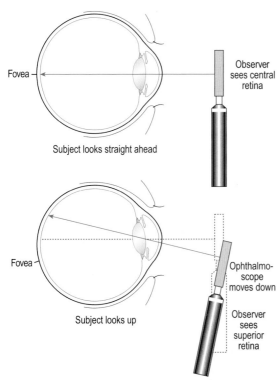

Fovea ───────────►

Observer
sees central
retina

Subject looks straight ahead

Fovea ─

Ophthalmo-
scope
moves down

Observer
sees
superior
retina

Subject looks up

Fig. 6.70   Position of the patient's eye and the ophthalmoscope when examining the central and superior fundus.

When the patient is looking down it will be necessary to gently hold up the upper eyelid to view the inferior retina.

20. Finally, evaluate the macula using the smallest aperture. This observation is performed at the end so that the patient has a chance to adapt to the light; however, many patients still find the light uncomfortably bright, therefore dimming the illumination may be required to get an adequate view of the macula. The macula is located slightly below centre and approximately 2 DD temporal to the disc. You can either move the light in this direction or ask the patient to look directly into the light. You will often note a bright reflection from the cornea that obscures the view of the macula. This is minimised by using the smallest aperture beam and/or changing the shape of the light beam (a half

circle shape is available with some ophthalmoscopes), changing your angle of observation and/or getting as close to the eye as possible.

6.20.4 Recording

Lens: If there are no opacities record 'clear'. Record cortical (Fig. 6.27) and subcapsular (Fig. 6.25) cataracts by drawing them (Fig. 6.45). The undilated pupil can be recorded as a dashed line on this diagram. Nuclear cataracts just present as a nondescript opacity that makes the view of the fundus hazy and these should be diagnosed and graded using slit-lamp biomicroscopy (see section 6.6.4 No. 3).

Vitreous: Record any findings or abnormalities noted in the posterior vitreous such as posterior vitreous detachment, floaters or cells. If no abnormalities are detected, record 'clear'.

A description of the recording of fundus assessments is provided in section 6.19.5.

6.20.5 Interpretation

See sections 6.4 and 6.5. Note that the cup-to-disc ratio is generally judged to be smaller when using a direct ophthalmoscope (monocular image) compared to when examined stereoscopically with fundus biomicroscopy (Varma et al. 1992).

6.20.6 Most common errors

1. Not getting close enough to the patient when performing the technique, particularly when attempting to view the macula.

2. Using the cup pallor instead of the deflection of the blood vessels as the determinant of the edge of the cupping.

3. Assuming that any optic disc cupping or possible macular oedmea has been evaluated adequately with the direct ophthalmoscope's non-stereoscopic view.

4. Not having the patient view in different directions of gaze to obtain a better view of the non-central retina.

5. Not using a systematic method of viewing for assessing the posterior pole and as far peripherally as is possible.

6. Assuming that the periphery has been evaluated adequately with a direct ophthalmoscope.

6.21 MONOCULAR INDIRECT OPHTHALMOSCOPY

Monocular indirect ophthalmoscopy is typically used to provide an assessment of the retina without the necessity of pupil dilation. Its use was therefore higher in the past when fewer countries allowed optometrists to use mydriatic drugs. It is still used in patients where pupil dilation is not possible or advisable, patients who are not tolerant of the brighter light of a binocular technique, young children, and basic screenings. It has also been used, instead of direct ophthalmoscopy, by clinicians who are essentially monocular and cannot use their weaker eye with the direct ophthalmoscope.

Recent innovations are the Welch Allyn PanOptic and Keeler Wide-Angle Twin Mag, which are marketed as direct ophthalmoscopes with a much larger field of view. In reality, they are monocular indirect ophthalmoscopes that provide an erect view of the fundus. The field of view is close to 25° versus the typical direct ophthalmoscope field of view of 5° and the magnification is similar to that of a direct ophthalmoscope at 15×. The Keeler instrument provides a second magnification level of about 22× with a field of view of about 17.5°. The focusing wheel adjusts the focus in a continuous action with a range of −20.00 D to +20.00 D. The aperture dial has three spot sizes (micro, small, and large), a slit aperture, a red-free filter, and as an option an additional cobalt blue filter with an add-on corneal magnifying lens.

6.21.1 General fundus examination

See sections 6.19.1 and 6.20.1. The monocular indirect ophthalmoscopy is generally used for mid-peripheral assessment of the fundus.

6.21.2 Advantages and disadvantages

The monocular indirect ophthalmoscope (or PanOptic) allows a five times greater area of the fundus to be viewed than with direct ophthalmoscopy. With this instrument it is possible to view beyond the equator when the patient has dilated pupils. The monocular indirect ophthalmoscope is also easier to use than a direct ophthalmoscope for an essentially monocular clinician and can be used with young children and special populations because of the further proximity from the patient.

As it is a monocular technique, the MIO provides a 2-D view of the fundus and therefore is not as valid as stereo techniques at assessing some important fundus features such as cup-to-disc ratio, and depth or elevation of lesions. The image of some monocular indirect ophthalmoscopes is inverted and reversed as with indirect ophthalmoscopic techniques, although more recent instruments have an internal erecting system that produces an upright and unreversed image. It provides a relatively low magnification (5×) compared to fundus biomicroscopy and direct ophthalmoscopy (see Table 6.4), although it is larger than binocular indirect ophthalmoscopy (2×). Although the MIO and PanOptic provide a good view of the majority of the posterior pole, the view of the peripheral fundus and macula is limited. The MIO can be focused for an anterior segment assessment and the PanOptic has a +13.3 D add-on corneal magnifying lens that is inserted over the objective lens to view the anterior segment. While this is possible, it is rarely used as the view of the anterior segment with a slit-lamp is far superior.

6.21.3 Procedure

Familiarise yourself with the controls of the indirect ophthalmoscope. Learn how to vary the intensity of the light beam and its size and colour and how to focus the instrument.

1. Seat the patient comfortably in the examination chair with their head held upright and not back against the headrest. The chair should be raised to such a position that you can comfortably look into the patient's eye (from the patient's temporal

side) by bending over only slightly. This is important to avoid a long-term strain injury to your back.

2. Inform the patient that you are going to examine the health of their eyes.

3. Ask the patient to remove their spectacles. You should be able to continue to wear your own spectacles for this technique. Now dim the room lights.

4. Turn on the instrument rheostat, push the iris diaphragm lever fully to the left to maximally increase the aperture size and centre the red dot on the filter dial to position the open aperture for normal viewing. Make sure the front dust shield is down in the fully open position.

5. Hold the ophthalmoscope handle in your right hand and use your right eye to examine the patient's right eye. Your left hand and left eye should be used to examine the patient's left eye. Your thumb should be placed to allow you to manipulate the focusing lever. Both of your eyes should be kept open to relax your accommodation.

6. Instruct the patient to look up and temporally (usually at the corner of the room). Some practitioners find this places less strain on the examiner's back than if the patient looks straight ahead at a target such as the duochrome.

7. Place the rest against your forehead and approach the patient's eye from about 20 cm, viewing the red reflex.

8. At about 18 mm (3/4″) from the patient's eye, the fundus should come into view. The view can be stabilised by resting your other hand against the patient's brow and the head of the instrument.

9. Use the focusing lever to make the picture of the posterior pole clear. Match the aperture size with the patient's pupil diameter.

10. Assessment of the posterior pole is essentially the same as for direct ophthalmoscopy.

11. Examine the retina more peripherally. Have the patient look into various positions of gaze (up, up and right, right, down and right, down, down and left, left and up and left) while systematically sweeping across the retina. When the patient is looking down it will be necessary to gently hold up the upper lid to view the inferior retina.

PanOptic procedure

1. Seat the patient comfortably in the examination chair with their head held upright and not back against the headrest. The chair should be raised to such a position that you can comfortably look into the patient's eye (from the patient's temporal side) by bending over only slightly. This is important to avoid a long-term strain injury to your back.

2. Inform the patient that you are going to examine the health of their eyes.

3. Ask the patient to remove their spectacles. You should be able to continue to wear your own spectacles for this technique but it is recommended that you remove them. Now dim the room lights.

4. Look through the PanOptic with your thumb on the dynamic focusing wheel and focus on an object in the room that's at least 3 to 4 metres away so that it is clear and sharp.

5. Make sure that the aperture dial is set to the small aperture position. This setting is marked with a green indicator line on the dial. It is the ideal setting for a typical non-dilated pupil.

6. Turn the PanOptic on and adjust the light intensity rheostat to its maximum position.

7. Explain to your patient that the eyecup will touch their brow. Instruct them to try not to move their head and to look straight ahead.

8. Position yourself about 15 cm away at a 15 to 20 degree angle on the temple side of the patient. To keep your patient's head steady, you may want to rest your left hand on the patient's forehead.

9. Shine the light at the patient's eye and look for the red retinal reflex. Slowly follow the red reflex toward the patient and into the pupil.

10. The eyecup should be compressed about half its length to maximise the view. At this point, a large view of the entire optic disc and surrounding vessels should be visible.

11. After examining the right eye, repeat the procedure for the left eye.

6.21.4 Recording

See section 6.19.4.

6.21.5 Interpretation

See sections 6.4 and 6.5.

6.21.6 Most common errors

1. Assuming that the MIO provides the same view of the peripheral retina as the binocular indirect ophthalmoscope.

2. Assuming that a lesion or anomaly has been evaluated adequately with the indirect ophthalmoscope's non-stereoscopic view.

3. Not getting close enough to optimise the view.

4. Not matching the aperture stop to the pupil diameter. It is best to have the aperture stop less than wide open to avoid reflection from the edge of the pupil.

5. Moving around the fundus can be difficult as the centre of rotation is around the entrance pupil which is different from other fundus examination techniques.

6.22 HEADBAND BINOCULAR INDIRECT OPHTHALMO-SCOPY (BIO)

The recommended technique for quick and thorough assessment of the entire fundus (equatorial, midperipheral and peripheral regions) is with a headband binocular indirect ophthalmoscope with a +20 dioptre aspheric condensing lens through a dilated pupil. Although a general assessment of the posterior pole with this technique is helpful for overall appearance, these structures should be examined with fundus biomicroscopy (section 6.19).

6.22.1 Examination of the peripheral fundus

There are many fundus abnormalities in the peripheral retina that are missed with the traditional assessment of direct or indirect monocular ophthalmoscopy through an undilated or dilated pupil, including but not limited to retinal holes/tears and retinal detachments, intraretinal haemorrhages, exudates and infarcts, neovascularisation, retinal degenerations, vitreoretinal traction, naevi and tumours (Batchelder et al. 1997, Parisi et al. 1996, Siegel et al. 1990).

6.22.2 Advantages and disadvantages

The advantages of BIO include:

■ Quick assessment of the entire fundus periphery and vitreous (Table 6.4).

■ Stereoscopic viewing enabling depth perception.

■ Simultaneous viewing of approximately eight disc diameters (about 35°) of the fundus. Note that less than two disc diameters can be viewed with the direct ophthalmoscope, although the exact amount is dependent on ametropia and actual disc size.

■ Easy localisation of most lesions due to the very large field of view.

■ Improved view through media opacities.

■ Patient ametropia does not affect the view.

■ Different lenses can be used to create different magnifications. The +20 D or +22 D aspheric lenses are recommended for routine use. Lower-powered lenses (+14 D or +15 D) provide higher magnification and may be used if the patient is bedridden or in a reclined wheelchair such that fundus biomicroscopy is not an option. They are somewhat more difficult to manipulate as they must be raised farther from the patient's eye to get an image and of course have a smaller field of view. Smaller, higher-powered lenses (+28 D or +30 D) provide a larger field of view but are rarely used because of their low magnification. They may be considered by a clinician who has small hands and difficulty manipulating the larger +20 D lenses, during scleral indentation due to easier lens manipulation around the scleral indentor (section 6.23) and when the patient has small pupils.

■ Scleral indentation can be used in conjunction with BIO to further evaluate peripheral areas of the fundus such as the ora serrata in a dynamic manner (section 6.23).

■ A very quick assessment is possible. This is especially useful when examining the fundus in cyclopleged children and special populations.

The main disadvantages of BIO are:

■ The image is reversed and inverted, making interpretation and recording a challenge to learn initially.

■ Mydriasis is usually required.

■ Lower magnification is provided (≈3× compared to 9× to 18 × with fundus biomicroscopy and 16 × slit-lamp magnification, and 15× with direct ophthalmoscopy). For a more magnified three-dimensional view of a lesion identified with BIO, a lower-powered condensing lens may be used (+14 D or +15 D), but it is probably best to use indirect fundus biomicroscopy to perform a detailed evaluation of lesions (section 6.19).

■ It is recommended that the patient be placed in a supine position for the examination.

■ The potential exists for light toxicity with prolonged exposure (Bradnam et al. 1995).

Box 6.3   Summary of headband BIO procedure

1. Dilate the patient's eyes.
2. Recline the patient to approximately hip level.
3. Adjust the headband.
4. Adjust the eyepieces and mirror vertically so the spot of light is in the upper half of the field of view.
5. Adjust the illumination intensity.
6. Dim or turn off the room lights.
7. Ask the patient to look straight up to the ceiling.
8. Align the two reflections from the condensing lens with middle of the pupil.
9. Gradually pull the lens directly toward you until the fundus detail fills the entire lens.
10. Examine the fundus in a systematic, predetermined order (usually clockwise), filling the condensing lens as much as possible.

Yellow condensing lenses or yellow filters attached to clear lenses may be used and are recommended for students. They can also reduce patient glare and discomfort.

6.22.3 Procedure

A concise summary of the procedure is provided in Box 6.3.

1. Explain the test to the patient. For example: 'I am going to examine the health of the inside of your eyes with light from the head unit and a lens held close to your eye.' Obtain informed consent and instil an appropriate mydriatic (section 6.17).

2. Adjust the back and top of the headband of the instrument to allow for a comfortable fit. The fit may need to be readjusted as the eyepieces are adjusted.

3. Plug the instrument into the battery pack and turn it on. Release the lock on the headset and swing the housing unit down in front of your eyes until the eyepieces are as close as possible and approximately perpendicular to your line of sight

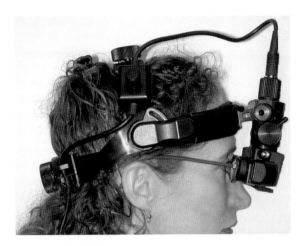

Fig. 6.71 Side view of the headband binocular indirect ophthalmoscope.

(Fig. 6.71). The closer the eyepieces are to the eyes, the larger the field of view.

4. Direct the ophthalmoscope light at your thumb or at a wall at arm's length, and adjust the eyepieces for your interpupillary distance so that the spot of light is exactly centred in the field of view for each eye. Adjust the mirror vertically until the spot of light is situated in the upper half of the field of view (±4° adjustment arm). This allows the

illumination beam to pass above the observation beam to minimise reflections during patient examination. Most instruments possess this adjustment.

5. Adjust the illumination intensity to low to medium low and the illumination beam to the largest spot size that can be used for the patient's pupil size. For a dilated pupil, use the largest spot size. A smaller spot size may be considered if the pupils are not fully dilated.

6. Ask the patient to remove any spectacles, and explain that you are going to recline the chair as at a visit to the dentist. Adjust the chair to the reclining position, so that the patient is at approximately hip level. The supine position allows you to stand approximately opposite the area of the fundus being viewed, optimising stereopsis

and the extent of viewing area while minimising back strain. Examination with the patient seated upright can also be performed if reclining is not possible. The inferior and superior fundi are more difficult to examine with a seated patient as the light source must be well above the patient's head to view the inferior peripheral fundus, and towards the patient's lap to see the superior peripheral fundus.

7. Dim or turn off the room lights.

8. Pick up the aspheric condensing lens with the white or silver edge of the lens casing toward the patient to minimise reflections and optical aberrations. Hold the lens between the index finger and the thumb. The little (or the third) finger can be used to retract the upper eyelid and allow for stable extension of the lens away from the patient's eye, while at the same time acting as a pivot, enabling the observer to tilt the lens in all planes merely by rocking the lens system. The other eyelid may be retracted with the thumb of the opposite hand. Alternatively, the little (or the third) finger of the opposite hand may be employed so that this second index finger can also be used to help stabilise the lens. The lens can be moved with critical control closer or further from the eye by increasing or decreasing the extension of the little finger stabilising on the patient's eyelids. Ambidexterity should be practised and is required for scleral indentation.

9. Novices will want to view the recognisable posterior pole first, so should ask the patient to look straight up to the ceiling if in supine position or over your shoulder if seated upright.

10. Direct the BIO light source so that it is centred on the patient's pupil. Introduce the condensing lens close to the patient's eye (2 to 4 cm) such that the external eye can be seen through the lens and with slight magnification. Centre the pupil in the condensing lens (observe the red reflex), and align the two reflections from the +20 D

lens surfaces with each other and in the middle of the pupil. Gradually move the lens away from the patient's eye (towards you) and fundus detail will become progressively magnified until the red reflex fills the entire area of the lens.

11. Keep the pupil centred in the lens at all times or the fundus view will be lost. Only slight misalignment of any part of the optical system will cause shadows, distortion, or complete loss of the view. Stabilisation of the lens with a finger from the second hand helps to minimise this fluctuation. When loss of the image occurs, move the lens towards the eye again, until the pupil can be recognised and centred, and pull the lens back towards you again to maximise the image in the lens.

12. Keep the headband unit at arm's length to the lens. When the examiner moves closer to the lens, difficulties with accommodation, convergence or loss of binocularity may occur, as will a smaller field of view.

13. If reflections from the condensing lens block visualisation of the fundus, displace the reflections by tilting the lens slightly. Excessive tilting, however, induces astigmatism and will distort the fundus image.

14. To view the different regions of the fundus, change position around the patient and tilt the lens so that the optical system formed by the patient's pupil and fundus, the condensing lens, and your pupils remain aligned along the widest part of the patient's pupil. To examine the superior fundus, for example, ask the patient to look upwards while you direct the illuminating beam toward the superior fundus. A 'full' lens image in this position will show approximately 8 DD of the fundus near the superior equator. Examine farther into the peripheral fundus by moving the light source anteriorly (toward the ora serrata), making sure the elements of the optical system remain in alignment so that the image continues to fill the lens as much as possible. To do this, you must bend along

the line of sight but in the opposite direction (i.e. towards the patient's feet). Because the image is reversed and inverted, attempting to shift the field of view in one direction will cause the image to move in the opposite direction. It helps to remember here that only the lens view is reversed and inverted; that is, if you wish to see more temporally, direct the light in that direction; more superiorly, direct the light towards the superior fundus and so on.

15. Stereopsis is achieved by imaging both of the examiner's pupils within the patient's pupil. This is facilitated by a large patient pupil with maximum dilation. During the examination of the patient's periphery, the patient's fixation is directed towards the sector that is to be examined. The pupil relative to the examiner's perspective is oval, with the long axis of this pupil perpendicular to the patient's line of sight. To maximise stereopsis in these situations, keep your two pupils aligned with this long axis. If the patient's pupil is very large or they are not looking too far off axis, stereopsis is still possible without this alignment with the long axis, but it is less likely and less consistently achieved.

16. It is advised that you examine the fundus in a systematic, predetermined order. Some clinicians elect to examine the regions of the equatorial and peripheral fundus before the posterior pole to allow the light-sensitive patient time to adapt (unless the posterior pole has just been examined with fundus biomicroscopy anyway). Direct the patient gaze towards each individual sector until all eight sectors of the fundus have been examined (plus the posterior pole). Moving clockwise in each eye is a good initial method.

6.22.4 Recording

The fundus image viewed through the condensing lens is a real image created between the patient and the examiner and the image is reversed and inverted. Therefore, when viewing the posterior

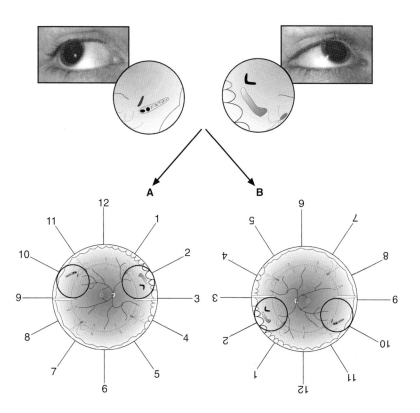

Fig. 6.72 Demonstration of recording methods for BIO and other indirect techniques. The top portion of the figure demonstrates the patient's position of gaze and diagrammatic representations of the view in the binocular indirect lens (+20 D). Option A represents mentally reversing and inverting the image seen and recording on the patient's chart. Asymmetric and complicated lesions are more difficult to interpret and document properly in this manner. Option B demonstrates how the examiner may draw the lesion exactly as it was seen and in the proper clock position, but with the recording paper turned upside down.

pole, what is seen to be superior in the view is actually inferior, nasal is temporal and temporal is nasal. When viewing the peripheral fundus, the area of the image that appears closest to you in the condensing lens (i.e. towards your thumb) is actually more anterior (peripheral) in the fundus. For example, when the patient is looking up above their head, the more peripheral retina will be seen at the bottom of the lens, and whatever appears to be located to your right within the lens is actually located to the left on the fundus. However, although the view of the superior fundus will be inverted and reversed, if you direct the light towards the superior fundus with the patient looking upwards, you will be looking at the superior fundus.

The most useful way to record fundus findings is with a sketch accompanied by brief explanatory notes. By convention, fundus details are recorded with two circles, one within the other. The inner circle represents the equator and the larger one surrounding it represents the ora serrata (Fig. 6.72). Note that although the outside circle is larger, the circumference of the ora serrata is actually less than the equator, the widest part of the globe. To draw a lesion, some examiners mentally reverse and invert the image as seen in the lens and then draw it in the correct location. Others place the examination form upside down to compensate for the reversed inverted image, and draw exactly what they see in the lens (while considering where the patient was looking and therefore the proper clock position; Fig. 6.72). Both methods take some practice to master. Determining the appropriate anterior-to-posterior location in the fundus can be facilitated by certain normal landmarks in the fundus (Fig. 6.73).

6.22.5 Interpretation

See sections 6.4 and 6.5. The various landmarks of the peripheral retina (Fig. 6.73) are rarely included in a fundus drawing but assist in identifying and documenting the location of any noted findings. There are many changes that can be noted in the peripheral retina, some of which are benign and

Fig. 6.73 Fundus drawing indicating peripheral landmarks. The ora serrata marks the termination of the retina (and the beginning of the pars plana); the equator is the widest part of the eye (represented here by a dotted circle) and is defined by the vortex vein ampullae. Other landmarks in the peripheral fundus include the long posterior ciliary nerves (LPCN) and arteries at the 3 o'clock and 9 o'clock positions of the fundus. The short posterior ciliary nerves (SPCN) are located approximately at the equator and may, like the vortex vein ampullae, be asymmetrical in each hemisphere.

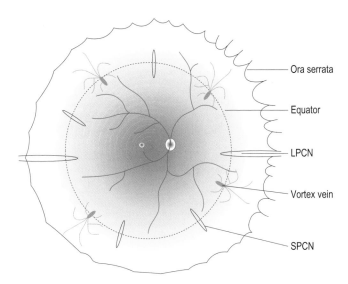

others that have quite a significant risk to vision if left undetected. Benign ocular findings include peripheral cystoid degeneration, which is present in essentially all patients over the age of 8 years. Disorders such as posterior vitreous detachment, white without pressure, lattice degeneration, vitreoretinal traction tufts, commotio retinae, pars planitis, retinal breaks, retinal detachment and others may be sight threatening and may go undetected without a dilated examination with BIO and possibly scleral indentation. Findings such as malignant melanoma can be life threatening.

6.22.6 Most common errors

1. Lack of practice. The image with the BIO relies on good technique and a stable view. All elements of the optical system must be maintained in alignment to obtain and maintain a steady image of the fundus. Your eyes, the oculars of the instrument, the illumination source, the patient's pupil, the condensing lens and the part of the patient's fundus that you wish to view must be synchronously aligned to maintain the 'full' lens image.

2. Recording incorrectly. Understanding and drawing the inverted and reversed image seen with BIO must be practised. Both the

anterior-to-posterior location as well as the 'clock' or 'sector' position of a lesion is important for accurate documentation.

3. Not reducing the intensity of the light source or using a yellow filtered lens to minimise patient photosensitivity.

4. Not adjusting the instrument properly, leading to diplopia, eyestrain or compromised stereopsis.

5. Starting the examination of a sector while already in the bent position. This not only limits the view of the periphery, but will cause you to miss sections of the equatorial fundus.

6.23 SCLERAL INDENTATION WITH HEADBAND BIO ASSESSMENT

Scleral indentation is an auxiliary examination technique used in conjunction with headband binocular indirect ophthalmoscopy. The primary use of scleral indentation is to enable a more detailed assessment of lesions detected with one of the other routine indirect techniques. Usually the detail is related specifically to the need for treatment of a retinal break of some sort. Scleral indentation may also be used to better understand an observed lesion. Examples include the thinning within and traction alongside lattice degeneration; the traction associated with vitreoretinal tufts; the layer separation in flat or bullous retinoschisis. Rarely, the clinician may elect to perform scleral indentation in all sectors if risk factors warrant a closer look when first examination with BIO noted no breaks. Generally, however, indentation is targeted to a previously identified lesion.

6.23.1 Assessment of the far peripheral retina

The assessment of the far peripheral fundus may be difficult in spite of a dilated pupil. Even when a sympathomimetic dilating agent (e.g. phenylephrine) is used in combination with a parasympatholytic agent (e.g. tropicamide), the ora serrata and pars plana can be limited optically by the orbital anatomy, iris, or crystalline lens. Pupils may dilate less well in patients who are older, diabetic, have darkly pigmented irides, have previously been treated with miotics or those who have had previous ocular surgery. Even when lesions are easily observed with fundus biomicroscopy and/or with BIO, closer examination may be required with higher magnification or with dynamic techniques to facilitate accurate diagnosis and the appropriate management. In addition to the more close examination of lesions detected by other methods, scleral indentation may be indicated in those patients where no break is detected on peripheral assessment, but when one is highly suspected. These situations include:

■ New symptoms of photopsia and/or floaters in the presence of highly suspicious signs including tobacco dust (RPE pigment) and/or haemorrhage in the vitreous.

■ History of retinal detachment in the fellow eye, especially with new symptoms.

■ Highly myopic patients where risk of peripheral retinal tears is greater.

6.23.2 Advantages and disadvantages

Scleral indentation provides a dynamic assessment of the peripheral fundus, allowing tissue separation and facilitating the detection of previously undetected tears. The technique also allows further examination of lesions detected with other methods, e.g. retinal breaks for the presence of fluid cuffs; lattice degeneration for the presence of breaks; vitreoretinal traction, etc. Disadvantages are that the technique is tricky to master as all of the elements of the optical system need to be aligned with the examiner's indentor, and these need to be aligned precisely on the lesion to be examined. Patient discomfort can also occur if the technique is not performed correctly.

6.23.3 Procedure

1. Perform binocular indirect ophthalmoscopy or dynamic fundus biomicroscopy of all sectors and determine the area(s) of the periphery requiring indentation. Note both the clock position and the anterior-to-posterior position (relative to the equator and ora serrata).

2. Explain the specific reasons for scleral indentation to the patient. For example: 'I am now going to apply a slight pressure to the outside of the eye to better view a region of the inside of the eye. You may note mild discomfort or a pressure-like sensation during the procedure.' Topical anaesthetic may be considered.

3. Recline the patient. Seated examination is not recommended.

4. Ask the patient to look in the opposite direction to the area to be viewed. Place the indentor tip on the fold of the eyelid (just beyond the tarsal plate) at the clock position on the globe where the lesion was localised. The indentor may be placed with the curve following or opposite the globe depending on patient anatomy.

5. Direct the patient fixation back toward the indentor and, as the patient moves their eye, have the indentor follow the globe back into the orbit. The indentor should be placed approximately 7 mm posterior to the limbus to indent the ora serrata, and 13–14 mm to indent the equator. If the orbital anatomy is obstructing the placement of the indentor, tilt

the patient's head slightly to facilitate manipulation of the instrument. For example, if the brow is prominent and in the way, tilt the head back somewhat. Maintain indentor position without pressure on the globe. Tangential pressure only is required.

6. Introduce the BIO light source. Note that 'on axis' indentor positioning can be determined in advance of introducing the condensing lens by noting a shadow in the red reflex in the pupil. When the lens is introduced, the optical system formed by the indented region of the fundus, the patient's pupil, the condensing lens and your pupils must be perfectly on axis to observe the indented retina. Do not apply pressure but gently roll the indentor laterally and forward and back. If the indentor is not seen, move the lens away in order to re-orient your view. You may need to alter the orientation so that the light is aimed directly at the indentor tip. Also check the anterior to posterior positioning of the indentor. If the elevated area is seen but not in the proper position, move the indentor in the opposite direction expected (away from the centre of the lens) as the view is reversed and inverted. Another way to obtain gross orientation is to remember that when the patient is looking into an extreme position of gaze and you direct your light source directly into their pupil, the equator should be in view. To extend the final 4–5 disc diameters between the equator and the ora serrata, you must bend away from the area being examined and direct the light up under the iris.

7. Observe all areas in question. For the more difficult temporal and nasal areas, the superior eyelid may be drawn downward or the inferior eyelid drawn upward with the indentor. If this is unsuccessful, the indentor may be disinfected and placed directly on the anaesthetised conjunctiva.

6.23.4 Recording

See section 6.22.4. Remember that the ora serrata and equator are located approximately 7 mm and 13–14 mm posterior to the limbus respectively.

6.23.5 Interpretation

There are many changes that can be noted in the peripheral retina, some of which are benign and others that have quite a significant risk to vision if undetected. Scleral indentation helps to identify such lesions. For example, retinal degenerations, breaks and shallow detachments are much more obvious with indentation. The contrast of a break is enhanced as the edge of the torn retina appears more whitened while the tear itself appears to open and become more red. Subtle breaks and traction may be missed without this technique. Fluid cuffs surrounding breaks are representative of sub-clinical or progressive retinal detachment and observation is facilitated with scleral indentation.

6.23.6 Most common errors

1. Lack of practice. The image with the BIO relies on good technique and a stable hand, and this is even more critical when performing scleral indentation. All elements of the optical system including the indentor must be maintained in alignment to obtain and maintain a steady image of the fundus. Often the indentor is placed too far anteriorly, so it cannot be seen.

2. Moving the indentor in the opposite direction to that which is needed to facilitate the view due to the reversed and inverted image orientation.

3. Inadequate dilation can cause the iris to obstruct the view of the far periphery.

4. Applying too much pressure to the globe or orbital rim, or placing the indentor too far anteriorly near the sensitive limbus or on the tarsal plate. This leads to patient discomfort and subsequent poor cooperation. If the indentor is not in view as expected, note your alignment and try again. Do not attempt to get the view by pressing harder on the indentor.

6.24 GOLDMANN 3-MIRROR UNIVERSAL EXAMINATION

The 3-mirror Universal contact lens has three mirrors for anterior chamber angle (gonioscopy), equatorial

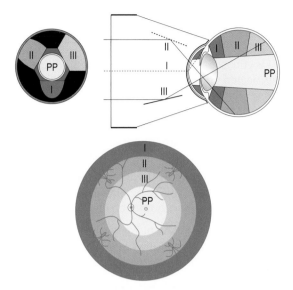

Fig. 6.74 Diagrammatical representation of the Goldmann 3-mirror contact lens, demonstrating the central lens for examining the posterior pole (PP); the thumbnail-shaped mirror angled at 60° and used for gonioscopic assessment of the anterior chamber angle as well as examination of the far-peripheral fundus in a dilated eye (I); the rectangular-shaped mirror angled at 66° and used to assess the peripheral fundus (II) and the trapezoidal-shaped mirror angled at 76° and used for examination of the equatorial fundus (III).

fundus and peripheral fundus examination and a central lens for posterior pole examination. The 'thumbnail' mirror (angled 59° to 64° from the horizontal plane) is used for gonioscopy (section 6.13), but can also be used to view the far peripheral fundus through a well-dilated pupil. The rectangular mirror (angled at approximately 66°) is used to examine more posteriorly to the thumbnail, but still in the fundus periphery. The third mirror is trapezoidal in shape (angled at approximately 76°) and is used to examine the equatorial fundus (Figs 6.53 and 6.74). Because of the limited field of view, the 3-mirror lens is not used for general assessment. Instead, it is employed when lesions are detected with other techniques such as BIO or indirect fundus biomicroscopy. This lens allows a stereoscopic view that is different from the indirect techniques. Note also that the central lens is an excellent tool for assessment of the macula (and disc), especially when fine stereopsis detail is critical (e.g. macula oedema).

6.24.1 Stereoscopic examination of the fundus

See section 6.19.1. The Goldmann 3-mirror lens allows for assessment of the macula (central lens) as well as targeted examination of previously located lesions in the periphery and midperiphery.

6.24.2 Advantages and disadvantages

Advantages include:

- The patient can remain at the biomicroscope and does not need to be placed into a supine position.

- The posterior pole, midperiphery and far periphery can be examined with the central lens and varied mirrors. The anterior chamber angle can also be examined with the thumbnail mirror (gonioscopy). This is why it is known as the 'Universal' lens.

- Due to the stereoscopic view that is essentially free of reflections, the central lens is very useful for examining for retinal thickening (oedema).

- With established slit-lamp skills, the technique is easier to learn than scleral indentation.

Disadvantages include:

- A dynamic view is not possible, nor is layer separation.

- The field of view is limited due to the size of the mirrors and central lens.

- Corneal anaesthesia is required.

- The patient's pupil must be widely dilated.

- Lesion localisation can be difficult as sector position as well as anterior-to-posterior positioning is important.

6.24.3 Procedure

1. Explain the specific reasons for using the lens. Inform the patient that it is a contact lens

used with local anaesthetic and a cushioning fluid between the lens and the eye. Explain that they may feel some pressure from the lens and will likely feel the lens on the eyelid, but will feel no discomfort with the instillation of anaesthetic. Obtain informed consent and dilate the patient's pupils (section 6.17).

2. Having determined the anterior-to-posterior positioning of the lesion to be evaluated, choose the mirror most likely to detect the lesion; that is, for a lesion at the ora serrata, use the thumbnail mirror; for a lesion in the peripheral retina, use the rectangular mirror; and for the midperiphery or equatorial fundus, use the trapezoidal mirror.

3. Prepare the patient at the slit-lamp and prepare the lens for insertion. Apply the lens to the eye (see section 6.13.3). Usually, the patient can maintain a primary gaze position for the examination of most areas of the fundus.

4. Rotate the lens such that the chosen mirror is positioned 180° from the lesion. To examine the posterior pole, use the central contact lens.

5. With the biomicroscope in a 'full-back' position, direct the slit-lamp light into the mirror of choice. Move the slit-lamp forward until the fundus is in focus, then rotate and tilt the lens to locate the lesion. If the lesion is more posterior to that portion of the fundus which is being viewed, tilt the lens away from the mirror; if more anterior (i.e. more peripheral), tilt the lens towards the mirror.

6. Once the lesion has been fully examined, remove the lens as indicated in section 6.13.3.

6.24.4 Recording

See sections 6.19.5 and 6.22.4. The fundus image viewed through the mirrors in the lens is a virtual and erect but reversed image. Record all observations.

6.24.5 Interpretation

See sections 6.4, 6.5 and 6.22.5. Subtle findings can be revealed with the different view afforded by the different light path and viewing with this lens.

6.24.6 Most common errors

1. Misinterpreting the location of the lesion to be examined. This is facilitated with scanning in the mirrors with rotation and tilting of the lens.

2. Using too little solution in the lens, causing bubbles behind the lens, limiting the view of the fundus.

3. Recording the location or dimension of the defect inappropriately. It is more difficult to compare defects with the size of the disc than with methods that can view all structures simultaneously or with the same lens/mirror.

6.25 DIGITAL IMAGING

A brief mention should be made of new imaging technologies. Imaging of the anterior eye, optic disc and fundus is becoming increasingly common in primary and secondary eye care. For fundus assessment, modern digital fundus cameras can produce a 2-D photograph of the posterior pole of the fundus through an undilated pupil (view the photographs in sections 6.4 and 6.5, which were virtually all taken through non-dilated pupils) and allow a significantly superior assessment compared to direct ophthalmoscopy and similar to that provided by a dilated fundus examination (Chow et al. 2006). It should be noted that 2-D fundus images provide slightly smaller assessments of cup-to-disc ratio than fundus biomicroscopy, although the reliability of assessments is similar (Hrynchak et al. 2003). The advantages that are brought about by using digital imaging are the speed with which the images can be examined (which mean that images can be examined immediately and a repeat photograph taken if necessary) and the ability to archive the images in an efficient, long-lasting and flexible fashion using a computer. The images can be shown to patients and can even be printed out and given to the patient. Computer manipulation also allows for the easy enhancement of images and automated measurements of diagnostic features within images. Finally, transmission of digital images through computer networks introduces the possibility of 'teleophthalmology', where the expert diagnostician is remote from the patient. With increasing technology and more widespread use, the quality of the images and storage facilities is improving while the cost is decreasing. Optic disc imaging techniques, such as scanning laser tomography with the Heidelberg Retina Tomograph (HRT) II, provides repeatable, objective and quantitative three-dimensional imaging of the optic nerve, that is particularly useful for individualised analysis of change or progression of the neural retinal rim and/or optic cup (Flanagan 2001).

6.26 THE PROBLEM–PLAN LIST

The problem–plan list is a system for recording a patient's diagnoses and the management plan for each diagnosis. If a diagnosis cannot be made, then the patient's problems (i.e. symptoms and/or signs) should be listed and a list of the further investigations required to attempt to obtain a diagnosis should be listed in the plan section.

6.26.1 Recording diagnoses and management plans

It is important to record a summary of your diagnoses and suggestions to the patient. This is useful for several reasons:

1. It is important legally to document all your diagnoses, treatment suggestions, suggestions of referral, etc. Similarly, it provides valuable support when dealing with patients who return with complaints that you failed to provide advice regarding the management of a certain condition.

2. It ensures that you must review the case history and discuss each of the patient's symptoms.

3. It ensures that you must review the record card and deal with any significant findings.

4. In subsequent examinations of the same patient, a review of the problem–plan list provides a thorough and complete summary of the examination without having to read the whole record card.

6.26.2 Advantages and disadvantages

The problem–plan list appears to be the only formal procedure that has been described to document a patient's diagnoses, treatment suggestions, further investigations necessary, comments made to the patient, etc. The problem–plan list is part of the problem-oriented examination.

6.26.3 Procedure

1. List each separate diagnosis in a column. Do not list the individual symptoms and signs that allowed the diagnosis. Order diagnoses with the most important first.

2. If a patient has symptoms for which no diagnosis has been made, include the symptoms in the problem list. Similarly, include any abnormal signs or test results for which a diagnosis was not yet possible in the problem list. By this method, any problems you do not immediately understand are highlighted and this prompts the consideration of further investigation.

3. For each problem, outline a plan or a series of actions to be taken in an adjoining column. Consider including the following forms of plan:
   a) Treatment plans.
   b) Further diagnostic procedures required.
   c) Counselling provided.

4. Counselling is a fundamental element in patient management. Effective counselling requires that all diagnostic and therapeutic plans be clearly stated to the patient in terminology that they can easily understand.

6.26.4 Recording

Examples of problem–plan lists are provided in Table 6.5.

Table 6.5 Two examples of problem–plan lists.

No.	Problem	Plan
(a)1	First time myope	Rx for b/board, TV, etc. Counselled to read & play s̄ Rx. Coun. Re: Typical progression & future changes in Rx.
2	Moderate protan	Coun. Re: Colour vision problems and effects on career choices.
(b)1	Hyperope and presbyope	Rx PALs (used previously). Coun. Re: Typical progression of presbyopia and future changes in Rx.
2	High IOP and large vertical CD ratio	Appt. made for full threshold visual fields and gonioscopy. Coun. Re: Reason for extra tests.

6.26.5 Most common errors

1. Listing signs and symptoms rather than diagnoses, when diagnoses are possible.

2. Ignoring and not listing an unexplained symptom.

3. Not providing a complete plan list for a given problem. For example, the treatment may be identified but not the counselling or vice versa.

6.27 PERSONAL LETTER OF REFERRAL OR REPORT

This is a referral letter or report written on headed notepaper that includes your practice address and contact information.

6.27.1 Referral letters and reports

Letters of referral to medical personnel or specialist clinicians are required to provide information regarding the reason and urgency of referral. Reports may be required to a referring colleague, teacher, general physician, etc. The categories of patients that require a report may be covered by legal or contractual obligations.

6.27.2 Advantages and disadvantages

The alternative to a personal letter is a form letter, with a standardised format and various boxes to fill in. Form letters can save time and if well designed may reduce the possibility of the omission of pertinent information. However, they are somewhat impersonal and restrictive and can lead to the inclusion of irrelevant information. Form letters can even lead to vital information being left off the referral, such as the optometrist's name and even the practice address (Lash 2003). Well-written referral letters are important to help develop a good relationship with secondary eye care personnel and increase the likelihood of feedback being obtained regarding referrals. A lack of feedback appears to be a significant problem in some areas (Steele et al. 2006), and without it the optometrist cannot learn from the process and improve the quality and appropriateness of referrals.

6.27.3 Procedure

1. Indicate to the patient that you will be sending a referral letter/report to another person or office. You should inform them of the reason for the referral or report.

2. Write the letter on headed notepaper that includes your practice address and contact information. The letter should ideally not be hand written, as this will make it less legible.

3. Include the date and the recipient's name and address at the top of the letter.

4. Begin the letter with the patient's name, address, date of birth (you may need to distinguish between several people with the

same name and even between two people with the same name and address), appointment date and file number (if applicable).

5. Remember that the person you are writing to is likely to be very busy, so that they want to read only essential information. Do not include information that is irrelevant to the referral as this could result in your letter not being read or being skim-read and misinterpreted.

6. A likely outline of a referral letter would be:
   a) Indicate the relevant symptoms and signs.
   b) Provide a diagnosis or tentative diagnosis if possible.
   c) Indicate if there is any urgency in the referral.
   d) If appropriate, you might indicate what further investigations or treatment you believe to be necessary.
   e) Request a reply regarding the outcome of the referral. This may require the patient's written consent.
   f) Indicate if you have copied the letter elsewhere (typically to the patient's general physician).

7. If referring a patient because of cataract (the most common referral letter, see Box 6.4) also include:
   a) The effect of reduced vision on the patient's lifestyle.
   b) Their willingness to undertake surgery.
   c) If a patient with cataract is at high risk of falling, this information could also be included as cataract surgery appears to reduce the risk of falls (Buckley & Elliott 2006).

8. A likely outline of a report would be:
   a) Thank the referring person (if applicable).
   b) Indicate the relevant symptoms and signs.
   c) Provide a diagnosis or tentative diagnosis if possible.
   d) If a diagnosis is not possible, indicate which tests were performed and any pertinent results.

   e) Indicate any management plan and the time of your intended follow-up appointment.

9. Make sure your spelling is accurate and grammar correct. Spelling and grammar checkers are available on all modern word processing packages.

10. Present the information at a level suitable to the recipient's knowledge. However, do not automatically assume that lay terms are appropriate in a letter to a non-medical person. It may be best to use the correct term with the lay term in brackets to avoid offence. For example, in a letter to a teacher, you may include a statement that 'David has myopia (short-sightedness). . .'

11. Sign the letter with your preferred title and qualifications.

12. Keep a copy of the letter for the patient's file. If the letter or report was not to the patient's GP, you may be required to send them a copy. If it is not a requirement, it is usually good practice to do so.

6.27.4 Recording

The style and content of referral letters and reports is likely to vary widely in different countries and areas within a country and because of a variety of other factors. Given this proviso, examples of a referral letter and report are given below (Boxes 6.4 and 6.5).

6.27.5 Most common errors

1. In a referral of a patient with cataract, failing to include information regarding the effect on a patient's lifestyle and their willingness to undertake surgery (Lash 2003).

2. Not including the patient's written consent for release of medical information back to you (Lash 2003).

Box 6.4   Example of a referral letter

21 April 2007
Dr John Smith
Bradford Health Centre
Ilkely Road
Bradford
Re: Mrs Mary Patient, 20 Anyold Street, Somewhere, Bradford. DOB 21-9-35.
File No. 1234.
Appointment date: 20 April 2007.
Dear Dr Smith
Mrs Patient complains of great difficulty reading and sewing and is unable to see well when outdoors on a sunny day. She has nuclear and posterior subcapsular cataracts in both eyes with visual acuities of 6/9 in each eye. However, her visual acuities in glare conditions are 6/18 in both eyes and her Pelli-Robson log contrast sensitivity scores are right eye 1.05 and left eye 1.10 and these latter clinical assessments represent a fairer reflection of her functional vision. Both eyes, and particularly both maculae, otherwise appear healthy. I have explained the situation to Mrs Patient and the options open to her and she wishes to be considered for cataract surgery.
Yours sincerely
David B. Elliott PhD, MCOptom, FAAO

Box 6.5   Example of a report

21 April 2007
Ms Joan Smith
Bradford Primary School
Ilkely Road
Bradford
Re: John Young, 20 Anyold Avenue, Somewhere, Bradford. DOB 27-8-93. File No. 4321.
Appointment date: 20 April 2007.
Dear Ms Smith
I saw John for his first eye examination today. He had no symptoms and his visual acuity was normal at 6/5 in both eyes. However, I found a problem with his colour vision in that John has deuteranopia (red-green colour deficiency) and will have difficulty differentiating between colours such as red, orange, yellow, brown and green. There are no effective treatments for this hereditary condition. I have discussed the restrictions that this will have on his future career with his family and have informed his GP as well as yourself. If you require any further information, please do not hesitate to contact me.
Yours sincerely
David B. Elliott PhD, MCOptom, FAAO

6.28 BIBLIOGRAPHY AND FURTHER READING

Alexander, L.J. (1994) *Primary care of the posterior segment*, 2nd edn. Norwalk: Appleton & Lange.

Bartlett, J.D. and Jaanus, S.D. (2001) *Clinical ocular pharmacology*, 4th edn. Boston: Butterworth-Heinemann.

Casser, L., Fingeret, M. and Woodcome, H.T. (1997) *Atlas of primary eyecare procedures*, 2nd edn, Norwalk: Appleton & Lange.

Doshi, S. and Harvey, W. (2003) *Investigative techniques and ocular examination*. Edinburgh: Butterworth-Heinemann.

Eskridge, J.B., Amos, J.F. and Bartlett, J.D. (1991) *Clinical procedures in optometry*. Philadelphia: J.B. Lippincott.

Jones, W.I. (1998) *Atlas of the peripheral ocular fundus*, 2nd edn. Boston: Butterworth-Heinemann.

Wallace, L.M. and Alward, M.D. (2006) *New colour atlas of gonioscopy*. American Academy of Ophthalmology.

6.29 REFERENCES

Albietz, J.M. (2000) Prevalence of dry eye subtypes in clinical optometry practice. *Optometry and Vision Science* **77**, 357–363.

Ang, R.T., Dartt, D.A. and Tsubota, K. (2001) Dry eye after refractive surgery. *Current Opinion in Ophthalmology* **12**, 318–322.

Ansari-Shahrezaei, S., Maar, N., Biowski, R. et al. (2001) Biomicroscopic measurement of the optic disc with a high-power positive lens. *Investigative Ophthalmology and Visual Science* **42**, 153–157.

Atkinson, P.L., Wishart, P.K., James, J.N. et al. (1992) Deterioration in the accuracy of the pulsair non-contact tonometer with use: need for regular calibration. *Eye* **6**, 530–534.

Batchelder, T.J., Fireman, B., Friedman, G.D. et al. (1997) The value of routine dilated pupil screening examination. *Archives of Ophthalmology* **115**, 1179–1184.

Bradnam, M.S., Montgomery, D.M., Moseley, H. et al. (1995) Quantitative assessment of the blue-light hazard during indirect ophthalmoscopy and the increase in the 'safe' operating period achieved using a yellow lens. *Ophthalmology* **102**, 799–804.

Brandt, J.D., Beiser, J.A., Kass, M.A. et al. (2001) Central corneal thickness in the Ocular Hypertension Treatment Study (OHTS). *Ophthalmology* **108**, 1779–1788.

Bron, A. (2001) Diagnosis of dry eye. *Survey of Ophthalmology* **45**, S221–S226.

Bron, A.J., Evans, V.E. and Smith, J.A. (2003) Grading of corneal and conjunctival staining in the context of other dry eye tests. *Cornea* **22**, 640–650.

Browning, D.J., Scott, A.Q., Peterson, C.B. et al. (1998) The risk of missing angle neovascularization by omitting screening gonioscopy in acute central retinal vein occlusion. *Ophthalmology* **105**, 776–784.

Buckley, J.G. and Elliott, D.B. (2006) Ophthalmic interventions to help prevent falls. *Geriatrics and Ageing* **9**, 276–280.

Celebi, S. and Aykan, U. (1999) The comparison of cyclopentolate and atropine in patients with refractive accommodative esotropia by means of retinoscopy, autorefractometry and biometric lens thickness. *Acta Ophthalmologica Scandinavica* **77**, 426–429.

Cho, P. (1993) Schirmer test. I A review. *Optometry and Vision Science* **70**, 152–156.

Chow, S.P., Aiello, L.M., Cavallerano, J.D. et al. (2006) Comparison of nonmydriatic digital retinal imaging versus dilated ophthalmic examination for nondiabetic eye disease in persons with diabetes. *Ophthalmology* **113**, 833–840.

Chylack, L.T., Wolfe, J., Singer, D. et al. (1993) The Lens Opacities Classification System III. *Archives of Ophthalmology* **111**, 831–836.

Classé, J.G. (1989) A review of 50 malpractice claims. *Journal of the American Optometric Association* **60**, 694–706.

Classé, J.G. (1992) Mydriasis: an eye-opening problem. *Journal of the American Optometric Association* **63**, 733–741.

Classé, J.G. and Rutstein, R.P. (1995) Binocular vision anomalies: an emerging cause of malpractice claims. *Journal of the American Optometric Association* **66**, 305–309.

Doughty, M.J. and Zaman, M.L. (2000) Human corneal thickness and its impact on intraocular pressure measures: a review and meta-analysis approach. *Survey of Ophthalmology* **44**, 367–408.

Efron, N., Morgan, P. and Katasara, S. (2001) Validation of grading scales for contact lens complications. *Ophthalmic and Physiological Optics* **21**, 17–29.

Ehlers, N., Bramsen, T. and Sperling, S. (1975) Applanation tonometry and central corneal thickness. *Acta Ophthalmologica (Copenhagen)* **53**, 34–43.

Emara, B.Y., Tingey, D.P., Probst, L.E. et al. (1999) Central corneal thickness in low-tension glaucoma. *Canadian Journal of Ophthalmology* **34**, 319–324.

Enyedi, L.B., Dev, S. and Cox, T.A. (1998) A comparison of the Marcus Gunn and alternating light tests for afferent pupillary defects. *Ophthalmology* **105**, 871–873.

Eshagian, J. (1982) Human posterior subcapsular cataracts. *Transactions of the Ophthalmological Societies of the United Kingdom* **102**, 364–368.

Farrell, J., Patel, S., Grierson, D.G. et al. (2003) A clinical procedure to predict the value of temporary occlusion therapy in keratoconjunctivitis sicca. *Ophthalmic and Physiological Optics* **23**, 1–8.

Flanagan, J.G. (2001) Imaging of the optic nerve. In: *Primary care of the glaucomas* (eds T.L. Lewis and M. Fingeret). Norwalk: Appleton & Lange.

Foster, P.J., Devereux, J.G., Alsbirk, P.H. et al. (2000) Detection of gonioscopically occludable angles and primary angle closure glaucoma by estimation of limbal chamber depth in Asians:

modified grading scheme. *The British Journal of Ophthalmology* **84**, 186–192.'

Fukuda, M. and Wang, H. (2000) Dry eye and closed eye tears. *Cornea* **19**, S44–S48.

Garway-Heath, D.F., Ruben, S.T., Viswanathan, A. et al. (1998) Vertical cup/disc ratio in relation to optic disc size: its value in the assessment of the glaucoma suspect. *The British Journal of Ophthalmology* **82**, 1118–1124.

Gaynes, B.I. (1998) Monitoring drug safety; cardiac events in routine mydriasis. *Optometry and Vision Science* **75**, 245–246.

Grey, R.H. and Hart, J.C. (1996) Screening for sight threatening eye disease. Stereoscopic viewing of the retina needed to identify maculopathy. *British Medical Journal* **312**, 440–441.

Gross, P.G. and Drance, S.M. (1995) Comparison of a simple ophthalmoscope and planimetric measurement of glaucomatous neuroretinal rim areas. *Journal of Glaucoma* **4**, 314–316.

Grosvenor, T.P. (2002) *Primary care optometry*, 4th edn. Boston: Butterworth-Heinemann.

Haicl, P. and Jankova, H. (2006) Prevalence of conjunctival concretions. *Ceská a Slovenská Oftalmologie* **61**, 260–264.

Harper, R.A. and Reeves, B.C. (1999) Glaucoma screening: the importance of combining test data. *Optometry and Vision Science* **76**, 537–543.

Healey, P.R. and Mitchell, P. (2004) Visibility of lamina cribrosa pores and open-angle glaucoma. *American Journal of Ophthalmology* **138**, 871–872.

Herndon, L.W. (2006) Measuring intraocular pressure-adjustments for corneal thickness and new technologies. *Current Opinion in Ophthalmology* **17**, 115–119.

Hrynchak, P., Hutchings, N., Jones, D. et al. (2003) A comparison of cup-to-disc ratio evaluation in normal subjects using stereo biomicroscopy and digital imaging of the optic nerve head. *Ophthalmic and Physiological Optics* **23**, 51–59.

Hurcomb, P., Wolffsohn, J. and Napper, G. (2001) Ocular signs of systemic hypertension: a review. *Ophthalmic and Physiological Optics* **21**, 430–440.

Iwama, T., Mishima, Y., Okamoto, N. et al. (1990) Association of congenital hypertrophy of the retinal pigment epithelium with familial adenomatous polyposis. *The British Journal of Surgery* **77**, 273–276.

Johnson, G.J. and Foster, P.J. (2005) Can we prevent angle-closure glaucoma? *Eye* 19, 1119–1124.

Johnson, M., Kass, M.A., Moses, R.A. et al. (1978) Increased corneal thickness simulating elevated intraocular pressure. *Archives of Ophthalmology* **96**, 664–665.

Jonas, J.B. (2005) Optic disk size correlated with refractive error. *American Journal of Ophthalmology* **139**, 346–348.

Jonas, J.B. and Budde, W.M. (2000) Diagnosis and pathogenesis of glaucomatous optic neuropathy: morphological aspects. *Progress in Retinal and Eye Research* **19**, 1–40.

Jonas, J.B., Kling, F. and Grundler, A.E. (1997) Optic disc shape, corneal astigmatism, and amblyopia. *Ophthalmology* **104**(11), 1934–1937.

Jonas, J.B., Budde, W.M. and Panda-Jonas, S. (1999) Ophthalmoscopic evaluation of the optic nerve head. *Survey of Ophthalmology* **43**, 293–320.

Kaufmann, C., Bachmann, L.M. and Thiel, M.A. (2004) Comparison of dynamic contour tonometry with Goldmann applanation tonometry. *Investigative Ophthalmology and Visual Science* **45**, 3118–3121.

Kawasaki, A., Moore, P. and Kardon, R.H. (1996) Long-term fluctuation of relative afferent pupillary defect in subjects with normal visual function. *American Journal of Ophthalmology* **122**, 875–882.

Kersten, R.C., Ewing-Chow, D., Kulwin, D.R. et al. (1997) Accuracy of clinical diagnosis of cutaneous eyelid lesions. *Ophthalmology* **104**, 479–484.

Kim, J. (2000) The use of vital dyes in corneal disease. *Current Opinion in Ophthalmology* **11**, 241–247.

Klein, B.E.K., Klein, R. and Linton, K.L.P. (1992) Prevalence of age-related opacities in a population: the Beaver Dam Eye study. *Ophthalmology* **99**, 546–552.

Korb, D. (2000) Survey of preferred tests for diagnosis of the tear film and dry eye. *Cornea* **19**, 483–486.

Koretz, J.F., Cook, C.A. and Kuszak, J.R. (1994) The zones of discontinuity in the human lens: development and distribution with age. *Vision Research* **34**, 2955–2962.

Kuszak, J.R., Peterson, K.L., Sivak, J.G. et al. (1994) The interrelationship of lens anatomy and optical quality. II. Primate lenses. *Experimental Eye Research* **59**, 521–535.

Lam, B.L. and Thompson, H.S. (1990) A unilateral cataract produces a relative afferent pupillary defect in the contralateral eye. *Ophthalmology* **97**, 334–338.

Lash, S.C. (2003) Assessment of information included on the GOS 18 referral form used by optometrists. *Ophthalmic and Physiological Optics* **23**, 21–23.

Laursen, A.B. and Fledelius, H. (1973) Variations of lens thickness in relation to biomicroscopic types of human senile cataract. *Acta Ophthalmologica* **57**, 1–13.

Levatin, P. (1959) Pupillary escape in disease of the retina or optic nerve. *Archives of Ophthalmology* **62**, 768–779.

Little, S.A. and Bruce, A.S. (1994) Repeatability of the phenol-red thread and tear thinning time tests for tear film function. *Clinical and Experimental Optometry* **77**, 64–68.

McCaghrey, G.E. and Matthews, F.E. (2001) The Pulsair 3000 tonometer – how many readings need to be taken to ensure accuracy of the average? *Ophthalmic and Physiological Optics* **21**, 334–338.

Manthorpe, R. (2006) Sjögren's syndrome criteria. *Annals of the Rheumatic Diseases* **61**, 482–484.

Mapstone, R. (1977) Dilating dangerous pupils. *The British Journal of Ophthalmology* **61**, 517–524.

Matsumoto, T., Makino, H., Uozato, H. et al. (2000) The influence of corneal thickness and curvature on the difference between intraocular pressure measurements obtained with a non-contact tonometer and those with a Goldmann applanation tonometer. *Japanese Journal of Ophthalmology* **44**, 691.

Mitchell, P., Hinchcliffe, P., Wang, J.J. et al. (2001) Prevalence and associations with ectropion in an older population: the Blue Mountains Eye Study. *Clinical and Experimental Ophthalmology* **29**, 108–110.

Moss, S.E., Klein, R. and Klein, B.E. (2000) Prevalence of and risk factors for dry eye syndrome. *Archives of Ophthalmology* **118**, 1264–1268.

Nava-Castaneda, A., Tovilla-Canales, J.L., Rodriguez, L. et al. (2003) Effects of lacrimal occlusion with collagen and silicone plugs on patients with conjunctivitis associated with dry eye. *Cornea* **22**, 10–14.

Nguyen, T.P., Nishimoto, J.H., Nakamura, C.Y. et al. (1996) Comparison of carboxymethylcellulose vs. hydroxypropyl methylcellulose as a gonioscopic fluid. *Optometry and Vision Science* **73**, 466–472.

Nichols, K.K., Nichols, J.J. and Zadnik, K. (2000) Frequency of dry eye diagnostic test procedures used in various modes of ophthalmic practice. *Cornea* **19**, 477–482.

Nichols, K.K., Nichols, J.J. and Mitchell, G.L. (2004) The lack of association between signs and symptoms in patients with dry eye disease. *Cornea* **23**, 762–770.

Nucci, P., de Pellegrin, M. and Brancato, R. (1996) Atlantoaxial dislocation related to instilling eyedrops in a patient with Down's syndrome. *American Journal of Ophthalmology* **122**, 908–910.

Panchapakesan, J., Hourihan, F. and Mitchell, P. (1998) Prevalence of pterygium and pinguecula: the Blue Mountains Eye Study. *Australian and New Zealand Journal of Ophthalmology* **26** (Suppl 1), S2–S5.

Pandit, R.J. and Taylor, R. (2000) Mydriasis and glaucoma: exploding the myth. A systematic review. *Diabetic Medicine* **17**, 693–699.

Parisi, M.L., Scheiman, M. and Coulter, R.S. (1996) Comparison of the effective- ness of a non-dilated versus dilated fundus examination in the pediatric population. *Journal of the American Optometric Association* **67**, 266–272.

Raasch, T. (1982) Funduscopic systems: a comparison of magnification. *American Journal of Optometry and Physiological Optics* **59**, 595–601.

Saleh, T.A., McDermott, B., Bates, A.K. et al. (2006) Phenol red thread test vs Schirmer's test: a comparative study. *Eye* **20**, 913–915.

Shaikh, N.M., Shaikh, S., Singh, K. et al. (2002) Progression to end-stage glaucoma after laser in situ keratomileusis. *Journal of Cataract and Refractive Surgery* **28**, 356–359.

Siegel, B.S., Thompson, A.K., Yolton, D.P. et al. (1990) A comparison of diagnostic outcomes with and without pupillary dilatation. *Journal of the American Optometric Association* **61**, 25–34.

Slusser, T.G. and Lowther, G.E. (1998) Effects of lacrimal drainage occlusion with nondissolvable intracanalicular plugs on hydrogel contact lens wear. *Optometry and Vision Science* **75**, 330–338.

Steele, C.F., Rubin, G. and Fraser, S. (2006) Error classification in community optometric practice – a pilot study. *Ophthalmic and Physiological Optics* **26**, 106–110.

Tekiele, B.C. and Semes, L. (2002) The relationship among axial length, corneal curvature, and ocular fundus changes at the posterior pole and in the peripheral retina. *Optometry* **73**, 231–236.

Tonnu, P.A., Ho, T., Newson, T. et al. (2005) The influence of central corneal thickness and age on intraocular pressure measured by pneumotonometry, noncontact tonometry, the Tono-Pen XL, and Goldmann applanation tonometry. *The British Journal of Ophthalmology* **89**, 851–854.

Tucker, N.A. and Codere, F. (1994) The effect of fluorescein volume on lacrimal outflow transit time. *Ophthalmic Plastic and Reconstructive Surgery* **10**, 256–259.

Twelker, J.D. and Mutti, D.O. (2001) Retinoscopy in infants using a near noncycloplegic technique, cycloplegia with tropicamide 1%, and cycloplegia with cyclopentolate 1%. *Optometry and Vision Science* **78**, 215–222.

Varma, R., Steinmann, W.C. and Scott, I.U. (1992) Expert agreement in evaluating the optic disc for glaucoma. *Ophthalmology* **99**, 215–221.

Watkins, R., Panchal, L., Uddin, J. et al. (2003) Vertical cup-to-disc ratio: agreement between direct ophthalmoscopic estimation, fundus biomicroscopic estimation, and scanning laser ophthalmoscopic measurement. *Optometry and Vision Science* **80**, 454–459.

Whitacre, M.M. and Stein, R. (1993) Sources of error with use of Goldmann-type tonometers. *Survey of Ophthalmology* **38**, 1–30.

Wilson, G., Ren, H. and Laurent, J. (1995) Corneal epithelial fluorescein staining. *Journal of the American Optometric Association* **66**, 435–441.

Wolffsohn, J.S., Napper, G.A., Ho, S.M. et al. (2001) Improving the description of the retinal vasculature and patient history taking for monitoring systemic hypertension. *Ophthalmic and Physiological Optics* **21**, 441–449.

Wong, T.Y., Foster, P.J., Johnson, G.J. et al. (2003) Refractive errors, axial ocular dimensions, and age-related cataracts: the Tanjong Pagar survey. *Investigative Ophthalmology and Visual Science* **44**, 1479–1485.

Yamaguchi, M., Kutsuna, M., Uno, T. et al. (2006) Marx line: fluorescein staining line on the inner lid as an indicator of meibomian gland function. *American Journal of Ophthalmology* **141**, 669–675.

Yokoi, N. and Komuro, A. (2004) Non-invasive methods of assessing the tear film. *Experimental Eye Research* **78**, 399–407.

Yokoi, N., Mossa, F., Tiffany, J.M. et al. (1999) Assessment of meibomian gland function in dry eye using meibometry. *Archives of Ophthalmology* **117**, 723–729.

PHYSICAL EXAMINATION PROCEDURES

PATRICIA HRYNCHAK

7

7.1 RELEVANT CASE HISTORY INFORMATION

The case history can provide significant information about a patient's general health and can help the practitioner decide whether particular physical examination procedures are appropriate.

7.1.1 Observations and symptoms

1. Observation of physical features: Simple observation of the patient as case history is being taken can be useful. For example, obesity is a risk factor for hypertension and carotid artery disease.

2. Symptoms of transient loss of vision (amaurosis fugax) may indicate carotid artery stenosis and requires further investigation. Amaurosis fugax is a sudden onset, painless loss of vision in one eye that is described as a curtain coming down over the vision. The vision loss generally lasts greater than one minute (McCullough et al. 2004).

3. Symptoms of a red eye could indicate the need for a preauricular node assessment to exclude a number of conditions from the differential diagnosis. The duration and laterality of the red eye need to be investigated along with the quality of any discomfort and type of any discharge.

4. Undiagnosed pulsating, suboccipital headaches that subside during the day, particularly in an older patient, may suggest hypertension and thus the need for sphygmomanometry.

7.1.2 General medical history and family history

The medical history in a patient with a red eye may be important in the differential diagnosis. For example, a history of a recent upper respiratory tract infection could be suggestive of viral origin to the red eye; the history of a urogenital infection could be suggestive of Chlamydia; a history of sinusitis, local skin abrasions and insect bites may be uncovered in a person with preseptal cellulitis and a history of being scratched by a cat could be suggestive of Parinaud oculoglandular conjunctivitis.

A history of hypertension, cardiovascular disease, cerebrovascular disease, obesity, physical inactivity, heavy alcohol intake, smoking, diabetes mellitus and hyperlipidemia are important when considering if blood pressure measurement is indicated. When there is a positive family history, the risk of developing hypertension is increased two to four times (Conto 1994). The patient's medical history should also include the current medical care for systemic conditions, frequency of monitoring for the conditions, previous and planned investigations for the conditions, medications prescribed and compliance with medication use. For example, if a patient has been diagnosed as hypertensive, is taking medication regularly, was last seen 2 weeks ago with a blood pressure reading of 118/78 and will be seen again in 3 months then there would be little need for optometric testing. If, however, the patient was previously diagnosed with hypertension, stopped taking her medication 6 months ago due to an adverse reaction and has not seen her physician for follow-up it would be prudent to take a blood pressure reading and advise the patient accordingly even in the absence of abnormalities on the ocular fundus examination.

When considering if carotid artery assessment is indicated, a history of hypertension, hyperlipidemia, diabetes mellitus, coronary artery disease and smoking can be significant. If a patient has had one or more episodes of amaurosis fugax, it is important to determine if he has already sought medical care and if and what investigations have already been done or are being planned. It is not uncommon to determine that the patient has already seen his physician and that a carotid ultrasound or other investigations are being arranged. The patient is then presenting to determine if any additional information can be gained through a dilated fundus examination.

7.2 RELEVANT INFORMATION FROM OCULAR HEALTH ASSESSMENT

7.2.1 Slit-lamp biomicroscopy assessment

A number of observations are helpful in the slit-lamp biomicroscopic assessment of the patient with a red eye. The external eye should be examined for the pattern of conjunctival injection (e.g. circumlimbal injection suggests anterior uveitis, segmental injection suggests episcleritis), flare and cells in the anterior chamber (present in anterior uveitis), the presence and quality of any discharge (e.g. watery suggests allergic conjunctivitis, mucopurulent suggests bacterial conjunctivitis). Other features to investigate are conjuctival chemosis (e.g. allergic conjunctivitis), palpebral conjunctival papillae or follicles (papillae suggest bacterial and follicles suggest viral conjunctivitis), lid swelling (e.g. allergic conjunctivitis) and corneal abnormalities (e.g. corneal ulcers). The intraocular pressure is helpful in suspected cases of angle closure glaucoma and anterior uveitis when it would be elevated or decreased respectively.

7.2.2 Fundus examination

The ocular fundus features of hypertension include narrowing and straightening of the arteries (grade 1), retinal arteries that indent/nick the retinal veins (grade 2), cotton wool spots, retinal haemorrhages and lipid exudates (grade 3) and optic nerve oedema with the features of grade 3 hypertensive changes (grade 4).

Ocular risk factors for haemodynamically significant carotid artery stenosis include emboli (Hollenhorst plaques), retinal vascular occlusions, peripheral retinal haemorrhages with dilated and tortuous veins (hypoperfusion retinopathy), microrubeosis iridis, ocular ischaemic syndrome, anterior ischaemic optic neuropathy, normal tension glaucoma and asymmetric diabetic retinopathy (Lawrence & Oderich 2002, Lyons-Watt et al. 2002).

7.3 PALPATING THE PREAURICULAR, CERVICAL, SUBMANDIBULAR AND SUBMENTAL LYMPH NODES

The presence of lymphadenopathy can provide information about the differential diagnosis of a red eye and this technique should be performed on every red eye work-up. Viral conjunctivitis, gonococcal conjunctivitis, chlamydial inclusion conjunctivitis, trachoma, severe bacterial lid conditions (preceptal cellulitis), Parinaud's oculoglandular conjunctivitis (cat-scratch disease, tularemia or tuberculosis), and upper respiratory infection and sarcoidosis can cause palpable nodes. The nodes may stay enlarged for weeks following the resolution of an ocular infection. A video clip of lymph node palpation is provided on the website .

7.3.1 Lymph nodes

The lymphatic system is composed of lymph vessels, lymph nodes and organs. It is a part of the circulatory system with the threefold purpose of:

1. immune system function to fight infection and cancer;

2. collecting and returning interstitial fluid to the blood thereby helping to maintain fluid balance and

3. absorbing lipids from the intestine and transporting them to the blood.

The lymph nodes are situated along the course of the lymphatic vessels. The nodes are bean-shaped organs containing large numbers of leukocytes and phagocytes which filter out infectious and toxic material and destroy it. When infection occurs, the nodes become enlarged and often painful and inflamed because of the production of anti-inflammatory lymphocytes and plasma cells (Gardner 1992).

The lymphatic system of the head and neck is important in infections of the eye. The preauricular lymph nodes receive lymph from the upper eyelid, the outer half of the lower eyelid and the lateral canthus. They are located 1 cm anterior and slightly inferior to the tragus of the external ear at the temporomandibular joint. The submandibular lymph nodes lie in close proximity to the submandibular gland and drain lymph from the medial portion of the upper and lower eyelids, the medial canthus and the conjunctiva. They also drain lymph from the submental nodes which are located under the tip of the chin. The mental nodes also drain anterior aspects of teeth, tongue and lower lip so if an oral infection is present then they may be enlarged and this should not be mistaken for a sign of an ocular infection. The superior cervical nodes are located inferior to the ear and superficial to the sternocleidomastoid muscle. They receive lymph from the occipital nodes as well as the preauricular and postauricular nodes (Gardner 1992). The skin and orbicularis oculi muscles drain into the deep cervical nodes near the internal jugular vein (Fig. 7.1).

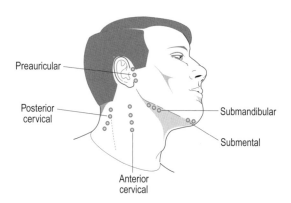

Fig. 7.1   The lymphatic system of the head and neck.

7.3.2 Advantages and disadvantages

Assessment of the lymphatic system by palpating the nodes is a quick and easy way of gaining information to aid in the differential diagnosis of a red eye. There are no complications or contraindications to performing this technique other than being gentle with patients who have node tenderness.

7.3.3 Procedure

Palpating the preauricular lymph nodes

1. Wash your hands thoroughly.

2. Stand in front of the seated patient.

3. Place the index and middle fingers of each hand in front of the tragus of the patient's external ears.

4. Slowly move your fingers in a circular motion to slide the patient's skin over the underlying bony structures of the temporomandibular joint and search for swollen lymph nodes. These will feel like a small pebble or bean under the patient's skin. A slight depression of the joint is the normal finding.

5. Compare the right and left sides to help determine whether a swollen node is present.

6. If lymphadenopathy is found, its laterality (right, left or bilateral), size (big or small), mobility, warmth and tenderness should be determined.

Palpating the cervical, submandibular and submental lymph nodes

1. All these lymph nodes are in the neck area (Fig. 7.1) and should be palpated using the tips of your index, middle and ring fingers of both hands (the submental can be palpated using just one hand). Slowly move your

fingers in a circular motion to slide the patient's skin over the underlying bony structures and/or muscle and search for swollen lymph nodes, which will feel like a small pebble or bean under the patient's skin.

2. In each case, if lymphadenopathy is found, its laterality (right, left or bilateral if appropriate), size (big or small), mobility, warmth and tenderness should be determined.

3. To assess the cervical nodes, palpate at the angle of the jaw and slowly move your fingers down, continuing to palpate to the base of the neck.

4. To assess the submandibular nodes, palpate just under the edge of the jawbone.

5. To assess the submental lymph nodes, palpate under the tip of the chin.

7.3.4 Recording

Record if the nodes are palpable (positive, +ve) or not (negative, −ve). The preauricular node is commonly abbreviated as PAN. If swollen nodes (lymphadenopathy) are found, describe their laterality (right, left or bilateral), size (big or small) and mobility (mobile or non-mobile) and indicate whether warmth and tenderness are present. Examples:

−ve PAN & neck lymph nodes.

+ve bilateral PAN small, mobile, non-tender, without overlying warmth.

+ve right PAN, large, tender and warm.

7.3.5 Interpretation

In the absence of disease there should be no palpable lymph nodes. Palpable lymph nodes (lymphadenopathy) are commonly seen in the following conditions:

1. Viral conjunctivitis: visible preauricular lymphadenopathy often greater on the side of the more involved eye and accompanied by ear, nose and throat symptoms.

2. Severe bacterial lid conditions such as preseptal cellulitis or infection in the medial canthal region: preauricular or submental lymphadenopathy.

3. Parinaud's oculoglandular conjunctivitis: often visible preauricular lymphadenopathy.

4. Chlamydial conjunctivitis or trachoma: preauricular lymphadenopathy.

5. Following the resolution of an ocular infection (several weeks).

6. Upper respiratory infection: cervical and submandibular lymphadenopathy.

Common causes of red eyes that would *not* involve lymphadenopathy include dry eye syndrome, fungal/bacterial/acanthamoebal keratitis, allergic conjunctivitis, bacterial conjunctivitis (other than gonococcal), recurrent corneal erosion, exposure and toxic keratopathy, pterygium, pinguecula, contact lens-related problems, superior limbic keratoconjunctivitis, episcleritis, blepharitis and angle closure glaucoma.

An awareness of the areas that the nodes drain is also important to rule out other causes of enlargement of the nodes. For example, if the submental and the submandibular nodes are swollen, the infection could be in the area drained by the submental nodes such as infections of the teeth, tongue and lower lip. This should be ruled out in the case history.

7.3.6 Most common error

1. Pushing too hard with patients who have lymphadenopathy as they may experience tenderness.

7.4 SPHYGMOMANOMETRY

A sphygmomanometer is a device to measure blood pressure, comprising of an inflatable cuff to restrict blood flow and a manometer to measure the pressure. Blood pressure is measured at the point when blood flow is just starting (systolic) and the point at which it is unimpeded (diastolic). A video clip of sphygmomanometry is provided on the website.

7.4.1 Blood pressure measurement

Hypertension is the most common cause of mortality in the developed world as a major contributing factor in stroke, heart attack, coronary artery disease and peripheral arterial disease (Hurcomb et al. 2001). Hypertension occurs in more than two-thirds of adults over the age of 65 and is the most common primary diagnosis by physicians. Systemic hypertension can be classified as primary (which has no known cause, 90–95%) or secondary (where the causative factor could be renal or endocrine disease or coarctation of the aorta, 5–10%; Hurcomb et al. 2001). Early hypertension is often asymptomatic but the patient may complain of suboccipital pulsating headaches that occur early in the morning and subside during the day or any other type of headache. Somnolence confusion, visual disturbances, and nausea and vomiting are only present in hypertensive emergencies (BP > 180/120) (Chobanian et al. 2003).

Optometrists often undertake blood pressure measurement when hypertensive retinopathy is detected on a fundus examination. However, some argue that because 30% of adults are unaware of their hypertension, more than 40% of hypertensives are not on treatment and two-thirds of patients on treatment are not being controlled to less than 140/90, blood pressure screening should be a routine part of optometric practice (Chobanian et al. 2003, Hurcomb et al. 2001). Since not all patients with hypertension develop retinopathy, blood pressure measurement is a more specific and reliable indicator for systemic hypertension than relying on fundus appearance alone (Wolffsohn et al. 2001). Even after 10 years, 70% of patients show either no retinopathy or only slight constriction and arteriosclerosis (Hurcomb et al. 2001). In the Beaver Dam Eye study the prevalence of retinopathy in the general non-diabetic population over the age of 40 years was 10.7% in those with systemic hypertension and 6.3% in normotensives (Hurcomb et al. 2001). It is therefore important to measure blood pressure before making a referral for medical management because referral based on fundus signs and other information obtained from an eye examination results in a significant over-referral rate (Hurcomb et al. 2001).

7.4.2 Advantages and disadvantages

The gold standard for the measurement of blood pressure is the auscultatory method using an arm cuff and mercury sphygmomanometer (Kikuya et al. 2002). Most devices for measuring blood pressure occlude a blood vessel in an extremity (usually the arm, wrist or finger) with an inflatable cuff then measure the blood pressure either by detection of Korotkoff sounds or oscillometrically (Beevers et al. 2001). In the auscultatory method, a stethoscope is used on the brachial pulse to detect Korotkoff Phase I sound (the systolic blood pressure) and the cessation of the Korotkoff Phase V sounds (the diastolic pressure) on the deflation of the cuff. In this method the sphygmomanometer used to measure the pressure can be mercury, aneroid or electronic with a digital display.

Mercury sphygmomanometers are accurate and affordable but have a limited future due to concerns about toxicity of mercury for users, personnel and the environment (WHO 2005). Aneroid devices are inexpensive and portable but the bellow-and-lever system used to measure pressure is subject to jolts and bumps which can lead to false readings (WHO 2005). Aneroid devices require regular calibration and should be checked against a mercury sphygmomanometer every 6 months. Hybrid devices use an electronic pressure gauge and display.

As an alternative to the auscultatory method, automated sphygmomanometers are very simple and easy to use. Automated devices were designed for self-measurement and may not be appropriate for the demands of clinical use (O'Brien et al. 2001). They can be reliable in that repeated measures are consistent (Sims et al. 2005). However, they lack accuracy and finger and wrist devices are not recommended due to inaccuracies caused by measurement distortion due to peripheral vasoconstriction (finger devices), the distal site of the reading, incomplete occlusion of the artery and the effect of limb position (finger and wrist) (O'Brien et al. 2001, Kikuya et al. 2002). Kikuya and colleagues (2002) showed that the wrist cuff devices could differ by more than ±10 mmHg (systolic) and ±5 mmHg (diastolic) from auscultation and Wong and colleagues (2005) showed average differences of 9.5 mmHg for systolic and 9.4 mmHg for diastolic readings. These devices cannot measure blood pressure in patients who have arrhythmias and in some other patients for reasons that frequently cannot be determined. It is important that if an automated device is used for blood pressure reading it has been validated using the published stand-ards for the evaluation of blood pressure devices either from the American Association for the Advancement of Medical Instrumentation or the British Hypertension Society (O'Brien et al. 2001). Periodic calibration is also recommended. Care should be taken not to apply the thresholds for standard sphygmomanometry to automated readings (O'Brien et al. 2001). It is likely that further technical advances will improve the accuracy of the automated devices and lead to more widespread use by primary care clinicians.

7.4.3 Procedure

1. Have the patient remain seated quietly with feet on the floor for at least 5 minutes before blood pressure readings are measured. Caffeine, smoking and exercise should have been avoided for 30 minutes prior to the blood pressure reading (Chobanian et al. 2003).

2. Describe the procedure to the patient: 'I am now going to measure your blood pressure. This involves wrapping a cuff around your arm and inflating it. You will feel the pressure on your arm increase but you shouldn't experience any pain.'

3. Ask the patient to remove any clothing covering the arm and ensure that any rolled up sleeve does not excessively constrict the arm.

4. Ask the patient to slightly bend their arm with the palm turned upwards and rest it on the chair armrest or nearby table. The arm should be at heart level.

5. Select a blood pressure cuff that encircles at least 80% of the arm to ensure accuracy (Chobanian et al. 2003). Typically two cuff sizes are required: large and regular adult.

6. Locate the brachial artery along the inner upper arm by palpation. Wrap the cuff smoothly and snugly around the arm, centring the bladder over the brachial artery (the artery arrow on the cuff should be pointing at the artery). The lower margin should be 2.5 cm above the antecubital crease (bend of the elbow).

7. Check that the cuff fits snuggly, but is not too tight or too loose. If it is difficult to insert a finger under the cuff edge it is too tight, if you can insert more than one finger it is too loose.

8. Before measuring the blood pressure, you should palpate the systolic pressure to avoid an artificially low reading caused by auscultatory gap (see section 7.4.6). Palpate the radial pulse at the wrist and inflate the cuff by pumping the bulb until the pulse disappears then continue to inflate the cuff until the reading is approximately 30 mmHg over the point where the pulse first disappears. Deflate the cuff smoothly at a rate of 2–3 mmHg per second until the pulse is felt again and note this reading. Then deflate the cuff rapidly and completely.

9. Insert the earpieces of the stethoscope into your ears so that they angle forward and are comfortable. Position the stethoscope head over the brachial artery between the lower cuff edge and the antecubital crease. Turn the chestpiece of the stethoscope so that the diaphragm side is transmitting and place it over the artery with light pressure, ensuring skin contact at all points. Heavy pressure may distort sounds.

10. Rapidly and steadily inflate the cuff to 20–30 mmHg above the palpated systolic pressure value determined in step 8. Release the air in the cuff by turning the manometer release valve to slowly and smoothly release air from the bladder at a rate of 2–3 mmHg per second.

11. Listen for the Korotkoff sounds. An audiotape of the sounds is available on the website 🖦. Note the systolic pressure at the onset of the first audible Korotkoff Phase I sound (soft tapping sounds). Determine the diastolic pressure at the cessation of the Korotkoff sounds (Phase V). Listen for 10–20 mmHg below the last sound heard to confirm disappearance, and then deflate the cuff rapidly and completely. Between Phases I and V are Phase II, which is a swishing, murmur, Phase III which is crisper sounds with increasing intensity and IV which is an abrupt muffling of sounds.

12. If a repeat reading is required, wait 1–2 minutes to permit the release of blood trapped in the forearm venous system.

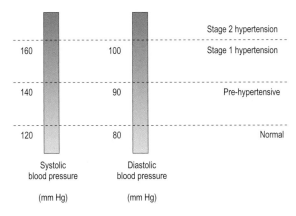

Fig. 7.2   Classification of hypertension in adults. From Chobanian et al. (2003).

7.4.4 Recording

Record the patient's position, the time and the arm used for the measurement. Record the cuff size if it was not the regular adult cuff that was used. By convention, record the systolic and diastolic reading to the nearest even number in mmHg. Examples:

120/80 right arm seated at 2.30 p.m.
132/84, left arm, seated @ 9.30 a.m., large adult cuff.
114/72, left arm, standing @ 4.00 p.m.
100/70, right arm, seated @ 2.30 p.m.

7.4.5 Interpretation

The Seventh report of the joint national committee on prevention, detection, evaluation and treatment of high blood pressure recently updated the classification of hypertension in adults over 18 years of age (Chobanian et al. 2003). The classification is shown in Figure 7.2. Two properly measured seated blood pressure readings on each of two or more separate office visits are required in order to place a person in the classification (Luo & Brown 2004).

Individuals suspected to be in the pre-hypertensive classification should be referred to a general physician for health-promoting lifestyle modifications. These modifications include weight control, increase in physical activity, and reductions in salt intake and alcohol consumption and smoking cessation. Stage 1 and 2 hypertension should be referred to a general physician to be treated with

pharmacological interventions, with most patients needing two or more antihypertensive medications to achieve a blood pressure of less than 140/90 (Chobanian et al. 2003).

A hypertensive emergency occurs when the systolic blood pressure is greater than 210 mmHg and the diastolic greater than 130 mmHg. There is evidence of progressive or impending target-organ damage and the blood pressure must be lowered immediately but carefully to prevent end-organ damage from lowering the blood pressure too quickly. This treatment normally requires hospitalisation. A hypertensive urgency is an increase in diastolic blood pressure to greater than 120–130 mmHg without end-organ damage which can be treated in office or in the emergency room with oral medications over several hours to lower the blood pressure. This usually occurs in patients who discontinue their treatment after achieving normal blood pressure (Chobanian et al. 2003, Luo & Brown 2004).

Hypertensive retinopathy is associated with twice the risk of coronary heart disease or myocardial infarction, independent of blood pressure and other coronary risk factors (Luo & Brown 2004). Therefore, retinopathy is an important indicator to be reported to the treating physician along with the blood pressure measured at the time of the ophthalmic examination.

7.4.6 Most common errors

1. Using the wrong cuff size: If you use too small a cuff for the size of the patient's arm, it leads to excessive loss of pressure from the cuff through the thick and compressible soft arm tissue and a falsely high blood pressure reading can be gained. You need to select a blood pressure cuff that encircles at least 80% of the arm to ensure accuracy (Chobanian et al. 2003). Typically, two cuff sizes are required in optometric practice: large adult and regular adult. Child size cuffs are also available, but unlikely to be used in optometric practice.

2. Ignoring the auscultatory gap: In some patients, particularly those with hypertension and when the cuff pressure is high, the sounds heard over the brachial artery disappear as the pressure is reduced and then

reappear at some lower level. This early, temporary disappearance of sound is called the auscultatory gap and occurs during the latter part of Phase I and Phase II. Because this gap may extend over a range as great as 40 mmHg, you could seriously underestimate the systolic pressure or overestimate the diastolic pressure, if you fail to gain an initial estimate of the systolic pressure after palpating the radial pulse at the wrist.

3. Using an incorrect arm position: The pressure in the arm increases as the arm is lowered from the level of the heart (phlebostatic axis); conversely, raising the arm above this position lowers the pressure measurement. The effect is largely explained by hydrostatic pressure or by the effect of gravity on the column of blood. Therefore, when measuring indirect blood pressure, the patient's arm should be positioned so that the location of the stethoscope head is at the level of the heart. This location of the heart is arbitrarily taken to be at the junction of the fourth intercostal space and the lower left sternal border. When the patient is seated, placing the arm on a nearby tabletop a little above waist level will result in a satisfactory position.

7.5 CAROTID PULSE AND AUSCULTATION WITH A STETHOSCOPE

If a blood vessel becomes partially occluded, as in atherosclerosis with or without accompanying thrombosis, the normal laminar flow is disrupted and turbulence develops. This turbulence results in vibrations that can be heard when listened for through the skin with a stethoscope (auscultation). In non-cardiac vessels this sound is termed a bruit. If a bruit is heard it indicates a stenosis (narrowing or blockage) at or proximal to the site of auscultation. A systolic bruit is generally first heard when the vessel is 50% occluded. At 70% to 80% reduction in diameter the bruit is heard in systole and in early diastole. If there is total occlusion of the vessel there may not be an audible bruit. Palpating the carotid arterial pulse gives the examiner an indication of the strength of the blood flow through the

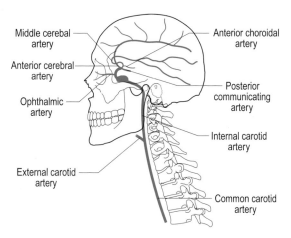

Fig. 7.3   The carotid artery.

arteries. This blood flow reflects the aortic pulsation that, if decreased, could be due to atherosclerosis of the vessel or a decreased stroke volume from the heart. Asymmetry between the right and left pulses could reflect a stenosis on the weaker side.

The right common carotid artery derives from the right brachiocephalic artery which branches off the aortic arch. The left common carotid artery derives directly from the aortic arch. The right and left common carotid arteries move up through the neck between the trachea and the sternocleidomastoid muscles and bifurcate into the internal and external common carotid arteries at the angle of the jaw. The first branch of the internal carotid artery is the ophthalmic branch, which supplies the globe and adnexa (Fig. 7.3). The carotid artery is palpated and auscultated in the fleshy area between the trachea and the sternocleidomastoid muscle.

7.5.1 Carotid artery assessment

Carotid artery occlusive disease may result in stroke, neurological disability or loss of life (Lyons-Watt et al. 2002). Ocular risk factors for haemodynamically significant carotid artery stenosis include transient loss of vision (amaurosis fugax), retinal emboli (Hollenhorst plaques), retinal vascular occlusions, peripheral retinal haemorrhages with dilated and tortuous veins (hypoperfusion retinopathy), microrubeosis iridis, ocular ischaemic syndrome, anterior ischaemic optic neuropathy, normal tension glaucoma and asymmetric diabetic retinopathy (Lawrence & Oderich 2002, Lyons-Watt et al. 2002). Symptomatic patients are more likely than non-symptomatic patients to have carotid artery stenosis and the most common symptom is amaurosis fugax. Amaurosis fugax is a sudden onset, painless loss of vision in one eye that is described as a curtain coming down over the vision. The vision loss generally lasts greater than one minute (McCullough et al. 2004).

In addition, systemic risk factors are additive to the risk of carotid artery disease. These include hypertension, hyperlipidemia, diabetes mellitus, coronary artery disease (including coronary artery bypass graft, peripheral vascular disease, a history of transient ischaemic attacks or cerebrovascular accidents), carotid bruit and smoking (Lyons-Watt et al. 2002).

Since ocular risk factors alone can be poor or unreliable predicators of carotid artery occlusive disease (studies show a range of 0 to 100%; McCullough et al. 2004), the additional information gained by the detection of a carotid bruit can be helpful in referring the patient with ocular signs to have carotid artery studies performed (duplex ultrasound scanning for carotid stenosis, carotid angiography; Lawrence & Oderich 2002).

7.5.2 Advantages and disadvantages

Palpating the carotid arterial pulse

Palpating the carotid arterial pulse is a straightforward technique requiring no equipment that gives the examiner an indication of the strength of the blood flow through the arteries. A difference between the right and left side could reflect a stenosis on the weaker side. If the examiner palpates the vessels too high on the neck the carotid sinus may be compressed. This may result in an increase in vagal tone, reflex bradycardia, a reduction in blood pressure and even syncope. Cardiac standstill is possible but very rare. Vigorous examination of the carotid arteries can also rarely cause embolisation of plaque and result in a cerebral stroke, especially in older individuals. As a result, palpation of the arteries should be performed with care and always unilaterally.

Carotid bruit

Auscultation for a systolic bruit is an easy rapid technique to gain information in the diagnosis of

significant carotid stenosis. 77% of patients with an audible bruit have been shown to have significant stenosis (Lawrence & Oderich 2002) on angiography. However, only about 57% of patients with significant stenosis (over 50%) will have an audible bruit (Lawrence & Oderich 2002). Combining a history of amaurosis fugax and ocular signs such as venous stasis retinopathy or other signs of ocular ischaemia with the presence of a bruit increases diagnostic accuracy significantly. More sensitive testing for carotid stenosis includes duplex ultrasound scanning or the carotid arteries and carotid angiography, which are arranged through a referral to a family physician or internist.

Another technique infrequently used to determine carotid insufficiency is ophthalmodynamometry. In ophthalmodynamometry the relative ophthalmic artery pressure is measured by applying pressure to the sclera while watching for the pulsation (diastolic pressure) and collapse (systolic pressure) of the arterial tree at the optic nerve head. The technique requires only the ophthalmodynamometer, which is small and portable, and a direct ophthalmoscope or a binocular indirect ophthalmoscope. There is concern with this technique that the ophthalmic artery may become permanently occluded when measuring the systolic pressure. The technique is also prone to error, with patient cooperation being crucial and may require an assistant to read the values. In addition, a clear ocular media is required for adequate visualisation of the retinal vasculature. The results are dependent on the intraocular pressure and are compared to the patient's brachial blood pressure to determine if the values are within normal limits (the diastolic should be within 45 to 60% of the diastolic blood pressure and the systolic should be within 57 to 70% of the brachial artery blood pressure).

7.5.3 Procedure

Carotid pulse

1. Inspect both sides of the patient's neck for significant prominent pulsations.
2. Explain the test to the patient: 'I am now going to place my fingers on your neck to check your pulse.'
3. Perform the test one side at a time. Never palpate the right and left common carotid pulses at the same time.

4. For the right carotid assessment, stand to the right of the patient and ask the patient to look to their left. For the left carotid assessment, stand to the left of the patient and ask the patient to look to their right. Adjust the headrest on the examination chair so that the patient's head is resting backwards with the chin slightly elevated.

5. Use the tips of the first and second fingers of one hand to gently palpate the pulse of the common carotid artery in the anterior triangle of the neck. Use the fingers of your left hand to palpate the right carotid artery and vice versa. Care should be taken not to palpate too high on the neck so as not to apply pressure on the carotid sinus.

6. Increase the pressure on the carotid artery until maximum pulsations are felt and then slowly reduce it.

7. Note the strength of the pulsations. Take note of any vibrations ('thrill').

8. Palpate the pulse on the contralateral side and make note of any differences between the carotid pulses on the right and left sides.

Carotid auscultation

1. Explain the test to the patient: 'I am now going to use a stethoscope on your neck to check your blood circulation.'

2. For the right carotid assessment, stand to the right of the patient and ask the patient to look to their left. For the left carotid assessment, stand to the left of the patient and ask the patient to look to their right. Adjust the headrest on the examination chair so that the patient's head is resting backwards with the chin slightly elevated.

3. Adjust the stethoscope so that the bell side of the chestpiece is clicked into position to transmit sounds through the stethoscope.

4. Insert the earpieces of the stethoscope into your ears so that they angle forward towards your face (Fig. 7.4).

5. Place the bell over the common carotid artery approximately 2.5 cm above the clavicle bone using gentle pressure.

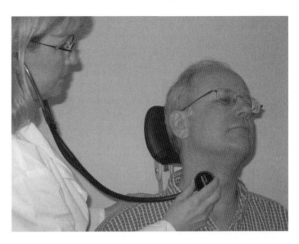

Fig. 7.4   Using the stethoscope to listen for carotid bruits.

6. Have the patient hold their breath in mid-expiration to prevent the breath sounds from distracting from your evaluation and listen for bruits for a few seconds. A bruit is a 'whooshing' sound heard superimposed on the sound of the pulse. Have the patient resume breathing.

7. Reposition the stethoscope two or three times further upwards on the neck to the bifurcation of the common carotid artery and then the internal carotid artery. Listen for bruits.

8. Repeat the procedure on the contralateral side.

7.5.4 Recording

Carotid pulse

The carotid pulse is graded according to the strength. Grade 0 is the absence of a pulse, Grade 1+ is a detectable but faint pulse, Grade 2+ is a stronger pulse but decreased in intensity, Grade 3+ is a normal pulse and Grade 4+ is a forceful pulse. Note if a 'thrill' or vibration is felt when palpating the arteries.

Carotid bruit

Bruits are recorded as present or absent. Additionally, if the artery is occluded by approximately 50%, a soft, early systolic bruit may be heard and if it is occluded by approximately 75%, a systolic and early diastolic bruit may be heard. Examples:

Carotid pulse: R 3+   L3+
Carotid bruit: R absent   L absent.

Carotid pulse: R 1+   L2+
Carotid bruit: R soft, systolic bruit   L absent.

7.5.5 Interpretation

The presence of a carotid bruit and/or weak or asymmetric carotid pulse with an ipsilateral ocular risk factor may be indicative of a potentially life-threatening cerebrovascular or cardiovascular disease. Referral should be made for an appropriate medical assessment. Note that the absence of a carotid bruit does not however rule out carotid stenosis as the artery could be nearly entirely occluded, resulting in the absence of turbulent flow sounds. An evaluation of symptoms, ocular and other systemic risk factors should be considered when deciding on referral for further assessment.

7.5.6 Most common errors

1. Inter-observer variability is high with this procedure so practice is required to obtain reliable results.

2. Interpreting as abnormal a bruit found in children or young adults. These are a result of the vessel elasticity in this age group and are benign.

3. Producing an iatrogenic bruit by placing too much pressure on the artery. Moving the bell over the skin, moving your fingers on the chestpiece or breathing on the tubing can also produce confusing sounds.

4. If too much pressure is put on the common carotid when it is partially occluded with atherosclerotic plaque, the vessel could become mechanically occluded producing a transient ischaemic attack.

5. It may be difficult to palpate the pulse or detect flow sounds in a patient with excessive neck tissue.

6. Palpating the carotid artery for the pulse at the level of the carotid sinus may result in an increase in vagal tone and bradycardia which may be substantial enough to result in syncope.

7.6 BIBLIOGRAPHY AND FURTHER READING

Casser, L., Fingeret, M. and Woodcombe, H.T. (1997) *Atlas of primary eyecare procedures*, 2nd edn. Norwalk: Appleton & Lange.

7.7 REFERENCES

Beevers, G., Lip, G. and O'Brien, E. (2001) ABC of hypertension: Blood pressure measurement. Part I-Sphygmomanometery: factors common to all techniques. *British Medical Journal* **322**, 981–985.

Chobanian, A.V., Bakris, G.L., Black, H.R. et al. (2003) Seventh report of the joint national committee on prevention, detection, evaluation and treatment of high blood pressure. *Hypertension* **42**, 1206–1252.

Conto, J.E. (1994) Cardiovascular disease. In: *Ocular manifestations of systemic disease* (ed. B. Blaustein). New York: Churchill Livingstone.

Gardner, M. (1992) *Basic anatomy of the head and neck*. Philadelphia: Lea & Febiger, pp. 183–186.

Hurcomb, P., Wolffsohn, J. and Napper, G. (2001) Ocular signs of systemic hypertension: a review. *Ophthalmic and Physiological Optics* **21**, 430–440.

Kikuya, M., Chonan, K., Imai, Y. et al. (2002) Accuracy and reliability of wrist-cuff devices for self-measurement of blood pressure. *Journal of Hypertension* **20**, 629–638.

Lawrence, P.F. and Oderich, G.S. (2002) Ophthalmic finding as predictors of carotid artery disease. *Vascular and Endovascular Surgery* **36**, 415–424.

Luo, B.P. and Brown, G.C. (2004) Update on the ocular manifestations of systemic arterial hypertension. *Current Opinion in Ophthalmology* **15**, 203–210.

Lyons-Watt, V., Anderson, S., Townsend, J. et al. (2002) Ocular and systemic findings and their correlation with hemodynamically significant carotid artery stenosis: a retrospective study. *Optometry and Vision Science* **79**, 353–362.

McCullough, H., Reinert, C., Hynan, L. et al. (2004) Ocular findings as predictors of carotid artery occlusive disease: is carotid imaging justified? *Journal of Vascular Surgery* **40**, 279–286.

O'Brien, E., Beevers, G. and Lip, G.Y. (2001) ABC of hypertension: blood pressure measurement.

Part IV. Automated sphygmomanometery: self blood pressure measurement. *British Medical Journal* **322**, 1167–1170.

Sims, A.J., Reay, C.A., Bousfield, D.R. et al. (2005) Low-cost oscillometric non-invasive blood pressure monitors: device repeatability and device differences. *Physiological Measurement* **26**, 441–445.

Wolffsohn, J.S., Napper, G.A., Ho, S.M. et al. (2001) Improving the description of the retinal vasculature and patient history taking for monitoring systemic hypertension. *Ophthalmic and Physiological Optics* **21**, 441–449.

Wong, W., Shiu, I., Hwong, T. et al. (2005) Reliability of automated blood pressure devices used by hypertensive patients. *Journal of the Royal Society of Medicine* **98**, 111–113.

World Health Organization (2005) *Affordable technology: blood pressure measuring devices for low resource settings*. Geneva: WHO library.

INDEX

References to illustrations are in *italics*.